Pediatric Nephrology

Editor

TEJ K. MATTOO

PEDIATRIC CLINICS
OF NORTH AMERICA

www.pediatric.theclinics.com

Consulting Editor
BONITA F. STANTON

December 2022 • Volume 69 • Number 6

ELSEVIER

1600 John F. Kennedy Boulevard • Suite 1800 • Philadelphia, Pennsylvania, 19103-2899

http://www.theclinics.com

THE PEDIATRIC CLINICS OF NORTH AMERICA Volume 69, Number 6
December 2022 ISSN 0031-3955, ISBN-13: 978-0-323-98719-6

Editor: Kerry Holland
Developmental Editor: Axell Ivan Jade M. Purificacion

The Pediatric Clinics of North America (ISSN 0031-3955) is published bimonthly by Elsevier Inc., 360 Park Avenue South, New York, NY 10010-1710. Months of issue are February, April, June, August, October, and December. Periodicals postage paid at New York, NY and additional mailing offices. Subscription prices are $263.00 per year (US individuals), $1028.00 per year (US institutions), $331.00 per year (Canadian individuals), $1074.00 per year (Canadian institutions), $395.00 per year (international individuals), $1074.00 per year (international institutions), $100.00 per year (US students and residents), $100.00 per year (Canadian students and residents), and $165.00 per year (international residents and students). To receive students/resident rare, orders must be accompanied by name of affiliated institution, date of term, and the signature of program/residency coordinator on institution letterhead. Orders will be billed at individual rate until proof of status is received. Foreign air speed delivery is included in all Clinics subscription prices. All prices are subject to change without notice. **POSTMASTER:** Send address changes to The Pediatric Clinics of North America, Elsevier Health Sciences Division, Subscription Customer Service, 3251 Riverport Lane, Maryland Heights, MO 63043. **Customer Service: 1-800-654-2452 (US and Canada). From outside of the US and Canada: 1-314-447-8871. Fax: 1-314-447-8029. For print support, E-mail: JournalsCustomerService-usa@elsevier.com. For online support, E-mail: JournalsOnlineSupport-usa@elsevier.com.**

Reprints. For copies of 100 or more, of articles in this publication, please contact the Commercial Reprints Department, Elsevier Inc., 360 Park Avenue South, New York, NY 10010-1710. Tel.: 212-633-3874; Fax: 212-633-3820; E-mail: reprints@elsevier.com.

The Pediatric Clinics of North America is also published in Spanish by McGraw-Hill Inter-americana Editores S.A., Mexico City, Mexico; in Portuguese by Riechmann and Affonso Editores, Rua Comandante Coelho 1085, CEP 21250, Rio de Janeiro, Brazil; and in Greek by Althayia SA, Athens, Greece.

The Pediatric Clinics of North America is covered in MEDLINE/PubMed (Index Medicus), Excerpta Medica, Current Contents, Current Contents/Clinical Medicine, Science Citation Index, ASCA, ISI/BIOMED, and BIOSIS.

PROGRAM OBJECTIVE

The goal of the *Pediatric Clinics of North America* is to keep practicing physicians and residents up to date with current clinical practice in pediatrics by providing timely articles reviewing the state-of-the-art in patient care.

TARGET AUDIENCE

All practicing pediatricians, physicians, and healthcare professionals who provide patient care to pediatric patients.

LEARNING OBJECTIVES

Upon completion of this activity, participants will be able to:
1. Review the causes for pediatric kidney disease, its risk factors, and its clinical manifestations.
2. Discuss applying a multidisciplinary approach to quickly diagnose and treat kidney disease and disease in a pediatric population.
3. Recognize the significance of traditional and novel assessment and monitoring techniques in diagnosing and managing pediatric kidney disease in a timely manner.

ACCREDITATIONS

Physician Credit

The Elsevier Office of Continuing Medical Education (EOCME) is accredited by the Accreditation Council for Continuing Medical Education (ACCME) to provide continuing medical education for physicians.

The EOCME designates this journal-based activity for a maximum of 13 *AMA PRA Category 1 Credit*(s)™. Physicians should claim only the credit commensurate with the extent of their participation in the activity.

All other healthcare professionals requesting continuing education credit for this journal-based activity will be issued a certificate of participation.

ABP Maintenance of Certification Credit

Successful completion of this CME activity, which includes participation in the activity and individual assessment of and feedback to the learner, enables the learner to earn up to 13 MOC points in the American Board of Pediatrics' (ABP) Maintenance of Certification (MOC) program. It is the CME activity provider's responsibility to submit learner completion information to ACCME for the purpose of granting ABP MOC credit.

DISCLOSURE OF CONFLICTS OF INTEREST

The EOCME assesses conflict of interest with its instructors, faculty, planners, and other individuals who are in a position to control the content of CME activities. All relevant conflicts of interest that are identified are thoroughly vetted by EOCME for fair balance, scientific objectivity, and patient care recommendations. EOCME is committed to providing its learners with CME activities that promote improvements or quality in healthcare and not a specific proprietary business or a commercial interest.

The planning committee, staff, authors, and editors listed below have identified no financial relationships or relationships to products or devices they or their spouse/life partner have with commercial interest related to the content of this CME activity:

Matthew D. Adams, MD; Arend Bökenkamp, MD; Olivia Boyer, MD, PhD; Per Brandström, MD, PhD; Caoimhe S. Costigan, BSc, BM BS, MRCPI; Emil den Bakker, MD; Minh Dien Duong, MD; Manpreet K. Grewal, MD; Dieter Haffner, MD; Sverker Hansson, MD, PhD; Emily Haseler, BM BCh; Abubakr A. Imam, MBBS, CHCQM; Priyanka Khandelwal, MD, DM; Larisa Kovacevic, MD; Tej K. Mattoo, MD, DCH, FRCP (UK), FAAP; Rajkumar Mayakrishnan, BSc, MBA; Nadia McLean, MBBS, DM; Dunya Mohammad, MD; Patrick Niaudet, MD; Kimberly J. Reidy, MD; Norman D. Rosenblum, MD, FRCPC, FCAHS; Sermin A. Saadeh, MD; Sami Sanjad, MD; Manish D. Sinha, PhD; Doreen Thomas-Payne, MSN, BSN, RN, PMHNP-BC; Rudolph P. Valentini, MD; Judith Sebestyen VanSickle, MD, MHPE, FAAP, FASN

The planning committee, staff, authors and editors listed below have identified financial relationships or relationships to products or devices they or their spouse/life partner have with commercial interest related to the content of this CME activity:

Shina Menon, MD: Consultant: Medtronic, Nuwellis, Inc.

Bradley A. Warady, MD: Consultant: Amgen Inc., Bayer AG, F. Hoffmann-La Roche, Reata Pharmaceuticals, Inc.

UNAPPROVED/OFF-LABEL USE DISCLOSURE

The EOCME requires CME faculty to disclose to the participants:

1. When products or procedures being discussed are off-label, unlabelled, experimental, and/or investigational (not US Food and Drug Administration [FDA] approved); and
2. Any limitations on the information presented, such as data that are preliminary or that represent ongoing research, interim analyses, and/or unsupported opinions. Faculty may discuss information about pharmaceutical agents that is outside of FDA-approved labelling. This information is intended solely for CME and is not intended to promote off-label use of these medications. If you have any questions, contact the medical affairs department of the manufacturer for the most recent prescribing information.

TO ENROLL

To enroll in the *Pediatric Clinics of North America* Continuing Medical Education program, call customer service at 1-800-654-2452 or sign up online at http://www.theclinics.com/home/cme. The CME program is available to subscribers for an additional annual fee of USD 324.00.

METHOD OF PARTICIPATION

In order to claim credit, participants must complete the following:

1. Complete enrolment as indicated above.
2. Read the activity.
3. Complete the CME Test and Evaluation. Participants must achieve a score of 70% on the test. All CME Tests and Evaluations must be completed online.

In order to claim MOC points, participants must complete the following:

1. Complete steps listed above for claiming CME credit
2. Provide your specialty board ID#, birth date (MM/DD), and attestation.
3. Online MOC submission is only available for the American Board of pediatrics' (ABP) Maintenance of Certification (MOC) program

CME INQUIRIES/SPECIAL NEEDS

For all CME inquiries or special needs, please contact elsevierCME@elsevier.com.

Contributors

CONSULTING EDITOR

BONITA F. STANTON, MD[†]
Professor of Pediatrics, Founding Dean, Robert C. and Laura C. Garrett Endowed Chair, Hackensack Meridian School of Medicine, President, Academic Enterprise, Hackensack Meridian Health, Nutley, New Jersey, USA

EDITOR

TEJ K. MATTOO, MD, DCH, FRCP (UK), FAAP
Professor of Pediatrics (Nephrology) and Urology, Wayne State University School of Medicine, Detroit, Michigan, USA

AUTHORS

MATTHEW D. ADAMS, MD
Assistant Professor, Department of Pediatrics, Wayne State University School of Medicine, Detroit, Michigan, USA

AREND BÖKENKAMP, MD
Department of Pediatric Nephrology, Emma Children's Hospital, Amsterdam University Medical Centers, Amsterdam, the Netherlands

OLIVIA BOYER, MD, PhD
Professor of Pediatrics, Pediatric Nephrology, Necker Enfants Malades Hospital, Université Paris Cité, Paris, France

PER BRANDSTRÖM, MD, PhD
Department of Pediatrics, Clinical Science Institute, Sahlgrenska Academy, University of Gothenburg, Pediatric Uro-Nephrologic Center, Queen Silvia Children's Hospital, Sahlgrenska University Hospital, Gothenburg, Sweden

CAOIMHE S. COSTIGAN, BSC, BM BS, MRCP
Doctor, Division of Nephrology, Clinical Fellow in Pediatric Nephrology, The Hospital for Sick Children, Toronto, Ontario, Canada

EMIL DEN BAKKER, MD
Department of Pediatrics, Emma Children's Hospital, Amsterdam University Medical Centers, Amsterdam, the Netherlands

MINH DIEN DUONG, MD
Department of Pediatrics, Division of Nephrology, Children's Hospital at Montefiore, Albert Einstein College of Medicine, Bronx, New York, USA

[†]Deceased.

MANPREET K. GREWAL, MD
Division of Nephrology and Hypertension, Department of Pediatrics, Children's Hospital of Michigan, Detroit, Michigan, USA; Department of Pediatrics, Central Michigan University College of Medicine, Mount Pleasant, Michigan, USA

DIETER HAFFNER, MD
Department of Pediatric Kidney, Liver and Metabolic Diseases, Hannover Medical School, Hannover, Germany

SVERKER HANSSON, MD, PhD
Department of Pediatrics, Clinical Science Institute, Sahlgrenska Academy, University of Gothenburg, Pediatric Uro-Nephrologic Center, Queen Silvia Children's Hospital, Sahlgrenska University Hospital, Gothenburg, Sweden

EMILY HASELER, BM BCh
Department of Paediatric Nephrology, Evelina London Children's Hospital, Guys & St Thomas NHS Foundation Trust, Kings College London, London, United Kingdom

ABUBAKR A. IMAM, MBBS
Division Chief, Nephrology and Hypertension, Department of Pediatrics, Sidra Medicine, Clinical Professor, College of Medicine, Qatar University, Associate Professor, Weill Cornell Medicine-Qatar, Doha, Qatar

PRIYANKA KHANDELWAL, MD, DM
Senior Research Associate, Division of Nephrology, Department of Pediatrics, All India Institute of Medical Sciences, New Delhi, India

LARISA KOVACEVIC, MD
Department of Pediatric Urology, Clinical Professor of Pediatrics, Michigan State University, Central Michigan University, Medical Director, Stone Clinic, Children's Hospital of Michigan, Detroit, Michigan, USA

TEJ K. MATTOO, MD, DCH, FRCP (UK), FAAP
Professor of Pediatrics (Nephrology) and Urology, Wayne State University School of Medicine, Detroit, Michigan, USA

NADIA MCLEAN, MBBS, DM
Consultant Pediatric Nephrologist, Cornwall Regional Hospital, St James, Jamaica, West Indies

SHINA MENON, MD
Assistant Professor, Department of Pediatrics, Division of Nephrology, University of Washington, Seattle Children's Hospital, Seattle, Washington, USA

DUNYA MOHAMMAD, MD
Assistant Professor of Pediatrics, Division Chief, Pediatric Nephrology, University of South Alabama, Mobile, Alabama, USA

PATRICK NIAUDET, MD, PhD
Emeritus Professor of Pediatrics, Pediatric Nephrology, Necker Enfants Malades Hospital, Université Paris Cité, Paris, France

KIMBERLY J. REIDY, MD
Associate Professor, Department of Pediatrics, Division of Nephrology, Children's Hospital at Montefiore, Albert Einstein College of Medicine, Bronx, New York, USA

NORMAN D. ROSENBLUM MD, FRCPC, FCAHS
Doctor, Division of Nephrology, Developmental and Stem Cell Biology Program, Research Institute, Staff Nephrologist and Senior Scientist, The Hospital for Sick Children, Professor, Department of Paediatrics, Physiology, and Laboratory Medicine and Pathobiology, University of Toronto, Toronto, Ontario, Canada

SERMIN A. SAADEH, MD
Department of Pediatrics, Pediatric Nephrology, King Faisal Specialist Hospital and Research Center, (KFSH&RC), Associate Professor, King Faisal University, Riyadh, Kingdom of Saudi Arabia

SAMI SANJAD, MD
Professor of Pediatrics (Nephrology), American University of Beirut Medical Center, Beirut, Lebanon

MANISH D. SINHA, PhD
Department of Paediatric Nephrology, Evelina London Children's Hospital, Guys & St Thomas NHS Foundation Trust, Kings College London, London, United Kingdom

RUDOLPH P. VALENTINI, MD
Professor of Pediatrics, Division of Nephrology and Hypertension, Department of Pediatrics, Children's Hospital of Michigan, Detroit, Michigan, USA; Department of Pediatrics, Central Michigan University College of Medicine, Mount Pleasant, Michigan, USA

JUDITH SEBESTYEN VANSICKLE, MD
Associate Professor of Pediatric Nephrology, Children's Mercy Kansas City, University of Missouri - Kansas City School of Medicine, Division of Pediatric Nephrology, Kansas City, Missouri, USA

BRADLEY A. WARADY, MD
Professor of Pediatric Nephrology, Children's Mercy Kansas City, University of Missouri - Kansas City School of Medicine, Division of Pediatric Nephrology, Kansas City, Missouri, USA

Contents

A good understanding of kidney function tests is essential for patient care. Urinalysis is the commonest used test for screening purposes in ambulatory settings. Glomerular function is assessed further by urine protein excretion and estimated glomerular filtration rate and tubular function by various tests such as urine anion gap and excretion of sodium, calcium, and phosphate. In addition, kidney biopsy and/or genetic analyses may be required to further characterize the underlying kidney disease. In this article, we discuss maturation and the assessment of kidney function in children.

Proteinuria and/or hematuria are common findings in ambulatory settings. Proteinuria can be glomerular and/or tubular in origin and it may be transient, orthostatic, or persistent. Persistent proteinuria may be indicative of a serious kidney pathology. Hematuria, which denotes the presence of an increased number of red blood cells in the urine, can be gross or microscopic. Hematuria can originate from the glomeruli or other sites of the urinary tract. Asymptomatic microscopic hematuria or mild proteinuria in an otherwise healthy child is less likely to be of clinical significance. However, the presence of both requires further workup and careful monitoring.

Postinfectious glomerulonephritis (PIGN) is a leading cause of acute glomerulonephritis in children. The presentation of PIGN can vary from asymptomatic microscopic hematuria incidentally detected on routine urinalysis to nephritic syndrome and a rapidly progressive glomerulonephritis. Treatment involves supportive care with salt and water restriction, and the use of diuretic and/or antihypertensive medication, depending on the severity of fluid retention and the presence of hypertension. PIGN resolves completely and spontaneously in most children, and the long-term outcomes are typically good with preserved renal function and no recurrence.

Nephrotic syndrome in children is mostly idiopathic in origin. About 90% of patients respond to corticosteroids; 80-90% have at least one relapse and 3-10% become corticosteroid resistant after the initial response. A kidney biopsy is seldom indicated for diagnosis except in patients with atypical presentation or corticosteroid resistance. For those in remission, the risk of relapse is reduced by the administration of daily low dose corticosteroids for 5-7 days at the onset of an upper respiratory infection. Some patients may continue having relapses through adult life. Many country-specific practice guidelines have been published, which are very similar with clinically insignificant differences.

Symptoms of urinary tract infection (UTI) in young children are nonspecific and urine sampling is challenging. A safe and rapid diagnosis of UTI can be achieved with new biomarkers and culture of clean-catch urine, reserving catheterization or suprapubic aspiration for severely ill infants. Most guidelines recommend ultrasound assessment and use of risk factors to direct further management of children at risk of kidney deterioration. The increasing knowledge of the innate immune system will add new predictors and treatment strategies to the management of UTI in children. Long-term outcome is good for the majority, but individuals with severe scarring can develop hypertension and decline in kidney function.

Vesicoureteral reflux (VUR) is the commonest congenital anomaly of urinary tract in children. It is mostly diagnosed after a urinary tract infection or during evaluation for congenital anomalies of the kidney and urinary tract. High-grade VUR, recurrent pyelonephritis, and delayed initiation of antibiotic treatment are important risk factors for renal scarring. The management of VUR depends on multiple factors and may include surveillance only or antimicrobial prophylaxis; very few patients with VUR need surgical correction. Patients with renal scarring should be monitored for hypertension and those with significant scarring should also be monitored for proteinuria and chronic kidney disease.

Congenital anomalies of the kidney and urinary tract encompass a broad spectrum of developmental conditions that together account for the majority of childhood chronic kidney diseases. Kidney abnormalities are the most commonly diagnosed congenital anomaly in children, and detection of this anomaly is increasing as a result of improved antenatal care and widespread access to more sensitive screening ultrasonography. Most paediatricians will encounter children with congenital kidney anomalies across a wide spectrum of disorders, and a broad understanding of the classification, investigation, and basis of management is important to appropriately direct their care.

The incidence of kidney stones in children is increasing. Approximately two-thirds of pediatric cases have a predisposing cause. Children with recurrent kidney stones have an increased higher risk of developing chronic kidney. A complete metabolic workup should be performed. Ultrasound examination is the initial imaging modality recommended for all children with suspected nephrolithiasis. A general dietary recommendation includes high fluid consumption, dietary salt restriction, and increased intake of vegetables and fruits. Depending on size and location of the stone, surgical intervention may be necessary. Multidisciplinary management is key to successful treatment and prevention.

Primary hypertension (PH) is most common during adolescence with increasing prevalence globally, alongside the epidemic of obesity. Unlike in adults, there are no data on children with uncontrolled hypertension and their future risk of hard cardiovascular and cerebrovascular outcomes. However, hypertension in childhood is linked to hypertensive-mediated organ damage (HMOD) which is often reversible if treated appropriately. Despite differing guidelines regarding the threshold for defining hypertension, there is consensus that early recognition and prompt management with lifestyle modification escalating to antihypertensive medication is required to ameliorate adverse outcomes. Unfortunately, many unknowns remain regarding pathophysiology and optimum treatment of childhood hypertension.

Hemolytic uremic syndrome is characterized by a triad of microangiopathic hemolytic anemia, thrombocytopenia, and acute kidney failure. Most cases are caused by Shiga-toxin-producing bacteria, especially Escherichia coli. Transmission occurs through ground beef and unpasteurized milk. STEC-HUS is the main cause of acute renal failure in children. Management remains supportive. Immediate outcome is most often. Atypical HUS represents about 5% of cases, has a relapsing course with more than half of the patients progressing to end-stage kidney failure. Most cases are due to variants in complement regulators of the alternative pathway. Complement inhibitors, such as eculizumab, have considerably improved the prognosis.

Pediatric vasculitis is a complex group of disorders that commonly presents with multisystem involvement. Renal vasculitis can be isolated to the kidneys or can occur as part of a broader multiorgan vasculitis. Depending on severity, renal vasculitis may present as acute glomerulonephritis (AGN) often associated with hypertension and sometimes with a rapidly deteriorating clinical course. Prompt diagnosis and initiation of therapy are key to preserving kidney function and preventing long-term morbidity and mortality. This review focuses on the clinical presentation, diagnosis, and treatment objectives for common forms of renal vasculitis seen in pediatric patients.

Acute kidney injury (AKI) is common in children and is associated with significant morbidity and mortality. In the last decade our understanding of AKI has improved significantly, and it is now considered a systemic disorder that affects other organs including heart, lung, and brain. In spite of its limitations, serum creatinine remains the mainstay in the diagnosis of AKI. However, newer approaches such as urinary biomarkers, furosemide stress test, and clinical decision support are being increasingly used and have the potential to improve the accuracy and timeliness of AKI diagnosis.

Chronic kidney disease (CKD) in children occurs mostly due to congenital anomalies of kidney and urinary tract and hereditary diseases. For advanced cases, a multidisciplinary team is needed to manage nutritional requirements and complications such as hypertension, hyperphosphatemia, proteinuria, and anemia. Neurocognitive assessment and psychosocial support are essential. Maintenance dialysis in children with end-stage renal failure has become the standard of care in many parts of the world. Children younger than 12 years have 95% survival after 3 years of dialysis initiation, whereas the survival rate for children aged 4 years or younger is about 82% at one year.

PEDIATRIC CLINICS OF NORTH AMERICA

SERIES OF RELATED INTEREST

Urologic Clinics of North America
www.urologic.com

THE CLINICS ARE AVAILABLE ONLINE!
Access your subscription at:
www.theclinics.com

Preface

A Gamut of Kidney Diseases in Children

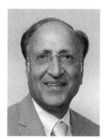

Tej K. Mattoo, MD, DCH, FRCP (UK), FAAP
Editor

The invitation to be the editor for this issue of *Pediatric Clinics of North America* brought back some nostalgic memories of my introduction to the journal during my residency training in pediatrics in Kashmir, India. It was an issue on neonatology, made available by one of our faculty mentors. My three other batchmates and I were mesmerized by its content and would look forward to the next issue of the journal that he generously kept sharing with us. Decades later, I feel honored to work together with many of my highly accomplished friends and former fellows to edit this particular issue on pediatric nephrology.

I am grateful to Dr Bonita Stanton, the former Consulting Editor of *Pediatric Clinics of North America*, who invited me to edit this issue but did not see it come to fruition because of her untimely demise earlier this year. My last communication with her in August 2021 was about the draft author list for various articles and this is what she had to say, "Wow!! I have never had the joy of reading a volume of *Pediatric Clinics of North America* with so many authors from other countries—this is just great! The more we can reach across continents for our academic partnerships, the stronger our profession will become." Bonnie's reply was so reflective of her excellence in academic medicine and passion for children all over the world, and I dedicate this issue to her memory.

Since the publication of the last issue of *Pediatric Clinics of North America* on pediatric nephrology 15 years ago, extraordinary advances have been made in diagnosis and management of children with kidney disease. Newer diagnostic tests, including genetic testing, and the availability of novel medications are opening new frontiers in the caring of children with kidney disease. Continuous renal replacement therapy is helping save many critically ill and hemodynamically unstable patients, including those on extracorporeal membrane oxygenation. The feasibility of long-term dialysis starting

Pediatr Clin N Am 69 (2022) xv–xvii
https://doi.org/10.1016/j.pcl.2022.09.016

at birth and significant improvement in kidney graft outcomes have greatly enhanced survival of pediatric patients with diseases that were considered fatal not so long ago.

Assessment of kidney function is at the core of clinical practice in nephrology. Drs Bakker, Bökenkamp, and Haffner, in their article, go over kidney maturation during the first two years of life, limitations with serum creatinine as the best available surrogate marker for renal function assessment, and the importance of estimated glomerular filtration rate in day-to-day patient care, particularly in ambulatory settings. The authors highlight the importance of next-generation sequencing in diagnosing a wide spectrum of kidney diseases, including chronic kidney disease (CKD) of unknown origin.

Proteinuria and/or hematuria are common presenting problems in ambulatory settings. The article by Drs Imam and Saadeh emphasizes the importance of urine sampling for evaluation of proteinuria, a stepwise approach for evaluation of patients with hematuria or proteinuria, the significance of persistent proteinuria, particularly when associated with hematuria, and a reminder that red-colored urine does not always mean hematuria.

Streptococcal infection remains the commonest cause for postinfection acute glomerulonephritis (PIGN). The article by Drs Duong and Reidy discusses other conditions that are associated with PIGN and highlights clinically relevant differences between postinfectious versus concurrent infection-associated glomerulonephritis and adult versus pediatric PIGN. The article also discusses the clinical presentation and management and ends with a reassurance that the long-term outcome in most patients is excellent.

Urinary tract infection (UTI) is common in younger children. In the article on UTI, Drs Brandström and Hansson highlight significant recent changes in the management of UTI in children. The authors discuss investigations and follow-up based on risk factors for recurrent UTI and kidney function deterioration and reiterate that even though the long-term outcome is good for most patients, those with severe scarring can develop hypertension and decline in kidney function. The article provides a detailed summary of some of the guidelines for febrile UTI in various parts of the world.

Renal anomalies constitute nearly a third of all antenatally diagnosed congenital anomalies and are the commonest cause of end-stage kidney disease in children. Drs Costigan and Rosenblum, in their article, discuss common congenital anomalies of the kidney and urinary tract (CAKUT), particularly those that are diagnosed antenatally. The authors review relevant aspects of kidney development and embryology and provide an outline for classification of CAKUT and a framework for investigation and key aspects of management of children with kidney anomalies.

Kidney stones in children are on the rise, and as mentioned in the article by Dr Kovacevic, about two-thirds of pediatric cases have a predisposing cause, with hypercalciuria and hypocitraturia emerging as the commonest causes of kidney stones in children. The article also discusses the clinical presentation, diagnosis, metabolic and genetic workup, medical and surgical management of kidney stones in children, as well as the prevention of kidney stone recurrence in children.

Hypertension in children is a growing problem across the globe. In their article, Drs Haseler and Sinha reiterate that despite differing guidelines in different countries, there is a consensus that early recognition and prompt management with lifestyle modification escalating to antihypertensive medication is required to ameliorate adverse outcomes. The authors affirm that out-of-office blood pressure measurements, preferably by 24-hour ambulatory blood pressure monitoring, is essential for the diagnosis and management of hypertension in children.

The article on hemolytic uremic syndrome (HUS) by Drs Boyer and Niaudet discusses in depth the clinical aspects of infection-induced and atypical HUS, focusing more on pathophysiology, clinical presentation, treatment, and prevention. The article elaborates on pathogenesis of atypical HUS, breakthroughs in its diagnosis, and the recent availability of lifesaving complement inhibitors, such as eculizumab, which has dramatically enhanced the survival of the affected patients.

In the article on renal vasculitis, Drs Grewal, Adams, and Valentini discuss the commonly used classifications for pediatric vasculitis and articulate multisystem presentation of the disease, approach to diagnosis, and treatment interventions. The authors assert a need for timely diagnosis and referral for possible renal biopsy, management of acute complications, such as hypertension and acute kidney injury (AKI), and an early initiation of therapy, which is essential for preserving kidney function and preventing long-term morbidity and mortality.

AKI is a common occurrence in children, particularly in inpatient settings. In the article on AKI, Drs Khandelwal, McLean, and Menon discuss the role of urinary biomarkers, furosemide stress test, and clinical decision support in helping improve the accuracy and timeliness of diagnosis of AKI. The article stresses the role of fluid overload with adverse outcomes and the importance of early intervention and long-term follow-up in those at risk of developing CKD. The authors elaborate on indications for various modes of dialysis and the limitations of each one of them.

In the article on CKD, Drs VanSickle and Warady discuss the emergence of congenital kidney anomalies as the leading cause of CKD in children and the importance of adequate nutritional support, including salt supplementation when indicated, for normal growth and development of young children with CKD. It elaborates on various dialysis modalities and options for kidney replacement therapy and renal transplantation in children with end-stage kidney disease. The need for a multidisciplinary team caring of such patients is emphasized.

My articles with Dr Sanjad and Dr Mohammad on nephrotic syndrome and vesicoureteral reflux, respectively, provide an overview of recent clinical advances in the management of these familiar conditions in children. The article on nephrotic syndrome is primarily about patients who respond to initial steroid therapy, and it underscores the futility of country-specific guidelines, which are remarkably similar with clinically insignificant differences. The article on vesicoureteral reflux defines risk factors for UTI and renal scarring in children, the importance of prompt treatment and prevention of recurrent pyelonephritis, as well as a need for "selective renal imaging" after the first febrile UTI and "selective antimicrobial prophylaxis" in those with recurrent UTI.

I would like to conclude by saying that it is not possible to cover the whole gamut of kidney disorders in children in a single issue. The topics presented here were selected mostly on the basis of their clinical importance, particularly in ambulatory settings. The articles are written by authors with remarkable expertise on the subject, and I owe them a lot of gratitude for their effort. I hope that you, the readers, will find these articles useful for education and patient care.

Tej K. Mattoo, MD, DCH, FRCP (UK), FAAP
Department of Pediatrics
Wayne State University School of Medicine
400 Mack Avenue
Suite 1 East
Detroit, MI 48201, USA

E-mail address:
tmattoo@med.wayne.edu

Assessment of Kidney Function in Children

Emil den Bakker, MD[a], Arend Bökenkamp, MD[b], Dieter Haffner, MD[c],*

KEYWORDS

- Estimated glomerular filtration rate • Proteinuria • Acute kidney disease
- Chronic kidney disease • Children • Diagnosis

KEY POINTS

- Kidney function, that is, glomerular filtration rate (GFR), at birth is only around 30 mL/min/1.73 m^2 and reaches adult values by the age of 2 years.
- A major limitation with serum creatinine is that it may not increase until the GFR has decreased by about 50%.
- Estimated GFR (eGFR) is the best surrogate for measured GFR, which is not possible during routine care in ambulatory settings.
- Urinalysis, sometimes with kidney ultrasound examination plays a central role in the workup of newly diagnosed kidney dysfunction.
- Kidney biopsy is essential in the diagnostic workup of some (acquired) glomerular diseases, suspected tubulointerstitial nephritis and kidney allograft dysfunction.
- Next generation sequencing is a powerful method to diagnose a wide spectrum of kidney diseases, including CKD of unknown origin.

WHAT IS KIDNEY FUNCTION?

The kidneys play a central role in water, electrolyte and mineral homeostasis, and elimination of water-soluble waste products. They synthesize renin, calcitriol, and erythropoietin, which are key regulators of blood volume and blood pressure, bone and mineral metabolism, and erythropoiesis, respectively. Kidneys also play an important

---

Contributions of the authors: All authors drafted the design of the article, wrote and revised it, and approved the final version.

COI statement: Authors declare no conflict of interest and received no funding related to the content of this article.

[a] Department of Pediatrics, Emma Children's Hospital, Amsterdam University Medical Centers, Meibergdreef 9, Amsterdam NL-1105 AZ, the Netherlands; [b] Department of Pediatric Nephrology, Emma Children's Hospital, Amsterdam University Medical Centers, Meibergdreef 9, Amsterdam NL-1105 AZ, the Netherlands; [c] Department of Pediatric Kidney, Liver and Metabolic Diseases, Hannover Medical School, Carl-Neuberg-Str. 1, Hannover 30625, Germany
* Corresponding author.
E-mail address: Haffner.dieter@mh-hannover.de

role in gluconeogenesis and insulin metabolism. The term "kidney function" is generally used as a synonym for the filtrating capacity of the kidneys—the glomerular filtration rate (GFR). Still, it must be kept in mind that each glomerulus is connected to a renal tubule, which processes the glomerular ultrafiltrate (primary urine) and is essential for fluid and electrolyte homeostasis.

Each day, some 150 L of urine containing physiologic amounts of electrolytes, amino acids, glucose, bicarbonate, and so forth are filtered. As an example, this means that 21,000 mmol of sodium (ie, the equivalent of 1.2 kg of kitchen salt) are filtered each day, whereas only about 10 gm of salt is excreted in the final urine/day. This illustrates that filtration and tubular regulation are essential for prevention of a severe and potentially life-threatening imbalance. Although low urine production may indicate kidney disease, renal failure can also present with excessive urine production (polyuria) reflecting renal-tubular damage. This is a potential pitfall in patients with tubulointerstitial nephritis, renal Fanconi syndrome or some congenital anomalies of the kidney and urinary tract (CAKUT). In these conditions, preserved diuresis may obscure dehydration and diminished kidney function.

MATURATION OF KIDNEY FUNCTION

- Nephrogenesis takes place until 36 weeks gestation (or 40 days after birth in a premature newborn)
- Creatinine at birth reflects maternal kidney function
- Kidney function at birth is around 30 mL/min/1.73 m^2 and reaches adult values between the age of 1 and 2 years.

Kidney development in humans takes place from the fifth week of gestation until approximately 35 to 36 weeks of gestation, a period vulnerable to any disruptive factors impairing renal development, for example, treatment of the mother with inhibitors of the renin-angiotensin-aldosterone system.[1,2] Important to note, nephrogenesis may continue up to 40 days after birth in preterm infants. Thereafter, kidney growth is only maintained by growth and maturation of already existing nephrons, numbering between 200,000 and 1.8 million per human being.[3] Consequently, any shortage in nephrons, either from prenatal kidney injury, renal hypo-dysplasia or postnatal loss of nephrons can only be compensated by compensatory hypertrophy of existing nephrons in order to maintain total GFR by increasing single nephron GFR (hyperfiltration).

In the fetus, electrolyte and fluid homeostasis is maintained by the placenta. Fetal renal blood flow is low, resulting in low GFR in utero, which steadily increases from approximately 0.5 mL/min around 20 to 25 weeks of gestation to approximately 4 mL/min at 40 weeks.[4] In parallel, fetal urine output increases from 5 to 50 mL/h and accounts for more than 90% of the amniotic fluid. Consequently, abnormal fetal kidney function during and after the second trimester can result in severe oligohydramnios, causing pulmonary hypoplasia and Potter's syndrome.[5] Fetal GFR is highly correlated with both gestational age and fetal body weight. GFR reference values for very preterm infants were published.[6] Creatinine clearance on day 3 in term infants is between 10 and 40 mL/min/1.73 m^2,[7] and even lower in preterm newborns.

Postnatal maturation of GFR is not linear and is best described by a sigmoid hyperbolic model. It doubles by 2 weeks of age, reaching approximately 50 mL/min/1.73 m^2 between 2 and 4 weeks of age, 90% of adult values (120 mL/min/1.73 m^2) at 1 year of age, and adult values around 2 years of age[8] (**Fig. 1**). This occurs more slowly in preterm infants. Thus, GFR in a given patient needs to be compared with age-appropriate reference values for interpretation. Drug dosing in newborns must consider the physiologically low GFR.[9]

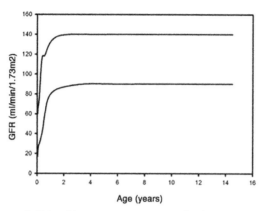

Fig. 1. Development of GFR with age. Presentation of 5th and 95th percentile of GFR measured by inulin clearance in healthy children. (*Reproduced from* den Bakker et al. with permission.[13])

As a rule of thumb, tubular functions mature in parallel with the GFR. These include an ability to maintain water, electrolyte, and acid-base homeostasis via regulation of the reabsorption of small molecules, such as water, sodium, potassium, phosphate, and bicarbonate, and excretion of titratable acid and ammonium into the urine.[10]

Serum creatinine values in the neonatal period change markedly after birth[11] (**Table 1**. As creatinine crosses the placenta and equilibrates between mother and child, serum creatinine levels on the first day of life mainly reflect the maternal kidney function. With increasing GFR, serum creatinine decreases in the following weeks and may take up to 3 months to reach the baseline. This must be considered when using serum creatinine levels as a measure of GFR in infants and neonates. In premature neonates, the decline in serum creatinine level is slower and may even increase in the first few days. This is most marked in extremely premature neonates. Therefore, serial measurements may be necessary to elucidate kidney function in premature infants. Interestingly, first day serum creatinine tends to be lower in

Table 1				
Reference values for serum creatinine levels in neonates				
	Serum Creatinine, Mg/dL			
	Term Infants	**Preterm 32 wk**	**Preterm 27 wk**	**Preterm 24 wk**
Postnatal age	Median (10–90th percentile)	Median (95% prediction interval)	Median (95% prediction interval)	Median (95% prediction interval)
Day 1	0.62 (0.49–0.79)	0.79 (0.50–1.29)	0.61 (0.38–0.98)	0.50 (0.31–0.81)
Day 3	0.48 (0.37–0.61)	0.86 (0.56–1.24)	0.87 (0.57–1.19)	0.90 (0.58–1.24)
Week 1	0.38 (0.31–0.50)	0.61 (0.39–1.17)	0.72 (0.45–1.30)	0.79 (0.49–1.41)
Week 2	0.35 (0.27–0.45)	0.44 (0.31–0.73)	0.51 (0.35–0.97)	0.57 (0.38–1.11)
Week 4	0.28 (0.23–0.36)	0.36 (0.28–0.50)	0.40 (0.29–0.59)	0.43 (0.31–0.69)

Modified from Boer et al.[11] for term and from van Donge et al.[64] for preterm neonates. For conversion to μmol/l multiply by 88.4.

extreme prematurity, most likely reflecting maternal renal function changes during pregnancy.

ASSESSMENT OF GLOMERULAR FILTRATION RATE

Serum creatinine and cystatin C are complementary markers of GFR.
- Large discrepancies between creatinine and cystatin C should prompt a search for a physiologic explanation.
- Calculation of an estimated GFR (eGFR) is required to quantify impairment of kidney function.
- Repeated assessments of eGFR are helpful for patient monitoring.

The GFR is defined as the plasma volume per unit of time that is entirely cleared from a marker molecule, which is freely filtered and neither secreted nor reabsorbed in the renal tubules (**Fig. 2**). GFR describes the volume of primary urine filtered by all glomeruli per unit of time and is the central parameter of global kidney function. It is measured in milliliter per minute and is standardized to the average adult body surface area of 1.73 m.[2] Because GFR measures the ultrafiltration capacity of the sum of all glomeruli, a loss of nephron mass may not be recognized as long as the filtration in the remaining nephrons is increased by higher filtration pressure. This "hyperfiltration" may cause progressive glomerular damage in the long run.[12]

Exogenous Clearance Methods

The most reliable way to measure GFR is by a clearance study using an exogenous marker (measured GFR, the "gold standard"). An ideal filtration marker passes freely across the glomerular barrier, is not protein bound, is neither reabsorbed nor secreted in the renal tubules, is not eliminated through another route and can be measured in serum and urine samples.[13] Examples of such markers are inulin, an inert polysaccharide, the radiocontrast agents iohexol and iothalamate, and radioactive markers such as ^{51}Cr-EDTA and ^{99m}Tc-DTPA.[14] The most used method at the moment is the plasma clearance of iohexol.[15] Unfortunately, the gold standard GFR measurements are too cumbersome for routine clinical use and are restricted to research studies or in selected cases if GFR estimation from serum creatinine or cystatin C is inconclusive.[16]

Endogenous Markers of Kidney Function

Endogenous markers must meet the same requirements as the exogenous markers. In addition, they must be produced at a stable and predictable rate.

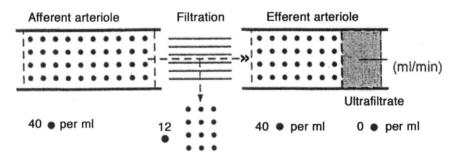

Fig. 2. Clearance that represents the volume/time from which all of the substance has been removed and excreted into the urine per unit of time. In the example the clearance is 12/40, that is, 30% of the plasma entering the afferent arteriole.

Creatinine

The most commonly used endogenous marker is creatinine. Creatinine (MW 113 Da) is a metabolite of creatine, which is stored in muscle cells as phosphocreatine where it serves as an alternative source of intracellular energy during peak energy consumption.[17] Creatinine leaks from muscle cells at a relatively constant rate, distributes over the total body water and is excreted exclusively by the kidneys, mostly by glomerular filtration but to a smaller extent also by tubular secretion.[18] The latter is problematic because tubular secretion is inversely proportional to GFR and may obscure a decline in GFR (**Fig. 3**). Another major limitation with serum creatinine is that it may not increase until the GFR has decreased by about 50%. Certain drugs such as trimethoprim interact with creatinine secretion and may mimic a decrease in kidney function.[19]

Historically, serum creatinine was measured using the colorimetric Jaffé reaction, which was less specific than enzymatic assays, in particular, in icteric samples. To overcome this problem, most modern assays are enzymatic and calibrated to the isotope dilution mass spectroscopy (IDMS) standard.[20,21] This needs to be considered when comparing creatinine measurements from different time periods or at different locations.

Cystatin C

Cystatin C is a low-molecular weight protein (MG 13.3 kDa) that is produced by all nucleated cells and is the most important inhibitor of extracellular proteinases. As opposed to creatinine, its volume of distribution is confined to the extracellular space, making it more suitable to detect rapid changes in GFR.[22] Following glomerular filtration, it is nearly completely reabsorbed in the renal tubules and catabolized, which means that it cannot be used to calculate "cystatin C clearance." The presence of cystatin C in urine indicates renal tubular dysfunction.[23] Unlike creatinine, the production rate of cystatin C is independent of muscle mass and is fairly constant throughout life.[24] Small amounts are metabolized in the liver.[25] Cystatin C can be measured quickly and reliably with standard automated immuno-assays. Previous calibration issues between different assays were solved by the introduction of a universal calibrator by the International Federation of Clinical Chemistry (IFCC).[26] However, cystatin C measurements are more expensive than the enzymatic assays for creatinine.

Urea

Urea is the end product of the hepatic urea cycle, which detoxifies ammonia. Even though urea is excreted primarily through glomerular filtration, it is a poor GFR marker

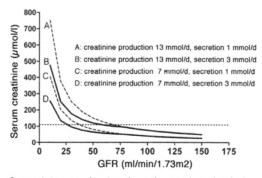

Fig. 3. The effect of creatinine production (muscle mass) and tubular secretion on serum creatinine concentration in relation to GFR from den Bakker and colleagues with permission.[13]

because there is significant renal tubular reabsorption in the presence of an antidiuretic hormone.[27] Serum levels of urea not only reflect GFR but also protein metabolism (catabolism) and hydration status. Yet, it is a useful marker in the classification of acute kidney injury (AKI), where an excessive increase of serum urea compared with creatinine indicates prerenal kidney failure.[28]

ESTIMATING GLOMERULAR FILTRATION RATE FROM ENDOGENOUS MARKERS

Increased serum creatinine or cystatin C indicate a diminished GFR. However, the correlation between the 2 is not linear (see **Fig. 3**), which makes it difficult to assess the degree of kidney function impairment based on the laboratory results. This is the reason why current guidelines recommend calculating an eGFR by using the endogenous GFR markers[29] in daily clinical practice.

The Concept of Estimated Glomerular Filtration Rate Equations

eGFR equations are developed using the correlation between measured GFR based on a gold standard technique and simultaneous marker concentrations, anthropometric data and potential other covariates reflecting the extrarenal factors affecting marker concentration such as sex, age, underlying diagnosis, or the use of specific medication. The endogenous marker must be in a steady state. Equilibration between the blood compartment and the total volume of distribution takes time and rapidly declining kidney function will result in overestimation of eGFR, whereas the opposite happens when kidney function improves.[30] Although several confounders are known and can potentially be corrected for, other factors are unknown and introduce bias and variability depending on the population studied. Moreover, the calibration of the creatinine and cystatin C assays in the local laboratory should be checked to choose the optimal eGFR equation. Hence, an eGFR equation reflects the analytical method and the population used for its generation, which may not be applicable to other populations (and most importantly) to a specific patient.[13] It must be borne in mind that the eGFR value is an *estimate* of the measured GFR bearing significant inaccuracy: Even with the best-performing equations, only some 90% of estimates fall within ±30% of measured GFR and some 40% within ±10%.[24,31,32]

A large number of equations have been developed, some in rather small populations and with crude statistical methods. Many of these have recently been compared in a large multicenter analysis.[31] Several equations stand out, some of which were developed by the Chronic Kidney Disease in Children (CKiD) consortium (often referred to as "Schwartz equations"), some by the group of Pottel and the European Kidney Function Consortium.

Creatinine-Based Estimated Glomerular Filtration Rate Equations

For creatinine, the CKiD consortium and Pottel's group have chosen different approaches to correct for age and sex-dependent differences in creatinine synthesis. Because muscle mass is related to height in children, the CKiD-based equations use height and a *coefficient k* to reflect age and sex-related differences in muscle mass. The most popular and convenient "bedside" Schwartz equation is calculated as follows:

- Schwartz equation for eGFR is [mL/min/1.73 m^2] = k × height [m]/serum creatinine [mg/dL], where k is constant at 41.4.[33] It has recently been revised, with variable sex and age-specific *k-values* up to the age of 25 years (**Tables 2** and **3**).[34] This new CKiD-U25 equation corrects the implausible "rise" in eGFR when

Table 2
Age-based *k* values for the CKiD-U25 equation and *Q* values for the FASage equation for calculation of estimated glomerular filtration rate

Age	*k* Value (CKiD-U25 Equation)		Q_{crea} (FASage Equation)	
	Female	Male	Female	Male
1	33.1	35.7	0.26	0.26
2	33.3	36.0	0.29	0.29
3	33.6	36.3	0.31	0.31
4	33.9	36.6	0.34	0.34
5	34.1	36.9	0.38	0.38
6	34.4	37.2	0.41	0.41
7	34.7	37.5	0.44	0.44
8	35.0	37.8	0.46	0.46
9	35.2	38.1	0.49	0.49
10	35.5	38.4	0.51	0.51
11	35.8	38.7	0.53	0.53
12	36.1	39	0.57	0.57
13	36.9	40.8	0.59	0.59
14	37.8	42.6	0.61	0.61
15	38.6	44.5	0.64	0.72
16	39.5	46.5	0.67	0.78
17	40.4	48.6	0.69	0.82
18	41.4	50.8	0.69	0.85
19	41.4	50.8	0.70	0.88
20	41.4	50.8	0.70	0.90
21–25	41.4	50.8	-	-

Age-specific and sex-specific *k-values* in the CKiD-U25 equation[34] and Q_{crea} in the FASage equation. Values for creatinine in milligram per deciliter and height in meter should be used. For conversion of CKiD-U25 to SI-units and centimeter, multiply by 0.884, and for the conversion of FASage to SI-units, multiply by 88.4. From Pottel and colleagues, with permission.[37]

switching from earlier versions of the CKiD equations to the adult chronic kidney disease (CKD)-Epi equation[35] at the age of 18 years.[36] For conversion of these equations to creatinine measured in micromoles per liter and height in centimeter, the *k* values need to be multiplied by 0.884.

- Pottel equation[37] relates the creatinine concentration in a given patient to 107.3 mL/min/1.73 m² (mean GFR in healthy children) and to the age-related or height-related Q_{crea} *value* (ie, the corresponding mean creatinine concentration in healthy children of the same age or height, respectively; see Table 2). Because this approach is used in adults too, equations following this principle are often referred to as "Full age spectrum" (FAS)-equations, and there is no leap in eGFR at transition to adult care.[24] The FASage equation, which uses Q_{crea} *values* based on age, is more versatile than FASheight because height is not always available for calculation. For this reason, FASage is particularly useful for direct laboratory reporting[38] and is calculated as follows:

FAS [mL/min/1.73 m²] = 107.3/Creat [mg/dL]/Q_{crea}; For creatinine in micromoles per liter, the Q value is multiplied by 88.4.

Table 3
Clinically relevant interactions affecting the choice of estimated glomerular filtration rate marker[7,19,38,40,65–70]

Condition	eGFRcys eGFRcreat	Pathophysiology
Glucocorticoids	Underestimate	Increased cystatin C synthesis
Hypothyroidism	Overestimate	Diminished cystatin C synthesis
Hyperthyroidism	Underestimate	Increased cystatin C synthesis
Severe obesity	Underestimate	Increased cystatin C synthesis
Neuromuscular disease/Spina bifida	Overestimate	Decreased creatinine production
Severe malnutrition	Overestimate	Decreased creatinine production
Active malignancy	Overestimate	Decreased creatinine production
Severe liver disease	Overestimate	Decreased creatinine production
Creatine supplement	Underestimate	Increased creatinine production
Drugs excreted via Organic Anion Transporter (eg, Trimethoprim)		Underestimate interaction with creatinine secretion
Urinoma		Underestimate recirculation of filtered creatinine

CYSTATIN C-BASED ESTIMATED GLOMERULAR FILTRATION RATE EQUATION

Cystatin C-based eGFR equations are as follows:

CKiDcys [mL/min/1.73 m^2] = 70.13 × (Cys/1.17)^−0.931[26,32]

FAScys [mL/min/1.73 m^2] = 107.3 / (Cys /0.82)[24]

Combining Creatinine-Based and Cystatin C-Based Equations

Creatinine and cystatin C have different characteristics in their extrarenal metabolism, and it is not surprising that the 2 are complementary when estimating GFR. Therefore, complex equations incorporating both markers (and even urea) have been developed.[32] Moreover, the arithmetical mean of a creatinine-based and a cystatin C-based eGFR has higher accuracy than either of the two.[39] Comparing the cystatin C-based and the creatinine-based eGFR is useful for conditions where 1 of the 2 markers may fail (**Table 3**).[40] In particular, a discrepancy of more than 40% is suspect for an analytical error or a significant physiologic interaction.[41,42]

Creatinine Clearance

Creatinine clearance calculated from timed urine collections and blood samples has long been considered the second-best method to assess GFR in the absence of a gold-standard measurement. In daily practice, however, precision and accuracy are disappointing due to incorrect urine collection and tubular creatinine excretion.[43] Therefore, creatinine clearance has largely been replaced by eGFR equations, as outlined above.

URINALYSIS

Dipstick analysis of a fresh and clean-voided midstream urine in older children allows evaluation of pH, specific gravity, protein, blood, glucose, ketone, leukocytes, and nitrite. It is well suited for rapid screening and can guide further investigations. The disadvantage, however, is that it does not provide precise quantitative results and can yield false-positive or false-negative results.

Specific gravity (normal range 1.001–1.035) varies widely under normal conditions, reflecting the hydration status of a child. In contrast, a low specific gravity in a child presenting with hypovolemia and/or hypernatremia suggests a concentrating defect (*vide infra*).

Urinary pH ranges between 5.0 and 8.0, depending on the acid–base balance of the body. A urinary pH above 5.5 in the setting of a metabolic acidosis suggests failure to acidify the urine. Still, pH needs to be measured formally by a pH-meter to make the diagnosis of distal renal tubular acidosis.[44]

Glucosuria in the absence of hyperglycemia (glucose >10 mmol/L) suggests a generalized or isolated tubular defect (ie, renal Fanconi syndrome and isolated renal glycosuria). The presence of generalized aminoaciduria and other signs of proximal tubular dysfunction, such as low molecular weight proteinuria, renal phosphate wasting, and hypercalciuria, further supports the diagnosis of Fanconi syndrome (*vide infra*).

Strip tests detect leukocyte esterase, which is expressed in neutrophils, and, if positive, suggests a urinary tract infection (UTI). However, it could be falsely negative. Therefore, urine microscopy for leukocyturia should be performed if a UTI is suspected. Of note, sterile leukocyturia may also be observed in patients with postinfectious glomerulonephritis or in the setting of lupus nephritis. A positive nitrite test suggests the presence of bacteria like *Escherichia coli* reducing nitrate to nitrite. It is negative if the infection is caused by nonnitrite-forming bacteria such as enterococcus. Nitrite may be falsely negative in infants and in patients with pollakiuria because urine must be incubated in the bladder for at least 4 hours for bacteria to produce nitrites from nitrates. For the same reasons, it may be negative in a catheter or suprapubic specimen. Therefore, a urine culture is required to confirm a diagnosis of UTI.

Strip tests also detect red blood cells (RBCs), myoglobin, and hemoglobin. Hematuria (>5 RBCs) should be confirmed by urine microscopy. Dysmorphic erythrocytes and RBC casts indicate glomerular hematuria from glomerulonephritis, hemolytic uremic syndrome (HUS), or Alport syndrome. Urine dipsticks are more sensitive to detect albumin than low-molecular weight proteins, such as alpha-1 microglobulin or retinol-binding protein (<40 kDa).[45] They are thus suitable to screen for glomerular proteinuria, whereas a negative urine dipstick does not fully exclude tubular proteinuria. Semiquantitative expressions of typical dipstick results are given in **Table 4**. Depending on urine concentration, urine protein may be falsely positive or negative. Therefore, a positive dipstick for proteinuria may require quantitative measurement by protein/creatinine ratio (*vide infra*). Moreover, orthostatic proteinuria should be sought, which is characterized by proteinuria in the upright but not in the recumbent position, that is, in the first morning urine sample. Other physiologic forms of proteinuria are febrile proteinuria and exercise proteinuria.

QUANTIFICATION OF PROTEINURIA

A positive dipstick for proteinuria is suggestive of glomerular damage, and it requires precise quantification before rendering diagnostic or therapeutic decisions. This can be done either by assessment of protein to creatinine ratio in a first morning spot urine or assessment of protein in a 24-hour urine sample. Both methods were shown to be reliable in children.[46] Reference values for urinary protein excretion are given in **Tables 5** and **6**. Alternatively, one may assess albumin to creatinine ratio in a spot urine

Table 4
Semiquantitative expressions of typical dipstick results

Dipstick Results	Proteinuria (mg/dL)
Negative	0 to <15
Trace	15 to <30
1+	30 to <100
2+	100 to <300
3+	300 to <1000L
If 4+	≥1000 mg

(normal value < 30 mg/g creatinine, microalbuminuria 30–300 mg/g creatinine, macroalbuminuria >300 mg/g) because this is the leading protein in most proteinuric diseases.[47] Albuminuria is also associated with the progression of CKD.[48] Finally, albumin-specific dipsticks or assessment of urinary albumin to creatinine ratio in spot urine should be used to detect microalbuminuria in children with increased risk for glomerular damage, for example, due to diabetes because this is less than the detection limit of standard urine dipsticks.[49,50]

ASSESSMENT OF TUBULAR FUNCTION

Fluid filtered by the glomerulus is mostly reabsorbed in the proximal and, to a lesser extent, in the distal renal tubule. This is highly regulated in order to maintain water and electrolyte homeostasis. In addition, the kidneys secrete acids (approximately 2–3 mEq/kg body weight in children), depending on the diet and body needs, in order to maintain acid–base homeostasis.

Acid–Base Balance and Anion Gap

Metabolic acidosis is defined as plasma pH < 7.35 and bicarbonate less than 22 mmol/L in children aged older than 2 years, and less than 20 mmol/L in neonates and infants aged younger than 2 years. The serum anion gap (SAG) is calculated as follows: $SAG = Na^+ - (Cl^- + HCO_3^-)$ and ranges between 8 and 16. The presence of metabolic acidosis in combination with a normal SAG suggests renal tubular acidosis or intestinal

Table 5
Reference values for urinary protein excretion

	24 h Collection (mg/m²/d)	Spot Urine[a] Protein/ Creatinine (mg/mg)	Spot Urine[a] Protein/ Creatinine (mg/ mmol)
Normal range			
1–6 mo	-	<0.7	<70
6–24 mo	<150	<0.5	<50
>24 mo	<150	<0.2	<20
Nephrotic	>1000	>2	>200

[a] Preferably a first morning void sample.

Table 6
Workup for kidney dysfunction in children

	Parameters	Comments
History	Birth history, drug exposure, surgery	Factors for increased renal risk
Physical examination	Height/length, head circumference, weight, blood pressure	Edema, dehydration, hypertension, short stature, malnutrition, rash, purpura, syndromic phenotype
Blood	Blood cell count Fragmentocytes	Anemia, thrombocytopenia Suspected hemolysis
Serum/plasma	Sodium, potassium, chloride Bicarbonate/blood gas analysis Calcium, phosphate Creatinine, urea Cystatin C Albumin C3 A ANA, ANCA, anti-dsDNA titer anti-GBM antibodies Antistreptolysine, anti-DNAse titer anti-PLA2R titer Parathyroid hormone	Life-threatening electrolyte disturbances Metabolic acidosis, anion gap Risk of tetany and rickets eGFR calculation, uremia eGFR, esp. in case of reduced muscle mass Nephrotic syndrome Postinfectious GN, MPGN, C3 glomerulopathy, lupus nephritis, aHUS Rapidly progressive GN, vasculitis, SLE Goodpasture syndrome Post-streptococcal GN Membranous GN CKD (not elevated in AKI)
Spot urine	Dipstick: • glucose, protein • leukocytes, nitrite • red blood cells, hemoglobin • myoglobin • pH • specific gravity • ketone Sodium, calcium, phosphate, creatinine, glucose ß2- microglobulin (or other low molecular weight proteins), amino-acids Microscopy (fresh urine): leukocytes, casts, dysmorphic erythrocytes Urine culture (clean urine)	Glomerular or tubular dysfunction Urinary tract infection Glomerular disease, hemolysis Rhabdomyolysis Distal renal tubular acidosis Urine concentration defect, polyuria Malnourishment Fanconi syndrome, nephrolithiasis, nephrocalcinosis Tubular dysfunction, Fanconi syndrome Urinary tract infection, glomerular hematuria Urinary tract infection
Calculations	eGFR Urine: protein and/or albumin/ creatinine ratio Urine: calcium/creatinine ratio FeNa T TmP/GFR (tubular maximum reabsorption of Pi per GFR) TRP SAG UAG	Kidney function Glomerular proteinuria Hypercalciuria, nephrocalcinosis Renal sodium wasting, extracellular volume contraction Hypophosphatemia, rickets, renal phosphate wasting (see text) Acidosis

(*continued on next page*)

Table 6
(continued)

	Parameters	Comments
Kidney ultrasound	Size, echogenicity, cysts, collecting system Duplex ultrasound	Enlarged (AKI) vs small kidneys (in most CKD), hydronephrosis/ obstruction CAKUT, cystic kidney disease, nephrocalcinosis, nephrolithiasis Renal venous thrombosis
Kidney biopsy	Light-, immunofluorescence, and electron microscopy	Specification of glomerular diseases, where histopathological confirmation of disease will likely have important implications for patient management
Genetic testing	Sanger or NGS Copy number variation analysis	Unclear diagnosis or suspected genetic cause, for example, tubular, metabolic or cystic kidney disease, Alport syndrome, atypical HUS (mutations in complement regulating genes), congenital nephrotic syndrome Syndromic phenotype

Further details are given in the text. Disease-specific workups are given in other articles in this special volume.

Abbreviations: aHUS, atypical hemolytic uremic syndrome; AKI, acute kidney injury; CAKUT, congenital anomalies of the kidney and urinary tract; CKD, chronic kidney disease; eGFR, estimated glomerular filtration rate; FeNa, fractional excretion of sodium; GN, glomerulonephritis; MPGN, membranoproliferative GN; NGS, next generation sequencing; PLA2R, phospholipase A2 receptor; Pi, phosphate; SAG, serum anion gap; TRP, fractional excretion of phosphate; UAG, urine anion gap.

bicarbonate losses. Metabolic acidosis caused by renal failure occurs due to reduced glomerular excretion of various acid anions and the SAG in such patients is increased. Finally, urine anion gap (UAG) can be calculated as follows: $UAG = (Na + K) - Cl$. A negative UAG in an acidotic patient indicates gastrointestinal losses of bicarbonate or renal loss of bicarbonate (eg, in proximal renal tubular acidosis), whereas a positive UAG (with normal SAG metabolic acidosis) suggests the presence of an altered distal urinary acidification (eg, in distal renal tubular acidosis).

Excretion of Sodium

Fractional excretion of sodium (FeNa) is a global test for tubular integrity and volume status. The results must be interpreted in the clinical context including plasma sodium and volume status. It is calculated as follows: $FeNa = (U_{Na} \times P_{cr})/(P_{Na} \times U_{cr}) \times 100$, where U_{Na} = urinary sodium; P_{cr} = plasma creatinine; P_{Na} = plasma sodium, and U_{cr} = urinary creatinine.

In clinical practice, both FeNa and U_{Na} may be applied to assess renal sodium wasting. In the setting of extracellular volume contraction, sodium and water are conserved and both FeNa and U_{Na} are low (FeNa <1% in children, 2.5% in neonates; U_{Na} <20 mEq/L in children, <30 mEq/L in neonates). In case of tubular dysfunction, both FeNa and U_{Na} will be inappropriately elevated (FeNa >2% in children, >2.5% in neonates; U_{Na} >30 mEq/L). Of note, these parameters are not reliable when sodium supplementation or diuretic therapy has been initiated.

Excretion of Phosphate

Usually more than 85% of filtered phosphate is reabsorbed in the proximal tubule. Suspected renal phosphate wasting can be assessed by calculating the tubular maximum reabsorption of phosphate per GFR (TmP/GFR) or percentage of tubular reabsorption of phosphate (TRP), although the latter is less reliable to detect renal phosphate wasting in children.[51] This can be done easily in the fasting and nonfasting state using a second morning spot urine and serum sample taken simultaneously using the following formulas: TmP/GFR $= P_p - (U_p/U_{cr}) \times P_{cr}$; TRP $= 1 - [(U_p/P_p) \times (P_{cr}/U_{cr})]$, where P_p = plasma phosphate, U_P = urinary phosphate, U_{cr} = urinary creatinine, and P_{cr} = plasma creatinine. Age-related norm values, an algorithm for the workup for tubular phosphate wasting[52] and an online calculator are given elsewhere.[51]

Excretion of Calcium

Urinary calcium excretion can easily be evaluated by use of a spot urine and calculation of calcium to creatinine ratio ($U_{Ca/Crea}$). Values should be related to age-specific reference values,[53] and, if high, confirmed by 24-hour urine sample.[52] A urinary calcium excretion greater than 4 mg/kg/ d (0.1 mmol/kg/d) indicates hypercalciuria.

Tubular Concentration

Maximal urinary concentrating ability increases with age. Healthy infants usually achieve a urine osmolality greater than 300 mOsm/kg H_2O, whereas children aged older than 2 years and adults achieve values greater than 800 mOsm/kg H_2O.[54] This can be evaluated by a water deprivation test, which may only be performed under inpatient conditions and with careful monitoring of weight, urine output, serum sodium concentration, hematocrit and blood osmolality, especially in cases of pronounced polyuria. In complete diabetes insipidus, urine output remains unchanged and its osmolality does not increase. In this situation, desmopressin is administered. Persistent urine osmolality of less than 200 mOsm/kg H_2O in combination with a serum sodium concentration greater than 145 mmol/L suggests the diagnosis of nephrogenic diabetes insipidus.

Diagnostic Approach to the Child with Suspected Impaired Kidney Function

- The first critical step in a patient with severely impaired kidney function is assessment of potentially life-threatening conditions including electrolyte imbalances (hyperkalemia, hyponatremia, hypocalcemia), metabolic acidosis, fluid overload, and hypertension.

The key parameters for the recognition of impaired kidney function are serum creatinine and cystatin C, whereas urea is less reliable because it is strongly affected by fluid and protein intake. If possible, earlier measurements should be sought to determine the course of kidney function. As a rule of thumb, an increase in serum creatinine or cystatin C by 33% reflects a decrease in GFR by 25%, even if the measurement is still within the normal range. This is particularly important in patients with abnormal creatinine production such as neuromuscular disease, liver disease or active malignancy, in whom impaired kidney function can easily be missed.

The first critical step in a patient with severely impaired kidney function is the assessment of potentially life-threatening conditions that need immediate attention such as hyperkalemia, metabolic acidosis, severe hypertension or fluid overload impairing oxygenation and/or cardiac function, hyponatremia as well as hyperphosphatemia leading to hypocalcemia.

History should address fluid intake, extrarenal losses and urine output, past medical history, recent disease, and medication. Urine color may indicate highly concentrated urine or hematuria. If available, findings on prenatal ultrasound may be helpful for the recognition of CAKUT or cystic kidney disease. A positive family history may indicate hereditary kidney disease such as Alport syndrome or polycystic kidney disease. Review of the growth chart may point toward longer-standing CKD. De novo bed-wetting can be a symptom of polyuria (cf. above) in a child who was continent previously.

On physical examination, assessment of volume status and blood pressure is of utmost importance. Arthritis, exanthema, or vasculitic changes may point toward a systemic disease such as systemic lupus erythematodes or Henoch-Schonlein vasculitis where as petechiae and icterus may indicate HUS. Bilateral flank pain can occur in glomerulonephritis, whereas unilateral pain may point toward pyelonephritis or ureteral obstruction.

Macroscopic urine appearance may distinguish between glomerular hematuria (dark red or brown urine without blood clots) and postglomerular hematuria (light red with blood clots). This can be further substantiated by urine microscopy (*vide supra*). Microscopic analysis may be hampered in case of severe macroscopic hematuria. In this setting, determination of the ratio between the urine albumin and total protein concentrations may be helpful: In case of postglomerular bleeding, the albumin-total protein-ratio corresponds to the albumin content in serum, that is, around 50%, whereas in glomerular disease, the proportion of albumin is higher.[45] Nephrotic-range proteinuria points toward a glomerular cause, whereas lower-grade proteinuria is seen in tubulointerstitial disease. AKI and urologic disease commonly has little or no proteinuria.

To distinguish intrinsic and postrenal from prerenal kidney failure, urine sodium concentration, osmolality, and the FeNa are determined *(vide supra)*. Kidney ultrasound will identify obstructive uropathy (hydronephrosis) unless the patient is dehydrated, which may mask dilatation of the urinary tract. Kidney size may help distinguish between AKI and CKD. Normal-sized or enlarged kidneys suggest recent (and potentially reversible) kidney disease (eg, glomerulonephritis and HUS), whereas small hyperechogenic kidneys indicate irreversible kidney damage, either from CAKUT or acquired chronic damage. Nephrocalcinosis may point toward hyperoxaluria or other stone disease, cystic changes may indicate polycystic kidney disease and genetic testing may be needed.

Blood tests will determine the degree of kidney function impairment (ie, eGFR) and its metabolic consequences (eg, hyperkalemia, hyperphosphatemia, metabolic acidosis, anemia). Secondary hyperparathyroidism and/or hyporegenerative anemia points toward CKD, hemolytic anemia points toward HUS (Coombs-negative, fragmentocytes on blood smear) and systemic lupus erythematodes (Coombs-positive). In glomerulonephritis and HUS, the assessment of complement activation is a central step in the differential diagnosis (see **Table 6**). Elevated antistreptolysin and anti-DNAse titers support the diagnosis of poststreptococcal glomerulonephritis. The autoimmune panel should include ANA/antidouble strand DNA, antineutrophil cytoplasmatic antibodies (ANCA) screening, and anti-glomerular basement membrane (GBM) antibodies. If anti-GBM disease (Goodpasture syndrome) is suspected, this test needs to be performed immediately because these patients require therapeutic plasma exchange as soon as possible.

Indications for Further Workup

- Ultrasound-guided kidney biopsy is a safe but invasive diagnostic procedure.
- Indications for kidney biopsy are mostly acquired glomerular diseases, suspected tubulointerstitial nephritis, and kidney allograft dysfunction.
- Genetic testing has replaced kidney biopsy in certain cases of nephrotic syndrome and suspected Alport syndrome.

Kidney Biopsy

Histopathological evaluation by light microscopy in combination with immunofluorescence and electron microscopy is the gold standard for renal tissue analysis. Kidney biopsy has a central role in the diagnostic workup of (acquired) glomerular diseases, suspected tubulointerstitial nephritis and in kidney allograft dysfunction. It has no value in (hereditary) tubular disorders, CAKUT or cystic kidney diseases, including polycystic kidney diseases.[55] Severe complications (ie, bleeding necessitating transfusions, arteriovenous-aneurysms, infection) although rare in children (<1%) may occur. It requires sedation or general anesthesia in small children and hospitalization. Therefore, kidney biopsy is only performed if the procedure will likely yield important information for patient management (ie, diagnosis and/or prognosis).[56] It is often not diagnostic in advanced CKD because scarring may mask the original cause. Children presenting with acute nephritic syndrome, that is, glomerular hematuria and nephrotic range proteinuria, should be considered as candidates for a kidney biopsy, especially in case of decreased eGFR or concomitant hypertension, unless a diagnosis can be made on clinical grounds (eg, postinfectious glomerulonephritis). In children presenting with nephrotic syndrome at the typical age without signs of systemic disease or impaired renal function, minimal change disease is most likely and glucocorticoid treatment is started without prior kidney biopsy.[55,57]

Genetic Testing

More than 450 monogenic disorders have been shown to cause CKD in children, and in approximately 30% of children presenting with CKD a genetic cause has been identified.[58–60] This includes glomerular and tubular diseases as well as metabolic (eg, primary hyperoxaluria, cystinosis) and cystic kidney diseases and CAKUT. Genetic testing is recommended in the workup of children with CKD if there is an established heritability.[61] Yet, it should also be considered in children with a negative family history if the clinical phenotype does not allow a clear diagnosis (eg, in children with tubulopathies, cystic kidney diseases). Genetic testing is indicated in patients with congenital nephrotic syndrome and syndromic/hereditary forms of nephrotic syndrome because it helps avoid immunosuppressive therapy, which will be ineffective and lead to significant side effects.[57,62] In a number of diseases, medical therapies are based on genomic data (eg, sporadic X-linked hypophosphatemia, atypical HUS). At many centers, including ours, genetic testing has replaced kidney biopsy for the diagnosis of Alport syndrome.[63] A definitive molecular diagnosis will end the diagnostic odyssey often observed in children suffering from unexplained CKD, allow information about prognosis, the delivery of precision medicine, genetic counseling of the family (eg, family planning) and "presymptomatic" testing in relatives.

Genetic testing may be performed by single gene testing using the Sanger technique if a specific genetic cause is likely.[61] However, in most cases, a wider approach using next generation sequencing (NGS) technology (massive parallel sequencing) is advised, depending on the local setting and clinical presentation. This should include copy number variation analysis, especially in case of a syndromic phenotype.[60] In case of negative test results, genetic testing should be repeated after some time in view of the rapidly evolving field of genetics.

SUMMARY

A stepwise approach starting with urinalysis, followed by estimation of GFR and quantification of proteinuria is recommended for early detection of kidney disease in children. In addition, specific tests for tubular function, kidney biopsy, and/or genetic analyses may be required to further characterize the underlying kidney disease.

CLINICS CARE POINTS

- A normal serum creatinine values does not exclude acute or chronic kidney injury.
- Estimate glomerular filtration rate (eGFR) by creatinine and/or cystatin C based equations in any child presenting with presumed acute or chronic kidney injury.
- Take into account that eGFR of newborns is only about 30% of that of adults and increases to adult values by the age of 2 years.
- Assess imbalances of electolytes including hyperkalemia, hyponatremia, and hypocalcemia, as well as metabolic acodosis, fluid overload and hypertension in any child presenting with acute or chronic kidney injury.
- Consider performing a kidney biopsy and/or genetic testing in children with suspected significant glomerular disease.

REFERENCES

1. Iacobelli S, Guignard JP. Maturation of glomerular filtration rate in neonates and infants: an overview. Pediatr Nephrol 2021;36(6):1439–46.
2. Bullo M, Tschumi S, Bucher BS, et al. Pregnancy outcome following exposure to angiotensin-converting enzyme inhibitors or angiotensin receptor antagonists: a systematic review. Hypertension 2012;60(2):444–50.
3. Hinchliffe SA, Sargent PH, Howard CV, et al. Human intrauterine renal growth expressed in absolute number of glomeruli assessed by the disector method and Cavalieri principle. Lab Invest 1991;64(6):777–84.
4. Haycock GB. Development of glomerular filtration and tubular sodium reabsorption in the human fetus and newborn. Br J Urol 1998;81(Suppl 2):33–8.
5. Potter EL. Bilateral renal agenesis. J Pediatr 1946;29:68–76.
6. Vieux R, Hascoet JM, Merdariu D, et al. Glomerular filtration rate reference values in very preterm infants. Pediatrics 2010;125(5):e1186–92.
7. Veille JC, Hanson RA, Tatum K, et al. Quantitative assessment of human fetal renal blood flow. Am J Obstet Gynecol 1993;169(6):1399–402.
8. Bueva A, Guignard JP. Renal function in preterm neonates. Pediatr Res 1994;36(5):572–7.
9. Ku LC, Smith PB. Dosing in neonates: special considerations in physiology and trial design. Pediatr Res 2015;77(1–1):2–9.
10. Arant BS Jr. Developmental patterns of renal functional maturation compared in the human neonate. J Pediatr 1978;92(5):705–12.
11. Boer DP, de Rijke YB, Hop WC, et al. Reference values for serum creatinine in children younger than 1 year of age. Pediatr Nephrol 2010;25(10):2107–13.

12. Brenner BM, Lawler EV, Mackenzie HS. The hyperfiltration theory: a paradigm shift in nephrology. Kidney Int 1996;49(6):1774–7.
13. den Bakker E, Gemke RJBJ, Bökenkamp A. Endogenous markers for kidney function in children: a review. Crit Rev Clin Lab Sci 2018;1–21.
14. Soveri I, Berg UB, Björk J, et al. Measuring GFR: a systematic review. Am J Kidney Dis 2014;64(3):411–24.
15. Schwartz GJ, Furth SL. Glomerular filtration rate measurement and estimation in chronic kidney disease. Pediatr Nephrol 2007;22(11):1839–48.
16. Ebert N, Bevc S, Bokenkamp A, et al. Assessment of kidney function: clinical indications for measured GFR. Clin Kidney J 2021;14(8):1861–70.
17. Wyss M, Kaddurah-Daouk R. Creatine and creatinine metabolism. Physiol Rev 2000;80(3):1107–213.
18. Zhang X, Rule AD, McCulloch CE, et al. Tubular secretion of creatinine and kidney function: an observational study. BMC Nephrol 2020;21(1):108.
19. Delanaye P, Mariat C, Cavalier E, et al. Trimethoprim, creatinine and creatinine-based equations. Nephron Clin Pract 2011;119(3):c187–93 ; discussion c193-4.
20. Schwartz GJ, Kwong T, Erway B, et al. Validation of creatinine assays utilizing HPLC and IDMS traceable standards in sera of children. Pediatr Nephrol 2009; 24(1):113–9.
21. Hoste L, Deiteren K, Pottel H, et al. Routine serum creatinine measurements: how well do we perform? *BMC Nephrol* Feb 2015;16:21.
22. Christiadi D, Simpson C, O'Brien K, et al. Cystatin C kidney functional reserve: a simple method to predict outcome in chronic kidney disease. Nephrol Dial Transpl 2021. https://doi.org/10.1093/ndt/gfab188.
23. Herget-Rosenthal S, van Wijk JA, Bröcker-Preuss M, et al. Increased urinary cystatin C reflects structural and functional renal tubular impairment independent of glomerular filtration rate. Clin Biochem 2007;40(13–14):946–51.
24. Pottel H, Delanaye P, Schaeffner E, et al. Estimating glomerular filtration rate for the full age spectrum from serum creatinine and cystatin C. Nephrol Dial Transpl 2017;32(3):497–507.
25. Sjöström P, Tidman M, Jones I. Determination of the production rate and non-renal clearance of cystatin C and estimation of the glomerular filtration rate from the serum concentration of cystatin C in humans. Scand J Clin Lab Invest 2005;65(2):111–24.
26. Schwartz GJ, Cox C, Seegmiller JC, et al. Recalibration of cystatin C using standardized material in Siemens nephelometers. Pediatr Nephrol 2020;35(2):279–85.
27. Weiner ID, Mitch WE, Sands JM. Urea and Ammonia Metabolism and the Control of Renal Nitrogen Excretion. Clin J Am Soc Nephrol 2015;10(8):1444–58.
28. Carvounis CP, Nisar S, Guro-Razuman S. Significance of the fractional excretion of urea in the differential diagnosis of acute renal failure. Kidney Int 2002;62(6):2223–9.
29. KCW Group. KDIGO 2012 clinical practice guideline for the evaluation and management of chronic kidney disease. Kidney Int Supplements 2013;1–150.
30. Slort PR, Ozden N, Pape L, et al. Comparing cystatin C and creatinine in the diagnosis of pediatric acute renal allograft dysfunction. Pediatr Nephrol 2012;27(5):843–9.
31. Bjork J, Nyman U, Berg U, et al. Validation of standardized creatinine and cystatin C GFR estimating equations in a large multicentre European cohort of children. Pediatr Nephrol 2019;34(6):1087–98.

32. Schwartz GJ, Schneider MF, Maier PS, et al. Improved equations estimating GFR in children with chronic kidney disease using an immunonephelometric determination of cystatin C. Kidney Int 2012;82(4):445–53.

33. Schwartz GJ, Muñoz A, Schneider MF, et al. New equations to estimate GFR in children with CKD. J Am Soc Nephrol 2009;20(3):629–37.

34. Pierce CB, Munoz A, Ng DK, et al. Age- and sex-dependent clinical equations to estimate glomerular filtration rates in children and young adults with chronic kidney disease. Kidney Int 2021;99(4):948–56.

35. Levey AS, Stevens LA, Schmid CH, et al. A new equation to estimate glomerular filtration rate. Ann Intern Med 2009;150(9):604–12.

36. Pottel H, Bjork J, Bokenkamp A, et al. Estimating glomerular filtration rate at the transition from pediatric to adult care. Kidney Int 2019;95(5):1234–43.

37. Pottel H, Dubourg L, Goffin K, et al. Alternatives for the Bedside Schwartz Equation to Estimate Glomerular Filtration Rate in Children. Adv Chronic Kidney Dis 2018;25(1):57–66.

38. den Bakker E, Gemke R, van Wijk JAE, et al. Accurate eGFR reporting for children without anthropometric data. Clin Chim Acta 2017;474:38–43.

39. Leion F, Hegbrant J, den Bakker E, et al. Estimating glomerular filtration rate (GFR) in children. The average between a cystatin C- and a creatinine-based equation improves estimation of GFR in both children and adults and enables diagnosing Shrunken Pore Syndrome. Scand J Clin Lab Invest 2017;77(5):338–44.

40. Schreuder MF, Swinkels DW, Kortmann BB, et al. Discrepant results of serum creatinine and cystatin C as a clue to urine leakage after renal transplantation. Transplantation 2009;88(4):596–7.

41. den Bakker E, Gemke R, van Wijk JAE, et al. Combining GFR estimates from cystatin C and creatinine-what is the optimal mix? Pediatr Nephrol 2018. https://doi.org/10.1007/s00467-018-3973-8.

42. Grubb A. Non-invasive estimation of glomerular filtration rate (GFR). The Lund model: Simultaneous use of cystatin C- and creatinine-based GFR-prediction equations, clinical data and an internal quality check. Scand J Clin Lab Invest 2010;70(2):65–70.

43. Schwartz GJ, Work DF. Measurement and estimation of GFR in children and adolescents. Clin J Am Soc Nephrol 2009;4(11):1832–43.

44. Trepiccione F, Walsh SB, Ariceta G, et al. Distal renal tubular acidosis: ERKNet/ESPN clinical practice points. Nephrol Dial Transpl 2021;36(9):1585–96.

45. Bokenkamp A. Proteinuria-take a closer look! Pediatr Nephrol 2020;35(4):533–41.

46. Hogg RJ, Portman RJ, Milliner D, et al. Evaluation and management of proteinuria and nephrotic syndrome in children: recommendations from a pediatric nephrology panel established at the National Kidney Foundation conference on proteinuria, albuminuria, risk, assessment, detection, and elimination (PARADE). Pediatrics 2000;105(6):1242–9.

47. Kashtan CE, Gross O. Correction to: Clinical practice recommendations for the diagnosis and management of Alport syndrome in children, adolescents, and young adults-an update for 2020. Pediatr Nephrol 2021;36(3):731.

48. Ruiz-Ortega M, Rayego-Mateos S, Lamas S, et al. Targeting the progression of chronic kidney disease. Nat Rev Nephrol 2020;16(5):269–88.

49. Ambarsari CG, Tambunan T, Pardede SO, et al. Role of dipstick albuminuria in progression of paediatric chronic kidney disease. J Pak Med Assoc 2021;71(Suppl 2):S103–6.

50. Pugia MJ, Lott JA, Kajima J, et al. Screening school children for albuminuria, proteinuria and occult blood with dipsticks. Clin Chem Lab Med 1999;37(2):149–57.
51. https://gpn.de/service/tmp-gfr-calculator/.
52. Haffner D, Leifheit-Nestler M, Grund A, et al. Rickets guidance: part I-diagnostic workup. Pediatr Nephrol 2021. https://doi.org/10.1007/s00467-021-05328-w.
53. Matos V, van Melle G, Boulat O, et al. Urinary phosphate/creatinine, calcium/creatinine, and magnesium/creatinine ratios in a healthy pediatric population. J Pediatr 1997;131(2):252–7.
54. Knoers N, Lemmink H. Hereditary Nephrogenic Diabetes Insipidus. In: Adam MP, Ardinger HH, Pagon RA, et al, eds GeneReviews((R)). 1993. Available at: https://www.ncbi.nlm.nih.gov/books/NBK1177/.
55. Kidney Disease: Improving Global Outcomes Glomerular Diseases Work G. KDIGO 2021 Clinical Practice Guideline for the Management of Glomerular Diseases. Kidney Int 2021;100(4S):S1–276.
56. Feneberg R, Schaefer F, Zieger B, et al. Percutaneous renal biopsy in children: a 27-year experience. Nephron 1998;79(4):438–46.
57. Trautmann A, Vivarelli M, Samuel S, et al. IPNA clinical practice recommendations for the diagnosis and management of children with steroid-resistant nephrotic syndrome. Pediatr Nephrol 2020;35(8):1529–61.
58. Hildebrandt F. Genetic kidney diseases. Lancet 2010;375(9722):1287–95.
59. Arora V, Anand K, Chander Verma I. Genetic Testing in Pediatric Kidney Disease. Indian J Pediatr 2020;87(9):706–15.
60. Hay E, Cullup T, Barnicoat A. A practical approach to the genomics of kidney disorders. Pediatr Nephrol 2022;37(1):21–35.
61. Ayme S, Bockenhauer D, Day S, et al. Common Elements in Rare Kidney Diseases: Conclusions from a Kidney Disease: Improving Global Outcomes (KDIGO) Controversies Conference. Kidney Int 2017;92(4):796–808.
62. Boyer O, Schaefer F, Haffner D, et al. Management of congenital nephrotic syndrome: consensus recommendations of the ERKNet-ESPN Working Group. Nat Rev Nephrol 2021;17(4):277–89.
63. Savige J, Lipska-Zietkiewicz BS, Watson E, et al. Guidelines for Genetic Testing and Management of Alport Syndrome. Clin J Am Soc Nephrol 2022;17(1):143–54.
64. van Donge T, Allegaert K, Gotta V, et al. Characterizing dynamics of serum creatinine and creatinine clearance in extremely low birth weight neonates during the first 6 weeks of life. Pediatr Nephrol 2021;36(3):649–59.
65. Bökenkamp A, Laarman CA, Braam KI, et al. Effect of corticosteroid therapy on low-molecular weight protein markers of kidney function. Clin Chem Dec 2007;53(12):2219–21.
66. Fricker M, Wiesli P, Brändle M, et al. Impact of thyroid dysfunction on serum cystatin C. Kidney Int 2003;63(5):1944–7.
67. Knight EL, Verhave JC, Spiegelman D, et al. Factors influencing serum cystatin C levels other than renal function and the impact on renal function measurement. Kidney Int 2004;65(4):1416–21.
68. Kaliciński P, Szymczak M, Smirska E, et al. Longitudinal study of renal function in pediatric liver transplant recipients. Ann Transpl 2005;10(2):53–8.
69. Williamson L, New D. How the use of creatine supplements can elevate serum creatinine in the absence of underlying kidney pathology. BMJ Case Rep 2014;2014doi.
70. Delanaye P, Cavalier E, Radermecker RP, et al. Cystatin C or creatinine for detection of stage 3 chronic kidney disease in anorexia nervosa. Nephron Clin Pract 2008;110(3):c158–63.

Evaluation of Proteinuria and Hematuria in Ambulatory Setting

Abubakr A. Imam, MBBS[a],*, Sermin A. Saadeh, MD[b]

KEYWORDS

- Proteinuria • Albuminuria • Transient proteinuria • Orthostatic proteinuria
- Persistent proteinuria • Hematuria • Microscopic hematuria • Familial hematuria

KEY POINTS

- Hematuria by dipstick examination should be confirmed by urine microscopy.
- Proteinuria in a random urine specimen should be confirmed by the protein/creatinine ratio in the first-morning urine specimen.
- Exercise and febrile illness can cause transient proteinuria and/or microscopic hematuria.
- Patients with microscopic hematuria and proteinuria need further workup and/or careful monitoring.
- Genetic testing is making it possible to diagnose certain kidney conditions without a kidney biopsy.

INTRODUCTION

Proteinuria and hematuria are common urinary findings in ambulatory settings.[1–3] Their presence may be detected by routine urine testing during office visits or when children present with a history or symptoms that warrant urine testing. The presence of either one by itself or the two presenting simultaneously can have different clinical implications with a different set of investigations. Some of the conditions leading to proteinuria and/or hematuria can be benign and causes no harm or they may be indicative of a more serious kidney disease that requires prompt attention and management.[3,4] In this article, we review the approach for evaluating children presenting with proteinuria and/or hematuria in an ambulatory setting.

[a] Nephrology & Hypertension, Department of Pediatrics, Sidra Medicine, College of Medicine, Qatar University, Weill Cornell Medicine-Qatar, PO Box 26999, Doha, Qatar; [b] Department of Pediatrics - MBC 58, Pediatric Nephrology, King Faisal Specialist Hospital and Research Center, (KFSH&RC), King Faisal University, PO Box 3354, Riyadh 11211, KSA
* Corresponding author.
E-mail address: aimam@sidra.org

Pediatr Clin N Am 69 (2022) 1037–1049
https://doi.org/10.1016/j.pcl.2022.07.002
0031-3955/22/© 2022 Elsevier Inc. All rights reserved.

pediatric.theclinics.com

Proteinuria

Overview

The ability of any protein to cross the glomerular basement membrane (GBM) is related to its molecular size and charge. Large molecules such as globulins are not able to pass, whereas albumin is filtered in a very low concentration and low-molecular-weight proteins (LMWPs) are filtered easily. The molecular charge also determines the protein's ability to pass through the GBM. This is attributed to the presence of the negatively charged sialoproteins on the surface of glomerular endothelial and epithelial cells as well as the presence of glycosaminoglycans on the GBM, resulting in a repelling effect for the negatively charged molecules. Moreover, the proteins that can pass through the GBM are mostly reclaimed back by the tubules and into circulation, predominantly by the proximal tubules by endocytosis. Normally, approximately 60% of proteins in urine are from the plasma proteins and the rest are LMWP degraded in the tubules or secreted in the urine. Tissue proteins, such as Tamm–Horsfall protein (THP), are excreted normally from the cells lining the urinary tract or excessively in response to inflammation.[5]

Kidney pathology that changes the structure or function of the GBM may result in increased amounts of large proteins in urine. Also, disorders affecting the recycling system in the proximal tubules, or conditions that cause excessive secretion of THP from kidney tissues, might result in increased proteins in the urine. On the basis of these underlying mechanisms, the proteinuria is classified as *glomerular proteinuria* (glomerular defects), *tubular proteinuria* (defect in tubular reabsorption), or *secretory proteinuria* (excessive secretion from the kidney tissue).[5] In some instances, glomerular proteinuria can occur when there are reduced numbers of functioning nephrons resulting in hyperfiltration-induced GBM damage and an increased filtration of proteins from the remaining nephrons. Tubular proteinuria may also occur if there is an increase in the plasma concentration of LMWP that exceeds the re-absorptive capacity of the proximal tubules without actual defect in the tubules.[6] Diseases such as vesicoureteral reflux or Dent disease, may sometimes present with mixed tubular and glomerular proteinuria if there is associated focal segmental glomerulosclerosis (FSGS)[7–9] (**Table 1**).

Diagnosis of proteinuria

The commercially available urine dipsticks are often used for routine urine analysis (UA) in the ambulatory settings. They use a colorimetric chemical reaction to measure many substances semi-quantitatively and are designed to detect varying concentrations of urine albumin by a tetrabromophenol blue reaction at slightly acidic urine pH. False-positive results can occur if the dipstick is left in urine for a long time or in the presence of hematuria or pyuria. Highly concentrated urine or alkaline urine with pH > 7 might also give false-positive results. Dilute or acidic urine can give a false-negative test for protein. The dipsticks can detect levels of albumin as low as 5–30 mg/dL and the test results are shown as negative, trace, 30, 100, 300, or 2000 mg/dL. They are less sensitive in detecting globulins or LMWPs and will result in false-negative results. Therefore, to identify non-albumin or to measure total urine protein (including albumin), sulfosalicylic acid assays[4] or a quantitative 24-h urine protein excretion or first-morning urine protein/creatinine ratio must be performed.

Clinically, it is important to accurately quantify urinary protein excretion for diagnosis and management and for defining the prognosis in some children with chronic kidney diseases (CKDs).[10–13] 24-h urine collection is the most reliable method for measuring urinary protein excretion; however, it is neither convenient nor reliable in

Table 1
Types and causes of persistent proteinuria in children

Type	Glomerular (Albuminuria)	Tubular (LMWP)	Secretory (THP)
Cause	• Nephrotic syndrome • Focal segmental glomerulosclerosis • Acute GN ○ Postinfectious GN ○ Membranoproliferative GN ○ IgA nephropathy ○ Membranous nephropathy • Henoch Schönlein purpura • Systemic lupus erythematosus • Alport syndrome • Hemolytic uremic syndrome • Diabetic nephropathy • Sickle cell nephropathy • Hyperfiltration (single kidney, nephron loss)	• Reflux nephropathy • Pyelonephritis • Obstructive uropathy • Fanconi syndrome • Dent Disease • Lowe syndrome • Polycystic kidney disease • Medications (NSAIDs)	• Neonatal period (normal) • Urinary tract infections • Interstitial nephritis • Medications (NSAIDs)

Abbreviations: GN, glomerulonephritis; LMWP, low-molecular-weight proteins; NSAIDS, non-steroidal anti-inflammatory drugs; THP, Tamm–Horsfall protein.

pediatric patients, particularly in out-patient settings. Alternatively, a spot first-morning urine sample is used for protein-to-creatinine ratio, which has been shown to have a strong correlation with the 24-h collections.[14–16] In certain diseases, such as diabetes mellites or sickle cell disease, detection of very small quantities of albuminuria (known as microalbuminuria) is an early marker for kidney involvement.[17–19] Microalbuminuria helps diagnose kidney pathology before overt proteinuria by urine dipstick examination.

In children, proteinuria is defined as urinary protein excretion greater than 100 mg/m^2 per day or more than 0.2 mg protein/mg creatinine on spot urine.[14,15] However, urinary protein excretion in children is known to vary according to age, sex, and body size. In infants and neonates, owing to some degree of incomplete maturation of the kidney, up to 300 mg/m^2 is acceptable.[2] By the age of 2 years, the kidneys are fully matured and urine protein excretion is similar to older children and adults.[5] Nephrotic range proteinuria is significant proteinuria, more than 1000 mg/m^2 per day or urine protein-to-creatinine ratio greater than 2 mg protein/mg creatinine in spot urine.[2,15] This degree of proteinuria is required for the diagnosis of nephrotic syndrome and is discussed in more detail in another article.

Clinical evaluation
Most pediatric patients presenting with proteinuria in ambulatory settings do not need extensive laboratory workup. A good clinical evaluation and assessment for the clinical significance of proteinuria are helpful in diagnosing most such cases.

History. Special attention should be paid to symptoms related to the urinary system (such as gross hematuria, dysuria, or polyuria), body swelling, or symptoms related to systemic diseases (such as skin rash, joint pain, or joint swelling). Past medical history of similar presentations, recurrent urinary tract infections or medication history might give clues to the etiology. Detailed family history about CKDs and hypertension and a specific inquiry about genetic kidney diseases such as Alport syndrome, polycystic kidney disease, or nephrotic syndrome are helpful.

Physical examination. Assessment of growth should be done as short stature may indicate an undiagnosed underlying CKD. Blood pressure should be measured and interpreted according to the latest clinical practice guidelines published in 2017.[20] Hypertension in presence of persistent proteinuria may indicate glomerular diseases. Presence of edema (periorbital, pleural effusion, ascites, scrotal or lower extremities) may indicate the diagnosis of nephrotic syndrome. In such patients, assessment of the intravascular volume status is critical for immediate management. Although joint swelling may suggest connective tissue diseases such as systemic lupus erythematosus, characteristic skin rash description and distribution may point toward specific diagnoses such as Henoch Schönlein purpura.

Assessing the clinical significance of proteinuria. Transient and orthostatic proteinuria is very common in children.[21,22] Less commonly, however, more clinically significant, persistent proteinuria might be present.[23]

Transient proteinuria

It is usually a physiological increase in urine protein in response to certain triggers such as fever, vigorous exercise, seizures, and dehydration. It is confirmed by obtaining a good history and a negative urine dipstick for protein or normal value for urine protein-to-creatinine ratio after the resolution of the underlying trigger.[24] Exercise-induced proteinuria may take 24–48 h to resolve.

Orthostatic proteinuria

It is defined by an elevated urine protein excretion in the upright position, which returns to normal in a supine or recumbent position. Orthostatic proteinuria is one of the commonest causes of increased urine protein in otherwise healthy children, particularly adolescents. It is a benign condition without any clinical significance.[6] The exact mechanism is not clear and hemodynamic factors and the compression of the left renal vein have been suggested as possibilities.[25–27] It is confirmed by a negative urine dipstick for protein or normal urine protein-to-creatinine ratio in the first-morning urine and a positive dipstick for protein or elevated urine protein-to-creatinine ratio when the child has been upright.[22] Furthermore, it is not associated with hematuria or hypertension.[23]

Persistent proteinuria

It is characterized by the detection of proteinuria on multiple occasions, ie, not *transient* nor *orthostatic*, and is caused by a wide range of kidney diseases of glomerular or tubulointerstitial origin (see **Table 1**). Persistent proteinuria might be associated with hematuria, hypertension, abnormal kidney function, or other systemic symptoms.[23,28,29] This form of proteinuria should not be missed in the ambulatory settings as it could be indicative of a CKD.[2,30,31]

Although there is no need for a routine screening urinalysis in children, clinicians often obtain a urine specimen for testing, particularly in cases presenting with symptoms related to the kidneys or urinary system. Conditions for which a screening urinalysis is recommended are mentioned in **Box 1**.[32] Obtaining detailed history and performing a thorough physical examination are of great value in reaching the correct diagnosis.

Investigations

For children with confirmed transient or orthostatic proteinuria, who are otherwise asymptomatic with normal blood pressure and physical examination, no further investigations are required. However, further investigations are warranted in children with

---

Box 1
Conditions for which urinalysis is recommended during the routine office visit

Screening urinalysis in children with high risk for CKD
  Previous acute kidney injury (AKI)
  Congenital anomalies of the kidneys and urinary tract (CAKUT)
  Previous acute glomerulonephritis
  Hypertension
  Active systemic disease
  Prematurity and/or intrauterine growth retardation
  Family history of kidney disease

---

persistent proteinuria, particularly when associated with hematuria, hypertension, or systemic symptom (**Fig. 1**).

- Urine microscopy: It should be performed on a clean-catch fresh urine sample. It detects red blood cells (RBC; confirming the presence of hematuria), different types of casts (indicating renal parenchymal diseases), or urinary crystals, which could be helpful in making a diagnosis.
- Quantitative measurement of urine protein excretion: The first-morning urine collected soon after waking up is the best urine sample for spot urine protein/creatinine ratio. Collecting first-morning urine helps rule out the possibility of orthostatic elements for protein excretion and allows better comparisons during follow-up. The patient should void before going to bed the night before urine collection. For diagnosing orthostatic proteinuria, a second urine sample can be collected anytime during the day, and it will show an elevated protein/creatinine ratio as compared with normal ratio in the first-morning specimen. A 24-h urine collection is not warranted in most cases.

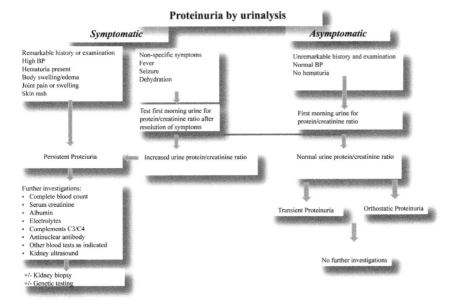

Fig. 1. Clinical approach to the child with proteinuria in ambulatory setting.

- Further investigations: Depending on clinical presentation, the severity of protein-uria, and the presence of hematuria, further investigations may be needed. These are shown in **Fig. 1** and elaborated below (under hematuria), and may include blood tests, kidney ultrasound examination, genetic testing, and/or a kidney biopsy.

Hematuria

Overview

Hematuria signifies the presence of blood in the urine. It could be visible (macroscopic or gross hematuria) or is seen only under the microscope (microscopic hematuria). Though there are variations in definition, the most agreed upon definition is the presence of more than 3–5 RBC per high-power field (HPF) in an uncentrifuged freshly voided midstream urine specimen,[33] and confirmed in two out of three appropriately collected urine samples.[33,34] Generally, $\geq$ 3 RBC/HPF is considered abnormal in adults, and $\geq$ 5 RBC/HPF is considered abnormal in children.

Urine turns red in color in presence of as little as 1 mL of blood in a liter of urine.[35] The intensity of redness can vary based on the amount of blood and location of bleeding; bright red or pink usually originates from the lower tract whereas brown or dark color results from oxidation of the heme pigment and is usually of a glomerular origin. Sometimes, there are other causes for red or dark discoloration, other than gross hematuria. These conditions are shown in **Box 2**, and they can easily be ruled out by the absence of increased RBCs on urine microscopy.

Our knowledge of the prevalence of hematuria in children is based on large screening studies done in the 1970s and it is estimated to be approximately 1–4%.[33,36] There is no recent large population-based study because a routine screening by urinalysis is not encouraged in most countries. The American Academy of Pediatrics no longer recommends a routine screening of healthy children with urinalysis during routine health surveillance visits.[37] This is because of a very high rate of false-positive results or transient abnormalities that lead to a low yield in detecting kidney problems in healthy asymptomatic children.[38,39] It is advisable to limit screening urinalysis to selected few patients who have a high risk for CKD as elaborated in **Box 1**.

Diagnosis of hematuria

Urine dipsticks are very sensitive to the presence of blood and detect as little as 150 µg/L of hemoglobin.[40] False-positive can result from the presence of free

---

Box 2
Causes of red urine discoloration

Food/dye:
  Food coloring
  Beetroot
  Blackberries
  Rhubarb

Medications:
  Rifampin
  Nitrofurantoin
  Metronidazole

Presence of pigment:
  Hemoglobin
  Myoglobin
  Urate crystals
  Porphyrins

hemoglobin following intravascular hemolysis, myoglobin following rhabdomyolysis, urine contamination with oxidizing agents, or concentrated urine. Urine test during or soon after menstruation will also give a positive test for blood. On the contrary, false-negative tests can result from very dilute urine, very acidic specimens (pH < 5), and the presence of reducing substances (such as ascorbic acid). The presence of hematuria by dipstick should be confirmed by microscopy of a fresh urine sample.

Besides confirming the presence of RBCs, urine microscopy can also be helpful in determining the origin of the bleeding. RBCs from a lower urinary tract bleeding are generally intact in shape (isomorphic). However, RBCs that have undergone the sheer stress of passing through the GBM are mostly denatured (dysmorphic; blebs and segments). A glomerular pathology should be suspected if more than 30% of RBCs are dysmorphic.[41]

Other components of microscopic examination can be helpful in making a diagnosis. Presence of RBCs with granular casts is suggestive of glomerular disease whereas the presence of RBCs with white blood cells is suggestive of infection or interstitial or glomerular inflammation. Presence of eosinophils makes the diagnosis of interstitial nephritis more likely. Neutrophils can be seen with infections and acute nephritis such as poststreptococcal glomerulonephritis (GN). The presence of crystals in the urine can be indicative of nephrolithiasis as the underlying etiology for hematuria, shape of crystals may also give some insight into the possible chemical composition of the kidney stone.

Causes of hematuria. Common causes of hematuria are as follows:

- *Microscopic hematuria:*
  - Transient: Strenuous exercise, fever, trauma, urinary tract infection, or urine collected by a catheter.
  - Persistent: with and without episodes of gross hematuria—IgA, Alport, thin basement membrane (TBM) glomerular disease, idiopathic hypercalciuria, subclinical acute post-infectious GN, nephrolithiasis, and nutcracker syndrome. Unlike adults, bladder cancer, which can present with microhematuria, is extremely rare in the pediatric population.
- Gross hematuria:
  - Without urinary system symptoms: post-infectious acute GN, other glomerulopathies, sickle cell trait, IgA GN, Alport syndrome, idiopathic hypercalciuria, and vasculitis.
  - With urinary system symptoms: Urethral irritation/trauma, cystitis, nephrolithiasis, and nutcracker syndrome

In general, the etiology of hematuria is attributed to glomerular and non-glomerular causes (**Table 2**) and can also be summarized based on anatomical location (**Fig. 2**). In children, the causes are more often glomerular rather than the urinary tract.[40] According to a recently published systematic review, isolated persistent microscopic hematuria in pediatrics is most often caused by familial hematuria, IgA nephropathy, or idiopathic hypercalciuria.[42]

Clinical Evaluation

Although the workup of isolated microscopic hematuria is often unrevealing, patients with persistent hematuria often require periodic monitoring for the development of proteinuria, hypertension, or other clinical signs or symptoms that warrant further investigations and management.

Table 2
Glomerular and non-glomerular causes of hematuria in children

	Glomerular	Non-Glomerular
Familial hematuria syndromes	Glomerulonephritis (GN)	Urinary tract infection
○ Autosomal dominant thin	Primary GN	Hypercalciuria
basement membrane (TBM)	○ Post-infectious GN	Kidney calculi
○ X-linked Alport (Male)	○ Membranoproliferative GN	Trauma
○ X-linked Alport (female)	○ Membranous nephropathy	Exercise-induced
○ Autosomal recessive Alport	○ Rapidly progressive GN	Chemical cystitis
	○ IgA nephropathy	(cyclophosphamide)
	Secondary GN	Coagulopathy
	○ Systemic lupus erythematosus	Vascular malformation
	○ Henoch Schönlein purpura	Nutcracker syndrome
	○ Polyarteritis nodosa	Urinary schistosomiasis
	○ ANCA-positive systemic vasculitis	Malignancy
	Hemolytic uremic syndrome	Menarche
	Renal vein thrombosis	Factitious
	Interstitial nephritis	
	Cystic kidney disease	

Adapted with permission.[40]

History

Blood at the onset or end of urination usually indicates a urethral or bladder origin, whereas dark brown or cola-colored urine throughout the stream is more indicative of an upper tract etiology. History regarding the onset of hematuria, any preceding events such as trauma or excessive exercise, upper respiratory tract or skin infections (recent or remote), renal colic or passage of stones, ingestion of medications or herbal supplements should be sought. Associated symptoms such as dysuria, abdominal or flank pain, and increase in frequency or urgency are suggestive of infection or stones.

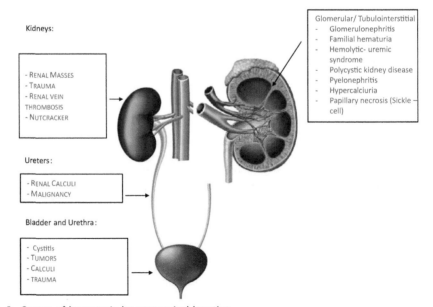

Fig. 2. Causes of hematuria by anatomical location.

Persistent microhematuria with episodes of gross hematuria precipitated by upper respiratory illness (URI) is suggestive of a glomerular disease such as immunoglobulin A (IgA) nephropathy. A history of skin rashes, joint pains, weight loss, fever, or edema would be consistent with a systemic illness. Gross hematuria in the neonatal period is suspicious for renal vein thrombosis and factors increasing the risk of this condition include maternal diabetes, dehydration, polycythemia, and umbilical catheters. Also, gross hematuria in a child with nephrotic syndrome is worrisome for renal vein thrombosis. A family history of hematuria, CKD, hearing loss, hypertension, stones, or coagulopathy can be very helpful. Menarche and the possibility of menstrual bleeding at the time of testing should be checked. In adolescents, social history of sexual activity and exposure of sexually transmitted diseases should also be explored.

Physical examination
Essential elements of physical examination are a measurement of vital signs (temperature, heart rate, and blood pressure), followed by systemic examination for pitting edema, skin rashes/purpura, lymphadenopathy, joint swelling/tenderness, abdominal mass, organomegaly, cardiac murmur, and loin tenderness.

Investigations
Fig. 3 provides a suggested road map for the workup of hematuria.

Patients with asymptomatic microscopic hematuria
Urinalysis with urine microscopy should be repeated three times to confirm the presence of persistent microscopic hematuria. The presence of febrile illness, vigorous activity, and menses can cause transient microscopic hematuria. In the presence of proteinuria, hypertension, and significant history or physical examination findings, a glomerular etiology for the hematuria and proteinuria is likely and would require further work up as shown in **Fig. 3**.

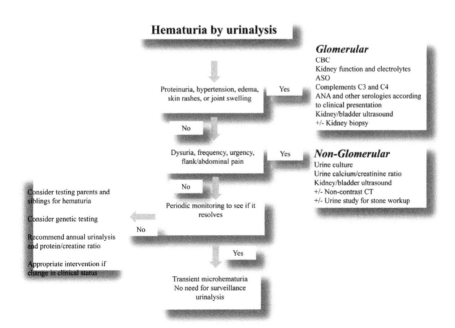

Fig. 3. Clinical approach to the child with hematuria in ambulatory setting.

Isolated asymptomatic hematuria with a known family history of hematuria is suggestive of familial hematuria. Screening immediate family members for hematuria might be useful in making the diagnosis.[43]

Patients with a family history of hematuria or impaired kidney function should be worked up further. Patients with a family history of isolated hematuria and normal kidney function can be given the tentative diagnosis of TBMs disease and generally don't require extensive investigations or biopsy for diagnosis. However, a reasonable approach would be annual screening with urinalysis and blood pressure measurement.[43]

Patients with gross hematuria with/without proteinuria

Thorough history and physical examination can help identify the source of bleeding in these cases. However, laboratory and radiological workup along with kidney biopsy, and/or genetic testing may be needed for diagnosis.

- Blood tests: These may include complete blood count (CBC), kidney function tests, serum complement studies (C3 and C4), antistreptococcal antibodies (ASO), other serologies such as antinuclear antibodies (ANAs), antineutrophil cytoplasmic antibodies (ANCAs) or anti-GBM antibodies, coagulation profile, hemoglobin electrophoresis, and other tests depending on the clinical presentation.
- Imaging: Kidney ultrasound is generally the first line imaging that helps diagnose congenital abnormalities of the kidney and urinary tract (CAKUT), kidney stones, nephrocalcinosis, tumors, and renal hematoma. Increase in kidney echogenicity is a marker of kidney parenchymal disease. Doppler ultrasound is useful in cases of hematuria suspected to be a result of renal vein thrombosis. Small stones may not be visible on ultrasound and in highly suspicious cases of nephrolithiasis a non-contrast computed tomography (CT) scan may be necessary. Other imaging studies such as MRI, MR angiography, or angiograms may be needed for diagnosis.
- Histopathology: Kidney biopsy is usually considered in cases suspicious of glomerulopathy that requires therapy or could lead to CKD. This may include the following:
  - Significant proteinuria, except in poststreptococcal GN
  - Persistent low complement C3
  - Unexplained change in kidney function or rapidly progressive GN
  - Systemic diseases such as systemic lupus erythematosus or ANCA-positive vasculitis
  - Family history of significant kidney disease suggestive of progressive forms of familial hematuria
- Genetic testing: In this era of precision medicine, and with better understanding of genetic causes for proteinuria or hematuria, genetic testing can be used in certain cases to establish the diagnosis without a kidney biopsy. For instance, genetic testing for pathogenic COL4A3–5 variants, is advised for patients with persistent hematuria, especially those with a family history of hematuria or kidney function impairment. It is also suggested that first-degree family members be tested because of their risk of impaired kidney function. Family members with COL4A3 or COL4A4 heterozygotes are advised against donating for kidney transplantation. Recent recommendations have also extended the scope of genetic testing to include patients with persistent proteinuria and steroid-resistant nephrotic syndrome because of suspected inherited FSGS and familial IgA GN, as well as for patients with kidney failure of unknown cause.[44,45]

SUMMARY

The presence of hematuria and/or proteinuria in the ambulatory setting requires individualized workup based on history, initial clinical findings, and laboratory workup. Most children do not need extensive laboratory workup. The differential diagnosis is wide, and a step-wise approach is required to identify the cause and guide the management. The availability of genetic testing to identify and confirm certain diseases associated with proteinuria and/or hematuria has decreased the need for kidney biopsy in some cases.

CLINICS CARE POINTS

- Urine may be red in color because of reasons other than hematuria.
- Microscopic hematuria or mild proteinuria in a healthy child should be confirmed on repeat urine testing.
- Spot urine protein-to-creatinine ratio is a validated test to quantify the amount of proteinuria.
- First-morning urine sample should be tested in children suspected of having orthostatic proteinuria.
- Proteinuria associated with hematuria or hypertension requires further evaluation.

DISCLOSURE

The authors have nothing to disclose.

REFERENCES

1. Mueller PW, Caudill SP. Urinary albumin excretion in children: factors related to elevated excretion in the United States population. Ren Fail 1999;21(3–4): 293–302.
2. Viteri B, Reid-Adam J. Hematuria and proteinuria in children. Pediatr Rev 2018; 39(12):573–87.
3. Norman ME. An office approach to hematuria and proteinuria. Pediatr Clin North Am 1987;34(3):545–60.
4. Mahan JD, Turman MA, Mentser MI. Evaluation of hematuria, proteinuria, and hypertension in adolescents. Pediatr Clin North Am 1997;44(6):1573–89.
5. Geary DF, Schaefer F. SpringerLink. Pediatric kidney disease. 2nd. Berlin, Heidelberg: Springer Berlin Heidelberg; 2016. p. 2016. Imprint: Springer.
6. Leung AK, Wong AH. Proteinuria in children. Am Fam Physician 2010;82(6): 645–51.
7. Cramer MT, Charlton JR, Fogo AB, et al. Expanding the phenotype of proteinuria in Dent disease. A case series. Pediatr Nephrol 2014;29(10):2051–4.
8. Bell FG, Wilkin TJ, Atwell JD. Microproteinuria in children with vesicoureteric reflux. Br J Urol 1986;58(6):605–9.
9. Ehlayel AM, Copelovitch L. Update on dent disease. Pediatr Clin North Am 2019; 66(1):169–78.
10. Warady BA, Abraham AG, Schwartz GJ, et al. Predictors of rapid progression of glomerular and nonglomerular kidney disease in children and adolescents: the chronic kidney disease in children (CKiD) Cohort. Am J Kidney Dis 2015;65(6): 878–88.

11. Ardissino G, Testa S, Daccò V, et al. Proteinuria as a predictor of disease progression in children with hypodysplastic nephropathy. Data from the Ital Kid Project. Pediatr Nephrol 2004;19(2):172–7.

12. de Sépibus R, Cachat F, Meyrat BJ, et al. Urinary albumin excretion and chronic kidney disease in children with vesicoureteral reflux. J Pediatr Urol 2017;13(6): 592.e591–7.

13. Fuhrman DY, Schneider MF, Dell KM, et al. Albuminuria, proteinuria, and renal disease progression in children with CKD. Clin J Am Soc Nephrol 2017;12(6): 912–20.

14. Huang Y, Yang X, Zhang Y, et al. Correlation of urine protein/creatinine ratios to 24-h urinary protein for quantitating proteinuria in children. Pediatr Nephrol 2020;35(3):463–8.

15. Abitbol C, Zilleruelo G, Freundlich M, et al. Quantitation of proteinuria with urinary protein/creatinine ratios and random testing with dipsticks in nephrotic children. J Pediatr 1990;116(2):243–7.

16. Carlotti AP, Franco PB, Facincani I, et al. [Protein/creatinine ratio in single urine samples for the semiquantitation of proteinuria in children with nephrosis]. J Pediatr (Rio J) 1998;74(5):404–10.

17. Ellis D, Becker DJ, Daneman D, et al. Proteinuria in children with insulin-dependent diabetes: relationship to duration of disease, metabolic control, and retinal changes. J Pediatr 1983;102(5):673–80.

18. Dharnidharka VR, Dabbagh S, Atiyeh B, et al. Prevalence of microalbuminuria in children with sickle cell disease. Pediatr Nephrol 1998;12(6):475–8.

19. McPherson Yee M, Jabbar SF, Osunkwo I, et al. Chronic kidney disease and albuminuria in children with sickle cell disease. Clin J Am Soc Nephrol 2011;6(11): 2628–33.

20. Flynn JT, Kaelber DC, Baker-Smith CM, et al. Clinical Practice Guideline for Screening and Management of High Blood Pressure in Children and Adolescents. Pediatrics 2017;140(3):e20171904.

21. Houser MT, Jahn MF, Kobayashi A, et al. Assessment of urinary protein excretion in the adolescent: effect of body position and exercise. J Pediatr 1986;109(3): 556–61.

22. Brandt JR, Jacobs A, Raissy HH, et al. Orthostatic proteinuria and the spectrum of diurnal variability of urinary protein excretion in healthy children. Pediatr Nephrol 2010;25(6):1131–7.

23. Chang-Chien C, Chuang GT, Tsai IJ, et al. A large retrospective review of persistent proteinuria in children. J Formos Med Assoc 2018;117(8):711–9.

24. Leung AK, Wong AH, Barg SS. Proteinuria in children: evaluation and differential diagnosis. Am Fam Physician 2017;95(4):248–54.

25. Shintaku N, Takahashi Y, Akaishi K, et al. Entrapment of left renal vein in children with orthostatic proteinuria. Pediatr Nephrol 1990;4(4):324–7.

26. Park SJ, Lim JW, Cho BS, et al. Nutcracker syndrome in children with orthostatic proteinuria: diagnosis on the basis of Doppler sonography. J Ultrasound Med 2002;21(1):39–45 [quiz: 46].

27. Gulleroglu K, Gulleroglu B, Baskin E. Nutcracker syndrome. World J Nephrol 2014;3(4):277–81.

28. Sellers EAC, Hadjiyannakis S, Amed S, et al. Persistent Albuminuria in Children with Type 2 Diabetes: A Canadian Paediatric Surveillance Program Study. J Pediatr 2016;168:112–7.

29. Wenderfer SE, Eldin KW. Lupus Nephritis. Pediatr Clin North Am 2019;66(1): 87–99.

30. Fathallah-Shaykh SA. Proteinuria and progression of pediatric chronic kidney disease: lessons from recent clinical studies. Pediatr Nephrol 2017;32(5):743–51.
31. Wong CS, Pierce CB, Cole SR, et al. Association of proteinuria with race, cause of chronic kidney disease, and glomerular filtration rate in the chronic kidney disease in children study. Clin J Am Soc Nephrol 2009;4(4):812–9.
32. Hogg RJ. Screening for CKD in children: a global controversy. Clin J Am Soc Nephrol 2009;4(2):509–15.
33. Dodge WF, West EF, Smith EH, et al. Proteinuria and hematuria in schoolchildren: epidemiology and early natural history. J Pediatr 1976;88(2):327–47.
34. Meyers KE. Evaluation of hematuria in children. Urol Clin North Am 2004;31(3): 559–73, x.
35. Bolenz C, Schroppel B, Eisenhardt A, et al. The investigation of hematuria. Dtsch Arztebl Int 2018;115(48):801–7.
36. Vehaskari VM, Rapola J, Koskimies O, et al. Microscopic hematuria in school children: epidemiology and clinicopathologic evaluation. J Pediatr 1979;95(5 Pt 1): 676–84.
37. Practice Co, Medicine A, Committee BFS. Recommendations for Preventive Pediatric Health Care. Pediatrics 2007;120(6):1376.
38. Kaplan RE, Springate JE, Feld LG. Screening dipstick urinalysis: a time to change. Pediatrics 1997;100(6):919–21.
39. Sekhar DL, Wang L, Hollenbeak CS, et al. A cost-effectiveness analysis of screening urine dipsticks in well-child care. Pediatrics 2010;125(4):660–3.
40. Yap H-K, Lau PY-W. Hematuria and proteinuria. In: Geary DF, Schaefer F, editors. Pediatric kidney disease. 2nd. Berlin: Springer Berlin Heidelberg; Imprint; 2016.
41. Shichiri M, Hosoda K, Nishio Y, et al. Red-cell-volume distribution curves in diagnosis of glomerular and non-glomerular haematuria. Lancet 1988;1(8591): 908–11.
42. Clark M, Aronoff S, Del Vecchio M. Etiologies of asymptomatic microscopic hematuria in children - systematic review of 1092 subjects. Diagnosis (Berl) 2015; 2(4):211–6.
43. Kashtan CE. Familial hematuria. Pediatr Nephrol 2009;24(10):1951–8.
44. Savige J, Lipska-Zietkiewicz BS, Watson E, et al. Guidelines for Genetic Testing and Management of Alport Syndrome. Clin J Am Soc Nephrol 2022;17(1):143–54.
45. Savige J, Storey H, Watson E, et al. Consensus statement on standards and guidelines for the molecular diagnostics of Alport syndrome: refining the ACMG criteria. Eur J Hum Genet 2021;29(8):1186–97.

Acute Postinfectious Glomerulonephritis

Minh Dien Duong, MD[a], Kimberly J. Reidy, MD[a],*

KEYWORDS

- Glomerulonephritis • Postinfectious glomerulonephritis
- Poststreptococcal glomerulonephritis • Complement pathway • Hematuria

KEY POINTS

- Postinfectious glomerulonephritis (PIGN) is a common kidney disease in children.
- Although bacterial, viral, and parasitic infections can all be associated with PIGN. *Streptococcal* infection remains the most common cause of PIGN in children.
- The classic presentation of PIGN includes glomerulonephritis with gross hematuria, hypertension, and edema with or without impaired kidney function.
- Glomerulonephritis with low complement C3 levels is typical of PIGN; C3 levels return to normal by 6 to 8 weeks.
- Most cases of PIGN resolve without recurrence with good long-term kidney outcomes.

INTRODUCTION

Acute glomerulonephritis (GN) is characterized by inflammation of the glomerulus, and classically presents with cola-colored urine and hypertension.[1] The leading cause of acute GN in children is postinfectious glomerulonephritis (PIGN), which is an immune-mediated glomerular injury triggered by an extrarenal infection.[2,3] The diagnosis of PIGN requires manifestations of GN and evidence of the prior infection.[2,3] One of the earliest forms of PIGN to be described is poststreptococcal GN (PSGN) caused by group A *Streptococcus*. Subsequently, it became clear that other strains of *Streptococcus* (groups C and G), as well as *Staphylococcus*, gram-negative bacilli, fungi, parasites and viruses can also cause acute PIGN. Thus, the broader term PIGN is now used more often, whereas PSGN remains the most common form of PIGN in children.[4–6]

HISTORY

As early as the eighteenth century, descriptions of edema and dark urine were noted following scarlet fever. In the 1800s, Wells recognized that there was blood in the urine

[a] Department of Pediatrics, Division of Nephrology, Children's Hospital at Montefiore, Albert Einstein College of Medicine, 3326 Bainbridge Avenue, Bronx, NY 10467, USA
* Correspondence author.
E-mail address: kreidy@montefiore.org

Pediatr Clin N Am 69 (2022) 1051–1078
https://doi.org/10.1016/j.pcl.2022.08.001   pediatric.theclinics.com
0031-3955/22/© 2022 Elsevier Inc. All rights reserved.

Abbreviations	
GN	Glomerulonephritis
PIGN	Postinfectiousglomerulonephritis
PSGN	Poststreptococal glomerulonephritis
RPGN	Rapidly progressive glomerulonephritis
SAGN	Staphylococcus related glomerulonephritis

and later Richard Bright described "Bright disease," which included edema (dropsy) and protein in the urine (detected by heating urine in a spoon). "Bright disease" likely represented many forms of kidney disease, of which PIGN was one form. In 1903, Clemens von Pirquet postulated that antibodies were the cause of nephritis following scarlet fever.[7,8]

EPIDEMIOLOGY

PIGN primarily affects children aged 3 to 12 years with the mean age of 6 to 8 years, and it is uncommon in children aged younger than 3 years.[5–7] The male:female ratio in patients with symptomatic PIGN is 2:1.[4] The true incidence and prevalence of PIGN are unknown given that most cases are subclinical and transient, and many studies have only focused on PSGN.[4,5] Subclinical PIGN may be 4 to 19 times more common than symptomatic disease.[9] PIGN remains the most common cause of gross glomerular hematuria in children.[10] The study by Carapeutis and colleagues found that the incidence of PSGN in children was 2 cases per 100,000 person-years in developed countries and 0.3 cases per 100,000 person-years in developing countries.[9] Epidemics and clusters of PSGN cases are reported in low income communities and rural areas.[4,11]

In developed countries, during the last few decades the incidence of PSGN has decreased because of better health care, including widespread use of antibiotics and improved socioeconomic and nutritional conditions.[4,5,7,11] However, PIGN remains one of the most common glomerular diseases in children in the United States.[4] In adults, PIGN is predominantly due to nonstreptococcal infections. The incidence of Staphylococcus-related GN (SAGN) has increased because of increased rates of methicillin-resistant Staphylococcus aureus (MRSA) infections. Staphylococcus is 3 times more common than Streptococcus in adults with PIGN.[11,12] In children, SAGN cases have been reported with a favorable prognosis.[13]

In developing countries, the incidence of PIGN including PSGN is also decreasing but it remains a common cause of kidney disease in children. The estimated global incidence of PSGN is 472,000 cases per year of which 77% cases are in low-income and moderate-income countries.[4] An estimated incidence of PSGN is more than 200 cases/million/year.[4] In low-income and moderate-income countries, PIGN is a frequent cause of severe acute kidney injury requiring dialysis and admission to pediatric intensive care unit.[4]

CAUSE

Although PIGN is associated with many causative agents, PSGN still accounts for 90% to 95% of PIGN cases.[3,4] Group A β-hemolytic Streptococcus is the most common but epidemics have been caused by group C or G Streptococcus.[11] A variety of nonstreptococcal agents including bacteria, viruses, fungi, and parasites has been reported to be associated with PIGN (**Table 1**).[1,14] Because nonstreptococcal GN cases are less common, there is a lack of data regarding their epidemiology, pathogenesis, and clinical course.[5] A study in India showed that PSGN was the predominant form of

Table 1
Causative agents for PIGN

Bacteria		Children
Infectious syndromes		
Pharyngitis or skin infections	Group A β-hemolytic Streptococcus (S pyogenes); most common Group C and G Streptococcus	>90%–95%
Bacterial endocarditis	Streptococcus viridans S aureus S epidermidis Enterococcus faecalis Escherichia coli Proteus Haemophilus	Uncommon
Pneumonia	Streptococcus pneumoniae Mycoplasma pneumoniae Legionella	Uncommon
Abscess (dental abscess, deep-seated abscess, osteomyelitis)	S aureus S viridans Gram-negative bacilli	Uncommon
Intraventricular shunt infections	S epidermidis S aureus Diphtheroids Pseudomonas	Uncommon

(continued on next page)

Table 1
(continued)

	Children
	Serratia
	Propionibacterium
Enterocolitis	Very rare
Yersinia enterocolitica	
Salmonella typhi	
Campylobacter jejuni	
Rickettsial disease	Very rare
Rocky Mountain Spotted fever	
Q fever: Coxiella burnetii	
Ehrlichiosis	
Others	Very rare
Neisseria meningitidis (mainly associated with membranoproliferative GN and subacute endocarditis)	
Brucella melitensis	
Treponema pallidum	
Borrelia	
Leptospira	
Mycobacteria (tuberculosis, avium, leprae)-associated with chronic GN	
Viruses	Very rare
Enterovirus: Coxsackie virus and Echovirus	
EBV, CMV[a]	
Hepatitis A	
Hepatitis B, and C[b]	
HIV[b]	

Rubella
Varicella
Paramyxoviruses: Measles and Mumps
Vaccinia
Parvovirus B19
Influenzae
Adenovirus
Dengue virus

| | Very rare |

Fungi

Coccidioides immitis
Histoplasmosis

| | Very rare |

Parasites

Malaria
• *Plasmodium malariae*
  •*Plasmodium falciparum*
  •*Plasmodium vivax*
Schistosoma mansoni and Schistosoma haematobium
Toxoplasmosis: Toxoplasma gondii
Filariasis: Wuchereria bancrofti
Trichinosis
Trypanosomes

[a] May be associated with nephrotic syndrome than acute GN.
[b] May be associated with tubulointerstitial disease than glomerular disease.
Modified from Refs.[1,14]

PIGN in 90% of cases followed by pneumonia, liver abscess, and mumps in about 10% of cases.[15] Among children with PIGN following viral infections, varicella and mumps are the most common causes.[16] In clinical practice, no clear evidence of infection is seen in up to 20% to 30% of patients with PIGN.[5,17]

SAGN with IgA-dominant deposits is rare in children but is well documented in adults with risk factors that include diabetes mellitus, obesity, age above 65 years, prolonged use of indwelling catheter and central lines, implants, and cardiac devices.[13,17] SAGN generally follows cellulitis, osteomyelitis or nosocomial infections due to *S aureus*. This contrasts with PIGN with staphylococcal endocarditis, deep visceral abscess, or shunt infection, which are usually caused by *Staphylococcus epidermidis*.[11,18]

PATHOPHYSIOLOGY

In acute GN, immune complex formation and deposition activate a common pathway of inflammatory response in glomeruli, which causes clinical features of acute GN. Immune complexes activate the complement system, stimulate inflammatory cell infiltration (including neutrophils, lymphocytes, monocytes), and cause glomerular cell proliferation. Narrowing of the endocapillary lumen leads to decreased glomerular filtration, which causes fluid and sodium retention with fluid overload. Decreased glomerular filtrate leads to an increase in renal tubular sodium and water reabsorption, which aggravates fluid retention. Depending on disease severity, a decreased glomerular filtration causes the accumulation of urea, creatinine, potassium, and other uremic toxins.[1]

Site and Course of Infection

PSGN has long been considered a consequence of streptococcal skin or pharyngeal infection. However, since the beginning of the twentieth century, other sites of infection have been found to be associated with PIGN. These include endocarditis, deep-seated visceral abscess (thoracic and abdominal cavities), central line infection, pneumonia, osteomyelitis, urinary tract infection, arthritis, and ventriculoatrial shunts[18] (**Table 2**). The site of infection leading to PIGN varies with climate and weather. Upper respiratory infections are seen more in winter and spring, whereas skin infection is seen more in summer and fall in tropical areas. In children, streptococcal pharyngitis has surpassed impetigo as a leading cause for PSGN. However, in the elderly population with PIGN, infections of the skin, lung and urinary tract are seen more often than pharyngitis.[11]

The term PIGN is usually used for all cases associated with infection, although in several circumstances, patients have GN in the setting of concurrent infection.[2] It has been proposed that the infection-related GN should be classified as PIGN versus concurrent infection-related GN.[19] To classify a GN as PIGN, it will typically meet 3 criteria: (1) Preceding infection, which resolves with or without antimicrobial therapy, (2) infection is followed by a latent period lasting more than several days and up to a few weeks, and (3) acute onset of features of GN after the latent period.[19] In contrast, infection-related GN has an ongoing infection.[17,19]

Pathogenesis

The nature of nephritogenic antigens that cause PIGN remains unknown because of the lack of a good animal model.[9,11] The fundamental pathogenic mechanism is the deposition of circulating immune complexes or formation of in situ immune complexes with nephrogenic antigen deposits within glomerular tufts. Immune complexes

Table 2
Site of infection associated with PIGN

	Site of Infection	Organism	Comment
Postinfectious GN			
Acute PSGN	URI, pharyngitis, tonsillitis, cellulitis	*Streptococcus* A or C (specific M types)	Onset of GN is between 7 and 21 d after infection
Other PIGN	Pneumonia, gastroenteritis	*S pneumoniae Klebsiella, Mycoplasma, Salmonella*	GN occurs during the acute infection. GN is usually mild and hematuria is a main manifestation
GN of concurrent infection			
Staphylococcal-related GN	Ischemic limb, cellulitis, endocarditis, osteomyelitis, shunts, pneumonia, central venous catheter infection	Coagulase-positive staphylococcus, often MRSA	The most common cause of GN from chronic bacterial infection
Other bacterial-related GN	Deep-seated abscess (thoracic, abdominal), osteomyelitis, endocarditis, shunts, central venous catheter infection	Gram-positive or gram-negative bacteria	Acute kidney injury is common
Viral infection	Liver (hepatitis B and C), systemic (HIV, CMV, parvovirus)	Hepatitis B, C, HIV, CMV, parvovirus	GN can be mitigated by antimicrobial therapy
Nonbacterial, nonviral infections	Viscera organ infection	Parasites, spirochetes, fungi	Rare in North America and Western Europe

Modified from Tibor Nadasdy, Lee A. Hebert, Infection-Related Glomerulonephritis: Understanding Mechanisms, Seminars in Nephrology, 31(4), 2011, 369-375. https://doi.org/10.1016/j.semnephrol.2011.06.008.

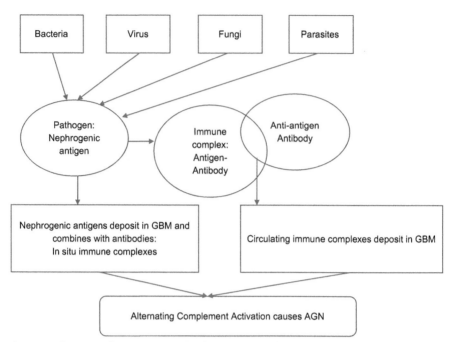

Fig. 1. Mechanisms of immune complex formation in infection-related acute GN. (*Modified from* Ref Balasubramania R, Mark SD. Postinfectious glomerulonephritis. Paediatr Int Child Health. 2017 Nov;37(4):240-247).

activate the alternative complement pathway, which leads to the recruitment of inflammatory cells and eventually presents with acute GN with low C3 levels (**Fig. 1**).[11] Autoantibodies against factor B (FB), which is the main enzyme for the regulation of the alternative complement pathway are known to increase during the acute phase of PIGN. The anti-FB antibody level is correlated with low plasma C3 levels and associated with an increased level of the terminal complement complex (serum C5b-9).[20,21] The mechanism of formation of anti-FB remains unknown but the hypothesis is that bacterial antigens may have molecular mimicry with FB and favor the formation of anti-FB antibodies.[20,21]

POSTSTREPTOCOCCAL GLOMERULONEPHRITIS
Nephritogenic Streptococcal Antigens

Despite intensive research of PSGN during the past century, the factors or pathogenic antigens of *Streptococcus*, which are responsible for PSGN remain obscure. One of the first putative nephritogenic antigens identified were M proteins. However, although group A *Streptococci* with M type strains is the most identified group causing PSGN, non-M strains group C and G *Streptococci* are also associated with PSGN. Within group A *Streptococcus*, M types 1, 2, 4, 12, 18, and 25 are associated with PSGN triggered by throat infection, whereas PSGN secondary to skin infection is linked with *Streptococcus pyogenes* M types 49, 55, 57, and 60.[8,17] Further evidence against M proteins as the primary antigen is the rarity of recurrent PSGN, given that the M protein types do not confer lifetime immunity. Similarly, streptokinase and streptococcal histone-like proteins have been proposed as nephritogenic streptococcal antigens but further studies were not conclusive.[8,9]

Two recently identified proteins that show nephritogenic activities in PSGN are as follows: (1) streptococcal glyceraldehyde phosphate dehydrogenase (GAPDH), also known as nephritis-associated plasmin receptor (NAPlr) and (2) streptococcal cationic proteinase exotoxin B (SPeB) and its zymogen precursor (zSPeB).[8,9,18] NAPlr and SPeB/zSPEB are 2 distinct antigens with pathogenicity determined by genetic background. They are present in S pyogenes and have been identified in kidney biopsies. High antibodies to these antigens are found in more than 90% of PSGN patients during the recovering phase.[14] Antibodies to GAPDH and SPeB persist at least 10 years and 1 year, respectively, after the acute PSGN.[9] NAPlr is isolated from group A and C Streptococci and seems to be the main antigen in the Japanese population. SPeB is a putative nephritogenic antigen in Latin America, the United States, and Europe.[8,9,14,18]

Host Predisposition

Host immune responses also play a role in PSGN.[17] Not every streptococcal infection leads to PSGN. Of all children with streptococcal infection, less than 2% show clinical signs of acute GN. About 20% to 40% of siblings of patients with sporadic PSGN will later develop clinical or subclinical PSGN. However, studies have not proven a specific association between human lymphocyte antigen and PSGN. Multiple factors may contribute to the genetic predisposition.[8]

Immune Complex Formation and Complement Activation

In PIGN, immune complexes accumulate in the glomeruli and activate the complement system and coagulation pathways leading to GN.[8,18] In the early phase of streptococcal infection, the circulating streptococcal antigens, including GAPDH and SPeB/zSPeB, deposit in the glomeruli. Subsequently, the host produces antibodies to these antigens, which appear in the circulation. These specific antibodies interact with the antigens present in glomeruli to form immune complexes in situ. As the antibody response fully develops, there is also formation of immune complexes in the circulation. The circulating immune complexes deposit in glomeruli. At later stage, in situ immune complexes stop forming whereas immune complexes continue to form between the circulating antigens and antibodies.[8,18]

NAPlr and SpeB nephritogenic antigens with or without bound specific antibodies interact with plasmin and cause damage to the glomerular basement membrane (GBM), activate alternative complement pathways, stimulate chemotaxis and mesangial cell interleukin 6 production, and stimulate inflammation via expression of adhesion molecules on the endothelium (**Fig. 2**).[9,14] They also promote the formation of immune complexes.[14]

GAPDH localization in glomeruli does not coincide with the distribution of IgG or complements. Because of its plasmin-binding activity, it stimulates local inflammatory reactions and metalloproteinase-mediated GBM degradation. SPeB is also a plasmin-binding receptor protein that can degrade fibronectin, activate matrix metalloproteinase, and release active kinin. With degraded GBM, in situ or circulating immune complexes can penetrate the GBM and accumulate as humps in the subepithelial space.[8,18] SPeB/zSPeB are cationic antigens that can penetrate the negatively charged GBM, thus promoting immune complex formation in situ.[8,18] The deposition of SPeB/zSPeB together with complements and IgG in the subepithelial humps is the hallmark lesion of PSGN.[8,18]

Complement activation is the main mechanism of inflammation in PSGN.[8] C3 activation in PSGN is predominantly via the alternative pathway. PSGN typically presents with low serum C3 level and glomerular deposits of IgG, C3, and C5.[4,22] C1q and C4 deposits of the classical alternative pathway are typically not seen in PSGN. However,

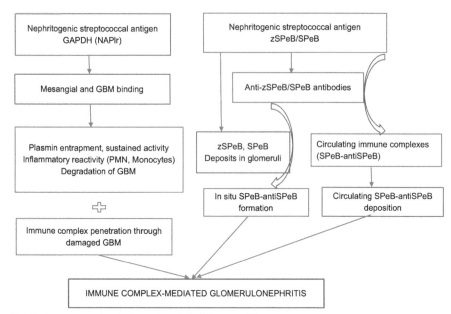

Fig. 2. Pathogenesis of PSGN. (*Modified from Ref.*[8])

in the first 2 weeks after the onset of PSGN, some patients may have low serum C1q, C2, C4 concentrations and the presence of circulating C1-inhibitor–C1r–C1s complexes because of the transient activation of the classical complement pathway.[4,22] In addition, the lectin-binding pathway is also found to be activated with deposition of mannan-binding lectin protein in some patients.[4,22]

Complement activation in PSGN is triggered by the deposition of NAPlr and SPeB/zSPEB antigens and plasmin activation, leading to C3 cleavage.[9,17] Complement activation recruits inflammatory cells and triggers a leukocyte-mediated injury.[14] The binding of immunoglobulin (Ig)-binding proteins of the streptococcal surface with C4BP (C4b-binding protein) interferes with the activation of the classical complement pathway and promotes activation of the alternative complement pathway.[8,17] In addition, complement regulatory proteins (FH and FHL-1) in the alternative complement pathway are removed by SPeB in PSGN.[8] SPeB is a protease and may modulate FH and FHL-1 recruitment during infection.[8]

Other Mechanisms in Poststreptococcal Glomerulonephritis

Cellular immune mechanisms may play a role in the pathogenesis of PSGN given the early presence of macrophages and T-helper cells in glomeruli.[18] There are reports of development of anti-IgG reactivity including IgG rheumatoid factor in the first few weeks of PSGN.[18] Production of anti-IgG autoantibodies may be in part due to streptococcal produced neuraminidase that can modify the host's IgG structure. Other autoantibodies such as antineutrophil cytoplasmic antibody (ANCA), antinuclear antibodies (ANA), and anticomplement antibodies may be present in PSGN but their role in the pathogenesis is not clear.[14]

IgA dominant staphylococcus infection-related glomerulonephritis

The pathogenesis of staphylococcal infection GN with IgA dominant deposits is not well understood. A superantigen (exotoxin toxic shock syndrome toxin, TSST-1) in

MRSA is thought to play an important role. It stimulates cytokine activity, IgA production, and IgA immune complex formation and deposition.[14] Staphylococcal superantigens are exoproteins that bind MHC class II molecules in antigen-presenting cells, leading to a massive proliferation of T cells with subsequent cytokine bursts causing increased IgA production.[18] Host-related factors also affect pathogenesis of staphylococcal GN. Diabetic patients with poststaphylococcal GN are frequently affected by subclinical mucosal infections and have a reduced IgA clearance, which increases IgA deposition in glomeruli.[20] SAGN is usually associated with soft tissue infections of ischemic limbs or osteomyelitis.[14] Data on staphylococcal GN in children are limited.[13]

Postinfectious glomerulonephritis with other microorganisms

Together with *Streptococcus* and *Staphylococcus*, other bacterial and nonbacterial microorganisms may cause PIGN. Pathogenesis of PIGN related to many of these microorganisms are not fully understood. PIGN secondary to intracellular virus and parasites may result from alterations of both cellular and antibody immunity.[9] More than one-third of these patients lack evidence of infection at the time of PIGN.[14]

CLINICAL PRESENTATION AND DIAGNOSIS

PSGN is the most common form of PIGN but the number of nonstreptococcal GN cases is increasing.[15] Preceding pneumonia, liver abscess, mumps, and gastroenteritis may be seen in 10% to 15% of PIGN cases in children.[5,15] The clinical presentation, clinical course, and outcome of patients with nonstreptococcal GN are generally similar to those with PSGN.[6] In most PIGN cases (70%–80%), there is a history of a preceding infection.[5,17] The timing of presentation varies depending on the organism. Classically, PIGN occurs 1 to 6 weeks after an infection. The site of infection depends on the population studied.[4,5,14] Clinical features of children with PIGN from 3 large cohorts are outlined in **Table 3**.[5,15,21] PIGN can present with one of the following.[4,6,14]

- *Subclinical glomerulonephritis:* This is up to 4 times more common than overt cases of PSGN. Patients with PIGN may present with asymptomatic urinary abnormalities including nonnephrotic range proteinuria, microscopic hematuria, and normal or mild elevated blood pressure.
- *Acute glomerulonephritis or acute nephritic syndrome:* This is the classic presentation of PIGN with an acute onset of gross hematuria (cola-colored urine) associated with hypertension, edema, and oliguria or anuria. Acute kidney injury with fluid overload may be present. Urine test shows hematuria, RBC casts, and non-nephrotic range proteinuria. Microscopic hematuria is seen in all cases with PIGN.
- *Rapidly progressive glomerulonephritis*: Rapidly progressive GN (RPGN) is a clinical syndrome characterized by signs of acute GN and a rapid decline in renal function. RPGN, which occurs in about 2% of children with PIGN, is characterized by the presence of epithelial crescents on renal biopsy.
- *Nephritic-Nephrotic syndrome:* In these cases of PIGN, nephrotic-range proteinuria, hypoalbuminemia, hyperlipidemia, and edema will be evident in addition to nephritis.

Diagnosis of Postinfectious Glomerulonephritis

The diagnosis is based on history, physical examination, and laboratory findings as well as a clinical course consistent with PIGN and, less often, kidney biopsy findings. Chronic GN should be on the differential diagnosis and be excluded. Clinical features

Table 3
Timing of kidney biopsy and pathologic features in PSGN[2]

	Early Biopsy	Typical Features	Late Biopsy (>4–6 wk)
Clinical features	Mild albuminuria and hematuria	Acute nephritic syndrome	Persistent hematuria and/or proteinuria
Light microscopy	Glomerular endocapillary proliferation may be focal and segmental	Diffuse global proliferation ("exudative" early on; lymphocytes, monocytes + mesangial and endothelial proliferation predominate later)	Mesangial proliferation
Immunofluorescence	C$_3$ and IgG, starry sky pattern	C$_3$ and IgG, starry sky or garland pattern	C$_3$ ± IgG, mesangial pattern
Electron microscopy	Mesangial, subepithelial (humps) ± deposits	Mesangial, subepithelial (humps), and ± subendothelial deposits	Mesangial ± rare subepithelial humps in the mesangial "notch"

suggesting chronic GN include anemia, alterations in bone mineral metabolism and parathyroid hormone, small echogenic kidneys on ultrasound, and/or long-standing hypertension with left ventricular hypertrophy on echocardiogram.[1]

Evaluation for PIGN should include the assessment of the following:

History

Presenting history

- Edema: Onset of edema: sudden for nephritic syndrome. Severity of edema: face, leg, ascites. Weight gain: previous weight, if available.
- Urine output (oliguria, anuria), frothy urine (protein), red urine (gross hematuria).
- Hypertensive symptoms: headache, vomiting, seizures, impaired consciousness (hypertensive encephalopathy).
- Symptoms of systemic disease: fever, skin rash (purpura), facial rash, photophobia, arthralgia, weight loss, mouth ulcers.
- Concurrent infections: abscess, shunt infection, hepatitis B, C, endocarditis. In PSGN, infectious symptoms are resolved before the development of nephritic syndrome. In contrast, infection-related GN may concur with persistent symptoms of infections such as fever or organ-specific symptoms.[1]

Past medical history

- Preceding streptococcal infection: upper respiratory tract infection, pharyngitis, impetigo, scarlet fever.
- Other infections such as *S aureus* infections (soft tissue infection, osteomyelitis), intra-abdominal abscess (liver), endocarditis, pneumonia, urinary tract infection, gastroenteritis, and viral infections (including varicella, mumps, dengue virus, adenovirus).
- Presence of ventriculoatrial shunt.
- Recent blood transfusion; hepatitis B or C infection.

Family history

- Autoimmune disease (systemic lupus erythematosus: SLE), GN (IgA nephropathy), deafness (Alport syndrome), PIGN.

Physical Examination

- Vital signs: tachycardia, hypertension, tachypnea (pulmonary edema), fever (concurrent infection).
- Signs of fluid retention: puffy face, ankle edema, ascites, pleural effusion.
- Signs of fluid overload with congestive heart failure or pulmonary edema: cardiomegaly, jugular venous distension, hepatomegaly, gallop rhythm, rales on lung examination.
- Signs of hypertensive encephalopathy: convulsion, altered mental status. Full neurologic examination including fundoscopy is required.
- Presence of ventriculoatrial or prosthetic vascular shunts.
- Signs of previous infections (impetigo or pyoderma) or current infections (fever, deep-seated abscess, osteomyelitis).
- Some systemic disease that may mimic PIGN and their clinical presentation is as follows:

SLE: malar rash, oral ulcers, arthritis, pericardial friction rubs, lymphadenopathy, hepatosplenomegaly.

ANCA vasculitis: lung and sinus involvements.

Goodpasture syndrome: pulmonary hemorrhage.

Henoch-Schonlein purpura or IgA vasculitis: joint, gastrointestinal, and skin involvements.

Laboratory and Radiologic Investigations

Urine tests

- Urinalysis: hematuria, proteinuria, WBC
- Urinary microscopy: dysmorphic red blood cells, RBC, and WBC casts.
- Urine protein/creatinine ratio (morning urine sample) for nonnephrotic or nephrotic-range proteinuria.

Blood tests

- Complete blood count (CBC), erythrocyte sedimentation rate (ESR), CRP. Anemia due to dilution secondary to fluid overload is commonly seen in patients with acute GN. Anemia is correlated with the degree of AKI and the eventual full recovery. CRP and ESR are elevated in PIGN due to inflammation from infections.[1,5,22]
- Basic metabolic panel, serum magnesium, and phosphate. Closely monitoring serum urea and creatinine, electrolytes are necessary to monitor for acute kidney injury and rapidly progressive glomerulonephritis (RPGN). Serum creatinine may be normal or elevated. Hyperkalemia and metabolic acidosis may be present if kidney function is impaired. Hyponatremia most often due to dilution may be present in PIGN.[1]
- Liver function tests might reveal low serum albumin level in cases with nephritic-nephrotic syndrome. Other abnormalities in liver function tests may be seen in viral or bacterial infections (hepatitis, liver abscess).
- Serum C3, C4. About 90% of patients with PIGN commonly present with low serum complement 3 and normal C4. However, in some cases there may also be low C4 due to involvement of classical and lectin complement pathways. C3 levels generally normalize in 6 to 8 weeks in most patients with PIGN. If recovery exceeds 3 months, an alternative diagnosis including C3 glomerulopathy should be considered.[4,6] Serum complements changes are different in other causes of acute GN[1]:
  - Low serum C3 and normal C4: Suggestive of PIGN (PSGN), membranoproliferative GN (MPGN) type 3, or C3 glomerulopathy/GN.
  - Low C3 and C4: Consider lupus nephritis, chronic bacteremia (shunt nephritis, endocarditis related GN), or MPGN type 1.
  - Normal C3 and C4: Consider ANCA vasculitis, Goodpasture syndrome, IgA nephropathy/IgA vasculitis, or Alport syndrome.

Evidence of streptococcal infection

- Throat culture for β-hemolytic streptococcus is positive in 15% to 20% of PSGN cases.[23]
- The streptozyme assay is preferred because it detects antibodies to 4 β-hemolytic streptococcal antigens (streptolysin O, DNAse B, streptokinase, and hyaluronidase) and improves the chance of detection of Streptococcal infection. It is positive in more than 80% of the cases.[23]
- Anti-DNAse B and antistreptolysin O (ASO) titers are positive in cases with recent streptococcal infection (Group A Streptococcus). ASO is only elevated in cases with streptococcal pharyngitis but elevated anti-DNAse B titers may be seen in

both pharyngeal and pyoderma infections with Group A *Streptococcus*. ASO is positive in up to 20% of healthy children. Elevated ASO is seen 60% to 97% in PSGN and is variable based on the studies. There is no correlation of ASO level and severity of clinical manifestations and low C3.[1]

- ASO titers peak approximately 2 to 4 weeks after pharyngitis and remain elevated for several months (6–8 months). They may be a false negative if checked early. ASO titer peak may be blunted in patients treated with antistreptococcal antibiotics.[1]

Evidence of PIGN cause other than streptococcal infection, if indicated: Hepatitis B surface antigen, antihepatitis B surface antibody, antihepatitis C virus antibody, mycoplasma antibody, epstein-barr virus (EBV) serology, cytomegalovirus (CMV) serology. Blood culture may be needed in selected patients.

Patients with atypical clinical presentation

- ANA, anti-Ds DNA, ENA
- ANCA
- Anti-GBM antibodies

Imaging studies

- Chest radiograph if there are concerns for pulmonary edema.
- Echocardiogram may be considered in cases with suspected long-term hypertension, heart failure, or to evaluate for bacterial endocarditis.
- Renal and bladder ultrasound is typically noncontributory but may be helpful in selected cases.

Indications for Kidney Biopsy

Most patients with PIGN do not require a kidney biopsy. Potential indications of kidney biopsy include the following:[4]

- RPGN in the acute phase as indicated by a sustained rapid increase in serum creatinine, or severe oliguria.
- Evidence of systemic disease: SLE, Henoch-Schonlein purpura, ANCA vasculitis.
- Atypical clinical course such as hypertension and edema lasting longer than 2 weeks and persistently low estimated glomerular filttration (eGFR) for greater than 4 weeks.
- Low serum complement greater than 12 weeks.
- Persistent proteinuria with urine protein creatinine (UPC) ratio more than 1 mg/mg: greater than 6 months.
- Persistent microscopic hematuria greater than 2 years.

Renal Histology

Poststreptococcal glomerulonephritis
In PSGN, the pathologic features are quite different when a kidney biopsy is performed early versus late (less than 2 weeks vs more than 4–6 weeks from onset, respectively; **Table 3**).[2,4]

Light microscopy. The typical light microscopy findings in PSGN are diffuse and global hypercellularity of endothelial and mesangial cells and infiltration of inflammatory cells in the glomerular tuft.[4,22] In the early phase, predominant neutrophils in glomeruli result in exudative appearance and subsequently, lymphocytes and monocytes increase along with mesangial and endocapillary hypercellularity.[4] The endocapillary hypercellularity causes a decrease in the capillary lumen that is associated with impaired kidney function. In severe cases with clinical RPGN, glomerular fibrinoid necrosis and cellular crescents in more than 50% of glomeruli are seen.[4] Subepithelial humps of PSGN may be visualized with trichrome stain under oil immersion. In both early or late phases, glomerular hypercellularity may be characterized with focal and segmental appearance.[4] In late phases, biopsies may demonstrate only mesangial hypercellularity because of resolving PSGN. PSGN is often accompanied with acute tubular injury, tubular protein reabsorption droplets, RBC casts, and interstitial nephritis.[24] However, interstitial inflammation and edema are usually mild. Vascular injury is unusual and should trigger investigation for other causes of GN or vasculitis.[4]

Immunofluorescence microscopy. The acute phase of PSGN demonstrates typically discrete granular deposits of C3 and IgG in a capillary loop and mesangial distribution, which is termed a "starry sky" appearance.[22] The term "garland pattern" indicates the presence of heavy and sometimes confluent capillary loop deposits without mesangial deposits.[21] Biopsies performed in the early clinical phase typically show C3 deposition and absence of IgG.[22] The late phase of PSGN or PIGN may reveal no significant immunofluorescence staining and a diagnosis is based on typical findings on electron microscopy.[24]

Electron Microscopy

The hallmark pathologic finding on electron microscopy is the subepithelial hump-shaped deposits with immune complexes. Electron dense deposits may occur in subepithelium and intramembrane.[22,24] Subepithelial humps are present in greater numbers in the acute phase and become scarce in the resolving or chronic phase.[24] Small mesangial and scattered subendothelial deposits are identified in nearly all cases with PIGN, especially in both acute and chronic phases.[24]

Other Forms of Postinfectious Glomerulonephritis including IgA-Dominant Staphylococcus Infection-Related Glomerulonephritis, Endocarditis, and Shunt Nephritis

S aureus, particularly MRSA can present with SAGN characterized by GN associated IgA deposits (**Table 4**).[2,12–14,17,24] Patients may have skin infections, cellulitis, osteomyelitis, septic arthritis, pneumonia, sepsis, postsurgical site infection, or IV line infection.[2,24] Endocarditis-related GN is less common in children.[2,6,23–25] Risk factors for infectious endocarditis in children are congenital heart disease and cardiac surgery.[2,23] In contrast, shunt nephritis is more common in children than adults and is seen in approximately 30% of children with ventriculoatrial shunt infection.[2,4,6] SAGN, endocarditis, and shunt nephritis may present with unique histopathologic features (see **Table 4**).

CLINICAL COURSE OF POSTINFECTIOUS GLOMERULONEPHRITIS

The patient's clinical course is one of the most important elements needed to support a diagnosis of PIGN. Clinical and abnormal laboratory findings in children with PIGN typically improve with time. If cases where improvement is not seen, a kidney biopsy should be considered to confirm the cause of acute GN. Studies of 3 cohorts of PIGN in children indicate that there is a similar clinical course between PIGN and PSGN (**Table 5**).[6,12] Clinical features of PSGN are summarized in **Table 6**.[1,15,22,23,26,27] The timeline of the recovery of clinical features and abnormal laboratory findings in PIGN are shown in **Table 7** . **Table 8** shows differential diagnosis of PIGN.

Table 4
Other forms of PIGN

	Clinical Features	Biopsy Findings
IgA-dominant staphylococcus infection-related glomerulonephritis (SAGN)	• GN with IgA deposits associated with S aureus, particularly MRSA • More common in older male adults but it has been reported in children • Associated with malignancy, IV drug use, alcoholism, and human immunodeficiency virus infection • Staph infection may involve skin, cellulitis, osteomyelitis, septic arthritis, pneumonia, sepsis, postsurgical site infection or IV line infection • Latent period between infections and clinical presentations is 4 wk on average • May have no free latent period • Infections can be occult and deep seated • Presents with Acute kidney injury, nephrotic range proteinuria in addition to gross or microscopic hematuria[2,24] • Low C3 is seen in 30%–70% of patients and serum C4 is normal[2] • ANCA is positive in cases with systemic symptoms[14]	• Light microscopy features include endocapillary hypercellularity with exudative lesions and mesangial hypercellularity • May have segmental necrotizing lesions, large capillary wall deposits resembling wire loops, and intracapillary hyaline pseudothrombi[17,24] • Acute tubular necrosis, often severe • On IF, mild-to-moderate IgA and moderate to strong C3 staining along capillary walls and mesangium • Codominant Ig A and IgG are seen in 40% of the biopsies[17] • On electron microscopy, the presence of epithelial hump is seen in 31% of SAGN cases[17]
Endocarditis-related GN	• Less common in children than adults	• Histopathology may be variable

(continued on next page)

Table 4 (continued)		
	Clinical Features	**Biopsy Findings**
	• In children, *S viridans* and *S aureus* represent more than 50% of the cases of bacterial endocarditis[23,25]	• Most common lesion is diffuse proliferative and exudative glomerulonephritis with endocapillary and mesangial hypercellularity
	• Risk factors for infectious endocarditis in children are congenital heart disease and cardiac surgery[2,23]	• May have infiltration of inflammatory cells/neutrophils[2,24,25]
	• Bacterial endocarditis is complicated by associated GN in 2%–60% of cases[2,24]	• Diffuse crescentic GN is very rare[25]
	• GN is usually seen within 7–10 d of clinical illness[2]	
	• Based on the studies in adults, the common presenting feature is AKI (30%–80%), followed by typical acute GN (9%), RPGN (6%), and nephrotic syndrome (6%)[6]	
	• Microscopic hematuria (97%) and proteinuria are common and may persist for weeks to months	
	• Hypocomplementemia (low both C3 and C4: 56%), high titers of rheumatoid factors, cryoglobulinemia, and sometimes positive anti-PR3 ANCA[6]	
	• Hypocomplementemia resolves when infection is eradicated	
	• Low serum complements are associated with renal prognosis and severity of infection	
	• In cases with crescentic GN or RPGN, steroid, and plasmapheresis may be considered[6]	

| Shunt nephritis | • Affects approximately 30% of children with ventriculoatrial shunt infection[2,6]
• Rarely seen with ventriculoperitoneal shunt[2,6]
• *S epidermidis* and *S aureus* most common associated infections[4]
• Typically is infection related and occurs during an active infection
• Typically present with gross and microscopic hematuria, variable levels of proteinuria and impaired kidney function[2,6]
• Hypertension is less common in shunt nephritis
• Recurrent fever, anemia, hepatosplenomegaly, and cerebral symptoms are suspicious symptoms of chronic shunt infection
• Both low C3 level (90%) and low C4 level (50%) that indicate activation of the classic complement system
• May have high rheumatoid factor titers and positive anti-P3 ANCA
• Low serum complements are normalized after the treatment of infection[2,6]
• Supportive laboratory findings are positive blood culture, elevated ESR, and high cryoglobulins[2] | • Histopathology is variable
• May have endocapillary proliferative or a membranoproliferative or crescentic GN[24]
• On immunofluorescence microscopy, will have dominant C3 staining with IgM, followed by IgG and IgA[24]
• May have a pauci-immune staining pattern with no immunoglobulin and complements[24] |

Table 5
Presenting features of childhood PIGN

Clinical Features	Dagan et al[5], 2016 n = 125	Gunasekaran et al[15], 2015 n = 72	Chauvet et al[21], 2020 n = 34
Study population	PIGN (Israel)	PIGN (India)	PIGN (France)
	PSGN: 85%	PSGN: 90.3%	PSGN:87%
Preceding infections (%)			
Pyoderma	5.6	80.6	0
URTI	25.6	–	–
Pharyngitis	44.8	5.5	25
Pneumonia	3.2	5.6	4
Mumps	–	2.8	–
Liver abscess	–	1.4	–
Gastroenteritis	11.2	–	–
Acute Otitis Media	–	–	9
Male (%)	74.4	72.2	
Age (years)	5.8 (±3.3)	6.7 (±2.7)	5.6 (4.7–7.7)
Hypertension (%)	82.4%	91.7	53
		19.4	
Edema (%)	59.2	88.9	44
Macroscopic hematuria (%)	16.8	65.3	71
Oliguria (%)	33.6%	69.4	
AKI (%)	70.16	20.8	79
Complications			
Hypertensive emergency (%)		19.4	
Congestive heart failure (%)		11.1	
Encephalopathy (altered sensorium and/or seizure) (%)		4.2	

Hypertensive retinopathy (%)		1.4
Required dialysis (%)	0.8 (pulmonary edema)	1.4 (RPGN)
High CRP (%)	81.5	
Low serum albumin (%)	22	
Anemia (%)	79	
Low serum C3 (%)	89	
Low C 4 (%)	23.8	
Hyperkalemia (%)	28.8	
Proteinuria (%)	92.8	100
Nephrotic range proteinuria (%)	32.5	33
Clinical presentations		
Nephritic syndrome (%)	41.1	
Nephrotic syndrome with nephritic syndrome (%)	22.9	33
Without nephritic or nephrotic syndrome (%)	51.6%	
Clinical course		
Follow up (months)	42 mo (±3)	
Blood pressure <95th percentile	99.2% at the last visit	98.3% at at 1 mo follow-up
Negative proteinuria	100% at the last visit	98.1% at 6 mo follow-up
Normal eGFR	100% at the last visit	85% at 1 mo follow-up 92.3% at 6 mo follow-up
Normalized complement	100% at the last visit	100% at 8 wk follow-up in PSGN group

Table 6
Clinical features of PSGN in children[1,2,15,22,23,26,27]

	Frequency (%)
Clinical features	
Recent infections	6.2%–51%
Pharyngitis	13%–89.2%
Pyoderma	
Hematuria (gross and microscopic hematuria)	100%
Gross hematuria	60%–80%
Edema	65%–90%
Hypertension	80%–90%
Hypertensive emergency	30%–35%
Encephalopathy	3%–5%
Congestive heart failure	6%–12%
Oliguria	50%–70%
Laboratory findings	
Abnormal urinalysis and microscopy	Dysmorphic RBCs, hematuria, RBC casts and WBC casts
Elevated blood urea nitrogen (BUN)	60%–65%
Impaired eGFR (elevated serum creatinine)	20%–30%
Hypoalbuminemia <3.5 g/dL	40%–46%
Proteinuria	60%–70%
Nephrotic range proteinuria	35%–50%
Low serum C3	90%–99%
Low serum C3 and C4	10%–16%
Evidence of streptococcal infection	
Elevated ASO	60%–97%
Elevated anti-DNAse B	65%–97%
4 antigens (DNAse B, Streptolysin O, hyaluronidase, and streptokinase)	80%
Streptococcal throat culture	<25%
Anti-NAPlr and anti-SPEB-zSPEB titers	Unavailable

Table 7
Timeline for the resolution of clinical features of PIGN[1,5,22]

	<1 Week (up to 10 Days)	1–2 Weeks	3–4 Weeks	6–8 Weeks (12 Weeks)	6 Months	18 Months (24 Months)
Gross hematuria	▓	▓				
Hypertension	▓	▓				
Edema	▓	▓				
Elevated serum creatinine	▓	▓	▓			
Low C3 (± low C4)	▓	▓	▓	▓		
Proteinuria	▓	▓	▓	▓	▓	
Microscopic hematuria	▓	▓	▓	▓	▓	▓

Table 8
Differential diagnosis of PIGN[1,2,14]

	Clinical Features that Differentiate it from PIGN	Renal Histology
MPGN	Associated with hepatitis B or lupus nephritis Persistent low complements	Glomerular basement membrane double contours
C3 glomerulonephritis or C3 glomerulopathy (Dense deposit disease: DDD)	Persistent low C3 but normal C4 over 2 mo Genetic analyses of the complement alternative pathway is needed	Only C3 staining on IF in C3 glomerulonephritis C3 staining and intramembranous dense deposit in DDD
Acute flare of IgA nephropathy	IgA nephropathy can be confused with IgA dominant GN Onset of GN in IgA nephropathy is 1–3 d after onset of infection (upper tract respiratory or gastrointestinal infections). GN is mild with gross hematuria IgA nephrology has normal complements	IgA nephropathy • Mesangial proliferative GN with IgA staining > C3. • Lack of glomerular neutrophils or subepithelial humps
Lupus nephritis (class III)	Systemic syndrome Low C3 and C4 Positive ANA	Full house on IF: C1q, C4, IgG, IgM
Pauci immune GN (ANCA vasculitis)	Systemic symptoms: fever, weight loss, arthralgia, purpuric rash Chronic sinusitis, epistaxis Dyspnea, saddle nose deformation (granulomatosis with polyangiitis) CXR: pulmonary infiltrate Positive ANCA (c-ANCA with granulomatosis with polyangiitis and p-ANCA with microscopic polyangiitis)	No deposits on IF
IgA vasculitis (Henoch-Schonlein purpura nephritis)	Characterized by IgA deposition on biopsy IgA vasculitis may present with staphylococcal infection with no latent period between infection episode and renal symptoms Palpable purpura, abdominal pain, joint pain/swelling	IgA staining

MANAGEMENT

There is no specific therapy for PIGN. The eradication of the involved infective micro-organisms by antibiotics or antiviral agent (HBV, HCV) and supportive therapy for acute nephritic syndrome are 2 main parts of the PIGN treatment. In typical PIGN, steroids or immunosuppressive agents are not indicated.[4,6]

Antibiotic Therapy

If an underlying bacterial infection is identified, appropriate antibiotics should be given. Such therapy does not change the course of GN given the cascade of glomerular inflammatory injury continues despite eradication of the microorganism.[6,9] Streptococcus Group A infection should still be treated promptly but the studies have failed to conclusively demonstrate that antibiotic treatment prevents the development of PSGN.[1,9] However, antibiotic therapy for streptococcal pharyngitis during epidemics prevents the transmission of nephritogenic strains of Group A Streptococcus and thus protects others against PSGN.[2,9] If clinical features of streptococcal infection (pharyngitis, pyoderma, or serologic evidence of streptococcal infection) are present at the onset of PSGN, oral penicillin V (10 days) or erythromycin in those with penicillin allergy is recommended.[2,4]

The mainstay of treatment in GN secondary to bacterial endocarditis and shunt infection is antibiotic therapy. Some reports suggest that a short-course of steroids may help improve renal function in cases with endocarditis-associated GN.[6,25] The removal of ventriculoatrial shunt is required in shunt nephritis.[6]

General Management

PIGN patients with subclinical disease can be followed as outpatients. If the patients present with RPGN, kidney biopsy, and immunosuppression may be indicated.[28] PIGN patients with severe edema, hypertension, fluid overload with acute pulmonary edema or congestive heart failure, oliguria and/or AKI require hospitalization.[1,14] Assessment of fluid balance, intravascular volume status, and kidney function are essential. In the acute phase (first 1–2 weeks) of PIGN, patients should be evaluated closely for complications. If serum creatinine greater than 50% of baseline, monitor serum creatinine every 12 hours for RPGN.[1] Nephrotoxic medications and intravascular volume depletion should be avoided to prevent further acute kidney injury.[6]

Fluid restriction

For edema and hypertension, fluid and salt restriction is recommended. If there is oliguria, daily fluid intake should be restricted to insensible fluid loss at 400 mL/m^2 plus urine output and additional losses (emesis, diarrhea). Low salt diet includes sodium less than 1 mEq/kg/d or less than 2 g/d in adults.[29] If there is impaired renal function, a low potassium diet may be needed. For admitted patients, daily weights, fluid balance, and vital signs should be monitored.

Treatment of fluid overload

In patients with significant edema, hypertension, cardiac failure, or pulmonary edema due to fluid overload, administration of a loop diuretic as well as fluid and salt restriction are needed. The starting intravenous dose of furosemide is 0.5 to 1 mg/kg/dose, which can be increased up to 2 to 5 mg/kg/dose (maximal 200 mg IV) depending on response.[23,29]

Hypertension

Furosemide is the preferred treatment of hypertension caused by salt and water retention. Depending on clinical course, other antihypertensive medications may be considered. Calcium channel blockers are often preferred. They are more effective when combined with fluid restriction and diuresis.[1] Angiotensin converting enzyme inhibitors or angiotensin receptor blockers are often avoided because of a risk of hyperkalemia and worsening of the glomerular filtration rate.[1] If patients have persistent or severe hypertension and are at risk of hypertensive encephalopathy, intravenous Nicardipine drip or Labetalol is indicated. Posterior reversible leukoencephalopathy, which is diagnosed by a brain MRI, may be seen in patients with acute PSGN. Patients present with altered mental status, visual changes, headaches, and/or seizures.[6,23] In a systemic review of PSGN in children, this complication occurred in 80% of cases with severe hypertension and in 20% of children with normal or increased BP in the absence of severe hypertension.[30]

Hyperkalemia
Patients with hyperkalemia are usually managed by low potassium-containing diet. Depending on severity, other treatments such as furosemide, potassium-binding exchange resins such as sodium polystyrene sulfonate (Kayexalate) or calcium polystyrene sulfonate (Patiromer), intravenous calcium gluconate, insulin infusion, and/or albuterol nebulization are indicated.[1,29]

Renal replacement therapy
Kidney replacement therapy (acute intermittent hemodialysis or continuous kidney replacment therapy) is indicated in patients with severe oliguria with AKI, severe hyperkalemia, uncontrolled hypertension, or pulmonary edema not responding to furosemide, and in patients with symptomatic uremia or blood urea nitrogen greater than 100 mg/dL.[1,4]

Immunosuppressive medications and plasmapheresis
The role of immunosuppressive agents in PIGN is controversial. Corticosteroid therapy with IV methylprednisolone pulses (10–15 mg/kg/dose or 500–1000 mg/dose) for 3 consecutive days followed by oral steroids is considered in PIGN patients with RPGN with extensive acute glomerular crescents GN on renal biopsy.[6,14] Recently, the efficacy of eculizumab administration in renal recovery in 2 cases with severe PIGN was reported.[31] The role of plasmapheresis, which has been tried in patients with RPGN, is not clear.[6]

PROGNOSIS

The overall long-term prognosis of PIGN is very good.[1,4] In the PSGN cohorts with a long-term follow-up (up to 10 years), less than 1% of patients develop end-stage kidney disease, 3% of patients have hypertension, and 5% to 20% have persistent urinary findings with hematuria and proteinuria.[1] Urinalysis and BP measurement should be performed quarterly for the first year and then annually. Recurrence of PSGN is very rare.[1]

Data on outcomes of nonstreptococcal PIGN data in children are limited. With early diagnosis and appropriate treatment with antibiotics, most patients with GN associated with shunt infection and bacterial endocarditis recover their renal function and normalize hypocomplementemia.[2,6] Persistent infection, tubulointerstitial changes, and preexisting kidney disease are features associated with progression of chronic kidney disease in patients with infection-related acute GN.[32] Although adults with IgA-dominant PIGN are treated with antibiotics, 41% of patients progress to end-stage kidney disease because most cases have an underlying diabetic nephropathy.[12]

CLINICS CARE POINTS

- Subacute glomerulonephritis is up to 4 times more common as compared with overt poststreptococcal acute glomerulonephritis.

- Chronic glomerulonephritis should be suspected in patients with anemia, kidney osteodystrophy, small echogenic kidneys, and left ventricular hypertrophy.

- Kidney biopsy is not needed in typical cases of postinfectious acute glomerulonephritis. Hypertension in acute glomerulonephritis is a result of salt and water retention, which should be restricted in such cases.

- Depending on the severity of fluid retention and hypertension, patients may need diuretics and/or antihypertensive medication.

- Steroid therapy is not indicated in typical cases and its use may aggravate hypertension.

DISCLOSURE

K.J. Reidy is a site investigator for Travere Therapeutics and Advicienne supported clinical trials unrelated to the content of this article. K.J. Reidy is supported by NIH, National Institutes of Health, United States R01 DK131176.

REFERENCES

1. VanDeVoorde RG 3rd. Acute poststreptococcal glomerulonephritis: the most common acute glomerulonephritis. Pediatr Rev 2015;36:3–12. PMID:25554106.
2. Kambham N. Postinfectious glomerulonephritis. Adv Anat Pathol 2012;19: 338–47. PMID:22885383.
3. Martínez-Maldonado M. Postinfectious glomerulonephritis. Am J Kidney Dis 2000;35:xlvi–xiviii. PMID: 10636819.
4. Balasubramania R, Mark SD. Postinfectious glomerulonephritis. Paediatr Int Child Health 2017;37(4):240–7. PMID: 28891413.
5. Dagan R, Cleper R, Davidovits M, et al. Post-Infectious glomerulonephritis in pediatric patients over two decades: severity-associated features. Isr Med Assoc J 2016;18:336–40. PMID: 27468526.
6. Hunt EAK, Somers MJG. Infection-related glomerulonephritis. Pediatr Clin N Am 2019;66:59–72. PMID: 30454751.
7. Mohammad D, Baracco R. Postinfectious glomerulonephritis. Pediatr Ann 2020; 49:e273–7. PMID: 32520369.
8. Rodríguez-Iturbe B, Batsford S. Pathogenesis of poststreptococcal glomerulonephritis a century after Clemens Von Pirquet. Kidney Int 2007;71:1094–104. PMID: 17342179.
9. Kanjanabuch T, Kittikowit W, Eiam-Ong S. An update on acute postinfectious glomerulonephritis worldwide. Nat Rev Nephrol 2009;5:259–69. PMID: 19384327.
10. Mishra K, Kumar M, Patel A, et al. Clinico-Etiologic Profile of Macroscopic Hematuria in Children: A Single Center Experience. Indian Pediatr 2022;59(1):25–7. PMID: 33506806.
11. Nast CC. Infection-related glomerulonephritis: changing demographics and outcomes. Adv Chronic Kidney Dis 2012;19:68–75. PMID: 22449343.
12. Nasr SH, D'Agati VD. IgA-dominant postinfectious glomerulonephritis: a new twist on an old disease. Nephron Clin Pract 2011;119. c18–25. PMID: 21659781.

13. Grosser DS, Persad P, Talento RV, et al. IgA-dominant infection-associated glomerulonephritis in the pediatric population. Pediatr Nephrol 2022;37(3): 593–600. PMID: 34453602.
14. Stratta P, Musetti C, Barreca A, et al. New trends of an old disease: the acute post-infectious glomerulonephritis at the beginning of the new millennium. J Nephrol 2014;27:229–39. PMID: 24777751.
15. Gunasekaran K, Krishnamurthy S, Mahadevan S, et al. Clinical characteristics and outcome of postinfectious glomerulonephritis in children in Southern india: a prospective study. Indian J Pediatr 2015;82:896–903. PMID: 25893528.
16. Wenderfer SE. Viral-associated glomerulopathies. Pediatr Nephrol 2015;30: 1929–38. PMID: 25752759.
17. Satoskar AA, Parikh SV, Nadasdy T. Epidemiology, pathogenesis, treatment and outcomes of infection-associated glomerulonephritis. Nat Rev Nephrol 2020;16: 32–50. PMID: 31399725.
18. Nadasdy T, Hebert LA. Infection-related glomerulonephritis: understanding mechanisms. Semin Nephrol 2011;31:369–75. PMID: 21839370.
19. Glassock RJ, Alvarado A, Prosek J, et al. Staphylococcus-related glomerulone-phritis and poststreptococcal glomerulonephritis: why defining "post" is impor-tant in understanding and treating infection-related glomerulonephritis. Am J Kidney Dis 2015;65:826–32. PMID: 25890425.
20. Noris M, Remuzzi G. Challenges in understanding acute postinfectious glomeru-lonephritisL are anti-factor B autoantibodies the answer? J Am Soc Nephrol 2020; 31:670–2. PMID: 32144171.
21. Chauvet S, Berthaud R, Devriese M, et al. Anti-factor B antibodies and acute postinfectious GN in children. J Am Soc Nephrol 2020;3:829–40. PMID: 32034108.
22. Eison TM, Ault BH, Jones DP, et al. Post-streptococcal acute glomerulonephritis in children: clinical features and pathogenesis. Pediatr Nephrol 2011;26:165–80. PMID: 20652330.
23. Rodríguez-Iturbe B, Najafian B, Silva A, et al. Glomerular disease: Acute postin-fectious glomerulonephritis in children. In: Avner ED, Harmon WE, Patrick N, ed-itors. Pediatric nephrology. 7th edition. Berlin: Springer; 2016. p. 959–75.
24. Khalighi M, Chang A. Infection-related GN. Glomerular Dis 2021;1:82–91.
25. Kannan S, Mattoo TK. Diffuse crescentic glomerulonephritis in bacterial endocar-ditis. Pediatr Nephrol 2001;16:423–8. PMID: 11405117.
26. Demircioglu Kılıc B, Akbalık Kara M, Buyukcelik M, et al. Pediatric poststrepto-coccal glomerulonephritis: clinical and laboratory data. Pediatr Int 2018;60: 645–50. PMID: 29729114.
27. Wong W, Morris MC, Zwi J. Outcome of severe acute poststreptococcal glomer-ulonephritis in New Zealand children. Pediatr Nephrol 2009;24:1021–6. PMID: 19096879.
28. Wenderfer SE, Gaut JP. Glomerular diseases in children. Adv Chronic Kidney Dis 2017;24:364–71. PMID: 29229167.
29. Rees L, Bockenhauer D, Webb N, et al. Acute nephritis (Acute nephritic syn-drome). In: Pediatric nephrology. 3rd edition. London: Oxford University Press; 2019. p. 220–3.
30. Orlando C, Milani GP, Simonetti GD, et al. Posterior reversible leukoencephalop-athy syndrome associated with acute postinfectious glomerulonephritis: systemic review. Pediatr Nephrol 2021. https://doi.org/10.1007/s00467-021-05244-z. On-line ahead of print. PMID: 34546419.

31. Chehade H, Guzzo G, Cachat F, et al. Eculizumab as a new treatment for severe acute postinfectious glomerulonephritis: two case reports. Front Med 2021;8: 663258. PMID: 34381795.

32. Oda T, Yoshizawa N. Factors affecting the progression of infection-related glomerulonephritis to chronic kidney disease. Int J Mol Sci 2021;22:905. PMID: 33477598.

Current Understanding of Nephrotic Syndrome in Children

Tej K. Mattoo, MD, DCH, FRCP (UK), FAAP[a],*, Sami Sanjad, MD[b]

KEYWORDS

- Children • Nephrotic syndrome • Minimal change • Glomerular disease • Edema
- Anasarca

KEY POINTS

- Children with nephrotic syndrome have edema and massive proteinuria.
- Steroid therapy is the standard of care.
- Kidney biopsy is needed in very few patients.
- Prognosis is excellent in most patients.
- Relapses may continue into adult life.

INTRODUCTION

Nephrotic syndrome (NS) in children is characterized by the presence of significant proteinuria, hypoalbuminemia, and edema. About 90% of the cases between 1 and 10 years of age and 50% of the cases above 10 years of age are idiopathic (INS) in origin.[1] Most patients with INS respond to corticosteroid therapy; 80% to 90% of patients relapse and nearly half of them have frequent relapses (FR) and may become steroid dependent (SD). Additional immunosuppressive therapy is needed in those with steroid resistance or FR/SD clinical course. The overall prognosis in those who respond to steroids is excellent. About a third of children with INS diagnosed during childhood, particularly those with more severe form of the disease, may have relapses during adult life. Many country-specific practice guidelines have been published and most of them are very similar with clinically insignificant differences. This chapter is focused primarily on steroid-sensitive INS; secondary NS and steroid resistant NS are not discussed here.

---

[a] Department of Pediatrics, Wayne State University School of Medicine, 400 Mack Avenue, Suite 1 East, Detroit, MI 48201, USA; [b] American University of Beirut Medical Center, Beirut, Lebanon
* Corresponding author.
E-mail address: tmattoo@med.wayne.edu

Pediatr Clin N Am 69 (2022) 1079–1098
https://doi.org/10.1016/j.pcl.2022.08.002
0031-3955/22/© 2022 Elsevier Inc. All rights reserved.
pediatric.theclinics.com

HISTORICAL ASPECTS

Edema, referred to as dropsy, from the Greek *hydrops* (water) has been documented in the medical literature from the times of Hippocrates about 2400 years ago. More than 500 years ago (1484), Cornelius Roelans of Belgium is credited with the first crude description in a child with NS: "The fifty-first disease of children is swelling of the whole body of the child.", very likely referring to nephrotic edema. Perhaps one of the best early descriptions of the NS was made 250 years later by the pediatrician Theodore Zwinger III of Basel in his *Paedoiatreia practica* of 1722. Despite this detailed clinical description of NS, Zwinger does not mention any associated urinary abnormalities. Almost 50 years later, Domenico Cotugno in his *De ischiade nervosa commentarius of* 1764, was the first to describe proteinuria upon boiling the urine of a 28-year-old man with dropsy and document albuminuria in NS and diabetic nephropathy. Fifty years later (1827), Richard Bright and others put together the triad of generalized edema, proteinuria, and kidney disease and thus are credited with describing NS in all its details. The term "nephrosis" was first mentioned by Friedrich von Muller of Marburg in 1905 (12). This term was popularized by Fritz Munk and for some time the term Munk's lipoid nephrosis was used to describe these cases. About the same time, Henry Christian and Louis Leiter in the United States pointed out the similarities of primary and secondary forms of severe proteinuric disease with edema, and introduced the terms "syndrome of nephrosis," or "nephrotic syndrome."[2,3]

EPIDEMIOLOGY

The overall incidence of NS in children is about 3/100,000 and ranges from 2% to 8% in various parts of the world. It is lowest in white children in Europe and North America and higher in South, Southeast and East Asian, Middle Eastern, and Northern African children. It is nearly twice as common in black as compared to white children. Its prevalence is about 16/100,000.[4–6] In younger children, it is more common in males (approximately 2:1). Only about 3% of patients have affected siblings,[7] and the incidence is 2 to 3 times higher in communities with a high rate of consanguinity.[8]

PATHOPHYSIOLOGY
Proteinuria

The underlying renal defect in NS is an increased glomerular basement membrane (GBM) permeability to albumin. Normally, very little (less than 0.1%) plasma albumin, which has a large molecular weight, crosses the glomerular filtration barrier and most of it is reabsorbed by the proximal tubular cells. Compared with a normal urine albumin excretion of usually less than 30 to 50 mg/24 h/1.73 m^2,[9] the albuminuria in NS may increase 100 to 200-fold. This massive albuminuria eventually leads to hypoalbuminemia. The increased catabolism of albumin in the renal tubular cells also contributes to hypoalbuminemia. Hypoalbuminemia causes a decrease in plasma oncotic pressure and edema (see below). The liver increases albumin synthesis but not enough to compensate for urine losses and increased catabolism.

The glomerular filtration barrier is made up of 3 layers (**Fig. 1**): (1) a thin fenestrated endothelial layer, (2) GBM, and (3) a visceral epithelial layer of cells known as podocytes. The podocytes have foot processes, which are very dynamic and functional cellular extensions that rest on the GBM. They are interconnected by the slit diaphragms to form the final component of the kidney permeability barrier.[6] Podocyte injury is at the core of significant proteinuria in NS. In view of its importance and as shown in **Table 1**, there is a trend to classify NS according to the underlying etiology for podocyte injury (podocytopathy).[10]

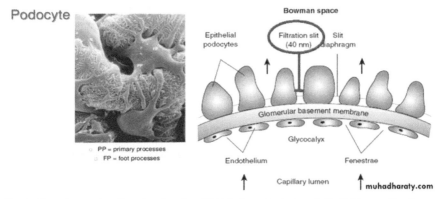

Fig. 1. The glomerular filtration barrier: (1) thin fenestrated endothelial layer, (2) glomerular basement membrane, and (3) a visceral epithelial layer of cells known as podocytes. (*From* Leeuwis JW, Nguyen TQ, Dendooven A, et al. Targeting podocyte-associated diseases. Advanced Drug Delivery Reviews 2010;62(14) pp 1325-1336.)

Previously it was believed that the INS is exclusively a T-cell dysfunction associated with a circulating factor or lymphokine. This hypothesis was based on the following clinical observations: (1) remission was commonly observed with measles infection whereby cell-mediated immunity was suppressed; (2) NS with minimal change is associated with Hodgkin's disease, which is a known T-cell disorder; and (3) patient response to corticosteroids and cyclophosphamide, which are inhibitors of T-cell function.[11] However, nearly 2 decades ago, it became obvious that B-lymphocytes also have a role in INS. The most compelling evidence is the sustained remission of NS following administration of rituximab, an anti-CD20 monoclonal antibody that depletes B cell population, and the occurrence of NS in some people with light chain gammopathy.[12–14] A recent study reported the presence of circulating nephrin autoantibodies in some children and adults with minimal change NS (MCNS). These were present during active disease and decreased significantly or were absent during treatment response.[15]

Table 1 Genetic and secondary causes of podocyte injury	
Intrinsic: Genetic Mutations	**Extrinsic: Podocyte Stress**
Nucleus: *WT1*, *PAX2*, and *LMX1B* mutations	Viral: infection or circulating viral protein
Cytoskeleton: *ACTN4, MYH9, INF2, ANLN, ARHGA24* mutations	Toxic: medication (pamidronate, interferon), toxin (puromycin amino nucleoside, adriamycin)
SD complex: *NPHS1, NPHS2, CD2AP, PLCE1, TRPC6* mutations	Lymphokine or another host protein: IFN-α, IFN-β, FSGS permeability factor
GBM: *LAMB2, ITGB4, ITGA3, COL4A/3/4/5* mutations	Mechanical: podocyte stretch (glomerulomegaly)
Mitochondria: *tRNA, COQ2, COQ6, COQ8* mutations	Acute ischemia with thrombotic microangiopathy
Metabolic, lysosomal: *GLA, OCRL, SCARB2, CFH, DGKE*	Immunologic: immune complex deposition or *in situ* formation (lupus, IgA nephropathy, membranous nephropathy)
	Metabolic: diabetes

Adapted and modified from Refs.[10,22]

Edema

As shown in **Fig. 2**, the initial trigger for edema formation is the decrease in plasma oncotic pressure below a critical level of 12 to 15 mm Hg, causing an imbalance in Starling's forces at the capillary end and resulting in net increase in plasma translocation into the interstitial spaces¶. Edema is sustained by compensatory mechanisms resulting from the decreased effective blood volume, which may be associated with (a) reduced glomerular filtration and increase in sodium and water reabsorption and (b) activation of homeostatic factors including the renin–angiotensin–aldosterone axis and antidiuretic hormone, and (c) a decrease in natriuretic peptide (ANP), all leading to salt and water retention in the distal renal tubules. This pathway for edema formation is known as the underfill hypothesis and applies to most children with INS. The overfill hypothesis implies that there is primary sodium and water retention with a rise in capillary hydrostatic pressure and hypervolemia, which causes intravascular fluid transudation into the interstitium. The underlying mechanisms are believed to be an activation of the epithelial sodium channels (ENaC) and Na-K ATPase in the distal renal tubules.[16,17]

DEFINITIONS

Nephrotic range proteinuria in children is defined by urine protein excretion of $\geq$40 mg/m² BSA/h, $\geq$1 gm/m² BSA/d, or greater than 50 mg/kg/d. However, it is neither

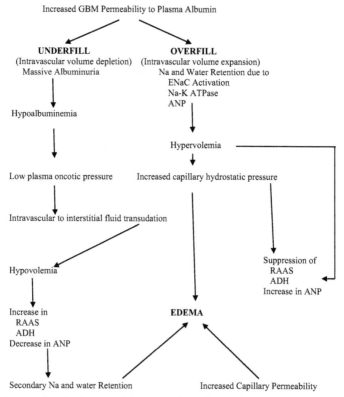

Fig. 2. Pathogenesis of edema and intravascular volume changes. ADH, antidiuretic hormone; ANP, atrial natriuretic peptide; ENaC, sodium epithelial channel; RAAS, Renin–angiotensin–aldosterone system.

practical nor necessary to have a timed urine collection for diagnosis. A random urine sample with ≥3+ protein (corresponding to ≥300 mg/dL) by dipstick examination or a protein/creatinine ratio of greater than 3 mg/mg is good enough for diagnosis. Serum albumin in patients with NS is usually less than 2.5 gm/dL.[18] Some commonly used definitions in INS are given in **Table 2**.

CLASSIFICATION

The 3 different classifications that have a strong bearing on clinical management of INS are based on the age of disease onset, underlying renal histopathology, and response to the initial steroid therapy.

Age of Disease Onset

According to the age of onset (not diagnosis), NS is classified as follows:

- Congenital: Birth to 3 months of age
- Infantile: Older than 3 months and up to 1 year of age
- Childhood: Older than 1 year of age
- Adult: Adult life

Most children with congenital or infantile NS have a genetic basis and poor outcome as compared with those with childhood NS.

Renal Histopathology

The International Study of Kidney Disease in Children (ISKDC) study, which included renal biopsy in 521 children with NS reported MCNS in about 76.4% cases, membranoproliferative glomerulonephritis in 7.5% and focal segmental glomerulosclerosis in 6.9% (FSGS). The remaining ∼10% cases had proliferative glomerulonephritis, pure

Table 2 Commonly used definitions in NS	
Remission	Urine dipstick negative or trace (<30 mg/dL) for protein on 3 consecutive days or urine protein/creatinine ratio ≤0.2 (mg/mg).
Partial remission	Decrease of proteinuria by ≥50% or urine protein/creatinine between >0.2 and <2 g/g
Relapse	Urinary dipstick showing ≥3+ proteinuria (corresponding to ≥300 mg/dL on urinalysis), P/c >2 g/g, for 3 d?
Steroid-sensitive NS	Remission during daily prednisone of 60 mg/m² BSA for 4 wk
Late responder	Remission at 6 wk of daily prednisone therapy for initial treatment
Steroid-resistant NS	
Early	No remission after first (initial) daily prednisone of 60 mg/m² BSA for 4 wk
Late	No response to standard steroid therapy for a relapse for 4 wk after initial response
Infrequent relapsing NS	1 relapse within 6 mo or ≤3 relapses within 12 mo after completion of initial steroid therapy
Frequent relapsing NS	≥2 relapses within 6 mo or ≥4 relapses within 12 mo after completion of therapy in steroid-sensitive NS
Steroid-dependent NS	≥2 relapses during steroid therapy or within 2 wk of its completion

(UPCR) based on a first morning void or 24-h collection.

diffuse mesangial proliferation, focal and global glomerulosclerosis, membranous glomerulopathy, and chronic glomerulonephritis.[1] However, the major limitation with this study was that it included cases with infantile NS and the data were collected from 24 participating centers with poorly defined patient inclusion and exclusion criteria. In another study, the ISKDC reported that about 95% of children with MCNS respond to steroid therapy as compared with 28% of those with other glomerular abnormalities,[18] indicating that the patients with INS who respond to the initial corticosteroid therapy have mostly MCNS but it also includes non-MCNS cases, notably FSGS. With increasing age, the risk for FSGS and membranous nephropathy increases. In adults, MCNS is prevalent in approximately 15% of patients with INS.

Response to Corticosteroids

More than 90% of children with INS respond to steroid therapy. A lack of response helps define the need for renal biopsy and subsequent clinical management, particularly immunosuppression. Response to initial steroid therapy is a better marker for long-term clinical outcome than the underlying renal histopathology, and steroid-sensitive patients have a much better prognosis compared with those with steroid resistance. Ethnic variations in response to corticosteroid therapy have been reported.[19,20] However, the possibility of socioeconomic and other factors contributing to these variations cannot be ruled out.

CLINICAL PRESENTATION

Patients with INS present with massive proteinuria, hypoalbuminemia, and edema. None of the other conditions that cause generalized edema in children is associated with significant ($\geq 3^+$) proteinuria (**Table 3**). The onset of INS is often preceded by upper respiratory tract infection (URI). Microhematuria is present in about 20% of cases. Depending on the severity, patients may also have oliguria or anuria, pulmonary congestion, fever, or sepsis. Hypertension is rare at presentation and its presence, or the presence of gross hematuria or other clinical findings as shown in **Table 3**, are suggestive of secondary NS. Some patients, particularly teenagers and older, may present with nephrotic-range proteinuria and hypoalbuminemia with no edema. The reason for the absence of edema in such patients, generally attributed to a decreased serum oncotic pressure due to hypoalbuminemia, is not known.

DIAGNOSIS

In addition to a good history and physical examination, certain investigations are necessary to confirm diagnosis and rule out the possibility of secondary NS.

Laboratory Tests

The laboratory tests that are commonly used in the diagnosis of INS are shown in **Table 4**.

Kidney Biopsy

Kidney biopsy is indicated in patients who present outside the usual age group (1–12 years) or show atypical clinical and laboratory findings (see above) suggestive of a secondary NS. The commonest reason for a kidney biopsy, regardless of age, is the lack of response to steroid therapy initially or later (late nonresponsiveness).

Table 3 Clinical presentation	
Causes of generalized edema in children	• Nephrotic syndrome • Congestive cardiac failure • Liver disease, • Protein malnutrition (kwashiorkor) • Kidney failure with severe fluid overload
Features indicative of secondary NS	
Clinical	• Gross hematuria • Hypertension • Skin rashes • Joint pain/tenderness • Worsening kidney function • AKI • Prolonged fever • Cardiac murmur • Hepatosplenomegaly • Lymphadenopathy • Syndromic features/dysmorphic • Age <1 or >12 y
Other	• High-risk patient: HIV • Abnormal serum C3 and or C4, positive ANA, positive hepatitis B surface antigen or hepatitis C antibody, high antistreptolysin O titer • Presence of renal cysts[56] • Associated with RTA[57]

Abbreviations: ANA, antinuclear antibodies; RTA, renal tubular acidosis.

Renal Imaging

Renal ultrasonography is not routinely needed as the findings are nonspecific. If performed, however, it will likely reveal enlarged, edematous kidneys with normal echoic pattern. In a study by Gershen and colleagues, it was found that increased echogenicity may be associated with resistance to corticosteroid therapy.[21] Renal ultrasound is indicated if the child has abnormal urinary sediment, gross hematuria, suspected renal vein thrombosis azotemia, and hypertension or if a kidney biopsy has been performed.

Genetic Testing

Routine genetic testing is not needed in the management of INS. It should be considered in children with steroid resistant nephrotic syndrome (SRNS) as close to 30% may have a monogenic cause for their disease and more than 70 genes have been identified to date.[22] The probability of finding a causative mutation is inversely proportional to the age at onset of the disease. Thus, the earlier the disease is diagnosed, the greater the relevance for genetic screening. As expected, mutations in recessive genes are in early-onset disease and mutations in dominant genes are more often implicated in adult-onset disease. A positive family history or consanguinity in any age group is highly suggestive of monogenic SRNS and recessive mutations are likely to be found on screening.[23] The presence of extra-renal manifestations or syndromic features would also be an indication for mutational analysis. Indications and benefits of genetic testing are elaborated in **Table 5**.

Table 4
Laboratory tests for idiopathic nephrotic syndrome

Routine Labs	Test	Interpretation
Urine	Urinalysis	3–4+ protein on urine dipstick
	Urine microscopy	20% of children have >3 RBC/HPF
	Protein/creatinine ratio	>2 mg/mg
Blood	CBC	WBC increase with suspected infection; elevated hemoglobin and hematocrit and platelet levels with hemoconcentration and intravascular volume depletion.
	Electrolytes	Hyponatremia, sometimes with mild hyperkalemia may be present
	BUN	intravascular volume depletion/AKI
	Creatinine	intravascular volume depletion/AKI
	Plasma albumin	<2.5 gm/dL
	Fasting lipids	Increased levels of TC, LDL, VLDL, and triglycerides, and normal or decreased HDL resulting in a high TC/HDL ratio
	Complement C3, C4, ANA[a]	Normal
	BSAg	Negative
	HCAb	
	Varicella titer	Those with negative titer need appropriate management with varicella infection and immunization.
Selected cases		
Blood test	ASOT CH50, Anti-dsDNA, ANCA, circulating immune complexes, Anti PLA2R HIV	Depending on clinical presentation, these tests may be needed to rule out the possibility of secondary NS; anti-PLA2R antibodies if membranous nephropathy suspected in an older child or adolescent
Skin test	Tuberculin test	To rule out tuberculosis before starting immunosuppression
Research purposes only	Urine biomarkers	Urine biomarkers that have shown promising results in differentiating FSGS from MCD include • uVDBP, • NGAL • A1BG, • CD-80 • A panel of 10 biomarkers [alpha-1 acid glycoprotein,

(continued on next page)

Table 4 (continued)		
Routine Labs	**Test**	**Interpretation**
		alpha-1 acid glycoprotein 2, alpha-1 microglobulin, alpha-1-B glycoprotein, fetuin-A, hemopexin, NGAL, prealbumin (transthyretin), thyroxine-binding globulin, and VDBP]. • Additional urine biomarkers that appear promising include transferrin, UBA52, calretinin, CD 14, C9, A1AT and a few more[58]

Abbreviations: A1BG, α 1B glycoprotein; BSAg, hepatitis B surface antigen; HCAb, hepatitis C antibody; HDL, high-density lipoprotein; LDL, low-density lipoprotein; NGAL, neutrophil gelatinase-associated lipocalin; TC, total cholesterol; uVDBP, urine vitamin D binding protein; VLDL, very low-density lipoprotein.

[a] Some centers do these selectively.

MANAGEMENT
Initial Management

The initial management of INS includes corticosteroid therapy, supportive care, parent education, and the treatment of complications, if present. Hospitalization should be considered in patients with anasarca, abdominal pain, fever, or for socio-economic considerations. About 5% of children undergo spontaneous remission within a week or two before treatment is initiated.[24] Spontaneous remission is also known to occur with the onset of measles or influenza B virus infection.[25] Such patients need close monitoring because a relapse is common and there is no evidence that their clinical course, including response to treatment, is any different as compared with the other children with INS.

Table 5 Indications and benefits of genetic testing in nephrotic syndrome	
Indications	• Congenital (<3 mo old) or infantile (<1 y) NS • SRNS, especially in patients younger than 2 y • History of consanguinity • Nephrotic syndrome associated with syndromic features • Positive family history of SRNS/FSGS
Benefits	• Sparing of immunosuppression • Avoidance of a kidney biopsy • Prenatal counseling in future pregnancies • Renal transplant planning for post-transplantation recurrence • Discovering rare monogenic causes of SRNS that are amenable to cure of coenzyme Q10 leading to deficiency, occurring in 1% of cases of familial SRN;.[23] coenzyme Q10 supplementation in these patients is effective for the treatment and cure of mitochondrial podocytopathies. ○ Cubulin and *MMACH* genes may present with SRNS that responds to vitamin B12 supplementation.[59]

Abbreviations: FSGS, Focal segmental glomerulosclerosis; SRNS, Steroid resistant nephrotic syndrome.

Corticosteroid therapy

Prednisone or its active metabolite prednisolone is the effective first-line therapy for INS. The first treatment regimen for corticosteroid administration for INS was established in 1979 by the ISKDC, which formed the basis for subsequent management protocols, including the current one. The ISKDC protocol consisted of prednisone 60 mg/m^2 per day for 4 weeks and 40 mg/m^2 3 days a week for another 4 weeks.[26] After the ISKDC study, many studies have been published in the quest for optimization of therapeutic response to corticosteroids with minimal side effects.

Some studies have shown that the administration of corticosteroids for longer than 2 to 3 months lowers the risk of relapse[27] whereas others have reported no significant benefit of increasing the duration of therapy beyond 2 to 3 months.[28–31] Based on recent data, the Cochrane Review concluded that the optimal duration of initial corticosteroid therapy should be 2 to 3 months and extending it for longer than 12 weeks does not significantly improve the outcome.[32] The most recent Kidney Disease: Improving Global outcomes (KDIGO) guidelines recommend a total of 8 or 12 weeks of prednisone or prednisolone for children diagnosed with INS.[33]

- Prednisone/prednisolone single dose at 60 mg/m^2/d or 2 mg/kg/d (maximum of 60 mg/d) for 4 weeks followed by alternate-day single daily dose 40 mg/m^2 or 1.5 mg/kg (maximum 50 mg on alternate days) for another 4 weeks.

Or

- Prednisone/prednisolone single dose at 60 mg/m^2/d or 2 mg/kg/d (maximum of 60 mg/d) for 6 weeks followed by alternate-day single daily dose at 40 mg/m^2 or 1.5 mg/kg (maximum 50 mg on alternate days) for another 6 weeks.

Four-week daily initial steroid therapy is not a drop-dead deadline for changing it to alternate days or defining steroid resistance. About 10% of patients with INS are known to achieve remission during the second month of daily steroid therapy.[18] In a patient who is in partial remission at the end of 4-week treatment, the daily treatment may be extended up to a total of 6 weeks and once in remission, the alternate-day regimen is the same as for those responding within 4 weeks. Administration of a high-dose oral methylprednisolone[34] or coadministration of a second immunosuppressant such as cyclosporin A[35] or anti-inflammatory agent such as azithromycin[36] is not helpful. Intravenous (IV) methylprednisolone in the beginning of steroid therapy is also not very helpful.[37] However, in a study using the French protocol in children with no response after 4 weeks of daily prednisone therapy, the administration of 3 intravenous pulses of methylprednisolone (1 g/1.73 m^2) induced remission in 10 of 22 (45%) patients.[38]

In a study by Saadeh and colleagues, underdosing and risk of frequent relapses was reported when the prescribed dose of corticosteroid was based on body weight as compared with the body surface area.[39] However later studies have not reported any significant difference in clinical outcome between the two regimens.[40,41]

Many country-specific practice guidelines about initial corticosteroid treatment in INS have been published. However, as shown in **Table 6** most of them are remarkably similar with clinically insignificant differences.

Diet

Protein: A relatively high protein intake of high biologic value is recommended, usually 130% to 140% of the normal daily allowance.

Sodium: All patients with NS have a positive sodium balance. This is generally attributed to a decrease in intravascular volume due to low plasma oncotic pressure,

Table 6
Initial corticosteroid therapy according to the various guidelines

Steroid Therapy	ISKDC[26] 1979	Canadian[60] 2014	Dutch[61,62] 2010	French[63] 2017	German[64] 2021	Indian[65]	Italian[66] 2017	KDIGO 2021
Total duration (weeks)	12–24	12–24	12	18	12	12	12	8 or 12
Dose and duration daily corticosteroid (weeks)								
• 60 mg/m² or 2 mg/kg daily	4	4–6	6	4	6	6	6	4 or 6
• 60 mg/m²/EOD	-	-	-	8	-	-	-	-
• 45 mg/m² EOD				2				
• 40 mg/m²/EOD (1.5 mg/kg)		8–20	6	-	6	6	6 (single dose)	4 or 6
OR 40 mg/m²/3 d per week (1.5 mg/kg)	4	-	-	-	-	-	-	-
• 30 mg/m²				2				
• 15 mg/m²				2				
Maximum dose (mg) while on daily/EOD corticosteroid	80/60	60/40	80/?	60/?	80/60	60/40	60/40	
Single or two divided daily doses	Divided	Single	Single		Single	Single or divided	Single or divided for daily/single for EOD	
Tapering	No	Yes	No	yes	No	No	No	

Abbreviation: EOD, every other day.

causing activation of the renin–angiotensin system and increased renal sodium absorption, as well as the activation of ENaC and Na-K ATPase in cases with intravascular expansion. A "no added salt" diet generally works in most cases, though a rigid sodium restriction to approximately 1 mEq/kg per day is recommended in severe cases.

Fluids: Fluid restriction is not easy particularly in ambulatory settings, and it may not be necessary unless there is moderate or severe hyponatremia. INS patients with severe edema may have an increased osmolal gap secondary to non-Na+ and non-K+ osmoles due to plasma volume contraction. Severe fluid restriction in such patients could increase their risk of prerenal failure.[42]

Diuretics

In ambulatory settings and depending on the severity of edema, a low-dose oral loop diuretic such as furosemide may be used alone or in combination with a distal tubular acting diuretic, such as amiloride or aldactone. In hospitalized patients, IV furosemide may be used with or without albumin, depending on the intravascular volume status. Patients with FeNa of ≥0.2% may receive a diuretic alone whereas it is safer to coadminister a diuretic with IV salt-poor albumin in those with FeNa of less than ,0.2%.[43] Diuretics should be discontinued promptly if the patient develops an intercurrent illness associated with fever, poor oral intake, vomiting or diarrhea because of an increased risk of thrombosis and acute kidney injury.

Albumin

IV albumin is reserved for patients with severe edema. Albumin infusion followed by IV furosemide is usually effective in refractory cases, but repeated infusions may be needed as the infused albumin is rapidly excreted in the urine. Patients, particularly those who may have hypervolemia, should be watched for complications such as hypertension, pulmonary edema, or congestive cardiac failure.

Infection risk assessment

Children with NS are at increased risk of pneumonia, peritonitis, or sepsis due to reduced cellular and humoral immunity, and the administration of immunosuppressant medications. *Streptococcus pneumoniae*, which used to be one of the commonest infections is uncommon nowadays because of the polyvalent pneumococcal vaccination.

The assessment of Varicella Zoster immune status should be included in the initial workup. Those susceptible need Zoster immunoglobulin, sometimes with acyclovir, depending on severity of the infection. No live vaccine should be administered during daily, high-dose steroid therapy or administration of alkylating agents. According to the American Academy of Pediatrics Red Book, 2021, the recommendations on live vaccines are as follows:[44]

- Children receiving ≥2 mg/kg/d of prednisone or its equivalent, or ≥20 mg/d (daily) if they weigh 10 kg or more for 14 days or more should not receive live-virus vaccines until 4 weeks after the discontinuation of treatment.
- Children receiving less than 2 mg/kg/d of prednisone (*daily or alternate days*) or its equivalent or less than 20 mg/d if they weigh 10 kg or more can receive live-virus vaccine during steroid treatment.

Killed vaccines such as pneumococcal conjugate (as well as 23-valent pneumococcal polysaccharide vaccine) can be given anytime. Live poliomyelitis vaccine should be substituted by inactivated vaccine and the live vaccine should not be given to siblings or other patient contacts during daily steroid treatment. Patients can have annual influenza vaccination.

Activity

We encourage physical activity as tolerated. This helps in mobilizing edema fluid and reduce the probability of venous thrombosis, muscle weakness, and osteoporosis.

Parent education

Parent education about daily urine dipstick testing at home helps monitoring for remission or relapse and thereby allows a prompt intervention and adjustments in corticosteroid administration. Education on dietary sodium restriction goes a long way in alleviating edema and may set up dietary lifestyle changes, which is particularly helpful in those who end up with a prolonged clinical course and are at risk of recurrent edema and or hypertension. Similarly, counseling on the risk of dehydration with gastroenteritis or poor oral intake due to abdominal symptoms, or increased risk of infection can be lifesaving.

Treatment of Relapse(s)

Approximately 80% to 90% of patients with INS relapse after initial response and 40% to 50% of these become steroid dependent (SD) and have frequent relapses (SD/FR). The current KDIGO recommendation for the treatment of a relapse is as follows:[33] Prednisone/prednisolone single dose at 60 mg/m^2/d or 2 mg/kg/d to a maximum of 60 mg/d until in remission for $\geq$3 days followed by 40 mg/m^2 or 1.5 mg/kg (maximum 50 mg on alternate days) for $\geq$4 weeks.

The two commonly used strategies for the management of children with FR/SD NS are given below.

Long-Term Low-Dose Corticosteroid

In FR/SD patients with no significant corticosteroid-related side effects, an alternate-day, low-dose corticosteroid for 6 months or longer may be used to sustain a remission.[45,46] The recommended dose is $\leq$ 0.5 mg/kg on alternate days. In a recent study, a daily administration of a low dose (0.2–0.3 mg/kg) over a 12-month period was reported to be more effective as compared with alternate days (0.5–0.7 mg/kg alternate day).[47]

Corticosteroid-Sparing Agents

In patients who need a high dose of corticosteroid to stay in remission or have steroid side effects, other medications that may be considered include calcineurin inhibitors (cyclosporin or Prograf), mycophenolate mofetil, levamisole, cyclophosphamide and rituximab. Further details about their use are listed in **Table 7**.

Prevention of Relapse

Relapses in INS are often precipitated by URIs. In a study of 36 children with FRNS on alternate-day, low-dose maintenance corticosteroid, it was shown that giving the same dose daily for 5 days significantly reduced the risk of a relapse (95% CI: -4.03 to -2.57; 36 participants).[48] These findings were validated by more studies[32,49,50] and this concept was later extended to children who are not on corticosteroids. Thus, in a study by Abeyagunawardena and colleagues[50] it was shown that a short course of daily corticosteroids (0.5 mg/kg/d) during a URI significantly reduces the frequency of URI-induced relapse in patients with steroid-responsive NS.[51] KDIGO currently recommends that for children with FRSD NS, who are currently taking alternate-day, low-dose corticosteroid or are off steroids receive daily corticosteroid

Table 7
Steroid-sparing medications for steroid-dependent/frequent relapsing nephrotic syndrome

Medication		Comments
CNI	Cyclosporin or tacrolimus	• Used for steroid-resistant as well as frequent relapsing/steroid-dependent cases. Generally used as first-line therapy for the latter. • CNIs are nephrotoxic, need to be given for a prolonged period of time, and nephrotic syndrome tends to recur when medication is stopped. • A minimum of 6 mo of treatment is required to determine whether the patient is responsive to the CNI. • Optimum duration of therapy with CNIs among responders is debatable although a minimum of 12–24 mo is frequently cited.[67] • Kidney biopsy to assess CNI-induced nephrotoxicity may be needed in selected cases after prolonged administration.[68]
Mycophenolate mofetil		• Fewer side effects as compared to CNI, CYP, and tacrolimus. • Is being increasingly used in frequent relapsing and steroid-dependent cases. • Recommended also for children who attain full remission on CNI treatment for ≥ 1 y, thus allowing for discontinuation of CNI.[67]
Levamisole		• An anthelminthic agent with low toxicity profile; it is not available in the USA.
CYP		• Generally avoided because of its toxicity but can be used effectively if other medications are not available. • Monitoring for side effects during administration is essential.
Monoclonal antibodies	Rituximab	• Chimeric anti-CD20 antibody that causes depletion of B cells. • Relatively new medication with potentially serious side effects and should be used cautiously and selectively. • May be considered in steroid-resistant as well as frequent relapsing/steroid-dependent cases. • Recent study by Basu and colleagues that included 176 pediatric patients with steroid-dependent nephrotic syndrome reported a higher 12-mo

(continued on next page)

Table 7	
(continued)	
Medication	**Comments**
	relapse-free survival rate in the rituximab group than in the tacrolimus group (90.0% vs 63.3%) as well as a lower 12-mo cumulative corticosteroid dose in the rituximab group.[69]
Ofatumumab abatacept, adalimumab fresolimumab	• Newer anti-CD20 monoclonal antibodies with little or no data on their use in nephrotic syndrome

Abbreviations: CNI, calcineurin inhibitor; CYP, cyclophosphamide; USA, United States of America.

0.5 mg/kg/d during URI or any other infections for 5 to 7 days to reduce the risk of a relapse.[33]

Other Supportive Care

Some patients with INS, particularly those with FR/SD clinical course, may need clinical intervention for the following:

Behavioral Issues
The occurrence of behavioral issues with steroid administration is not uncommon and these may include anxiety and depressive or aggressive behavior. It is worse in those with abnormal behavior at baseline. According to a study by Soliday and colleagues, the behavioral changes occur mostly at prednisone doses of 1 mg/kg every 48 hours or more.[52] Depending on the severity, an adjustment in steroid dosage, administration of a steroid sparing agent, or an appropriate referral should be considered in such patients.

Hypertension
Hypertension is rare at presentation in INS, particularly in those who respond to steroid therapy. A few patients may become hypertensive during steroid therapy, and the risk of hypertension increases in those who have recurrent relapses or become steroid resistant. Administration of CNI and the onset of CKD further increases the risk of hypertension in such cases. Angiotensin converting enzyme inhibitors or angiotensin II receptor blockers are preferred because of their additive antiproteinuric benefit and ability to slow progression of renal impairment. Other options include calcium channel blockers or beta-blockers.

Hypercoagulability
The risk factors for vascular thrombosis in NS include hemoconcentration, thrombocytosis, hypercoagulability, dyslipidemia, and hypovolemia. Low-dose aspirin or dipyridamole, or the administration of an anticoagulant may be needed in high-risk patients, particularly those with an episode of a thromboembolic complication. Prompt treatment of sepsis, prevention of intravascular volume depletion and hemoconcentration, regular ambulation, and avoidance of central catheters help reduce the risk of thromboembolism.

Hyperlipidemia
Hyperlipidemia is a common occurrence in INS and in the past its presence was included in the definition of NS. It is mainly a result of an increased hepatic synthesis

of cholesterol, triglycerides, and lipoproteins and a decreased catabolism of lipoproteins caused by decreased lipoprotein lipase. Patients can have increased levels of total cholesterol, low-density lipoprotein, very low-density lipoprotein , triglycerides, and normal or decreased high-density lipoprotein resulting in a high TC/HDL ratio. These resolve soon after the resolution of proteinuria and as such there is no need for routine administration of statins in INS but should be considered in those with refractory NS.[53]

NEPHROTIC SYNDROME IN ADULTS

Adults may have a new-onset INS or continue having relapses from the disease diagnosed during childhood. Recent literature shows that a more severe form of SS INS in childhood may continue into adult life. In a study that included 102 adults with NS in childhood, 43 (42.2%) experienced at least one relapse of NS in adulthood.[54] In another recent study, in 39 adult patients with a mean age of 22.8 (range 18.0–30.9) years with childhood-onset steroid sensitive nephrotic syndrome (SSNS) at a mean age of about 8 years (6–11.1) years, 12 (31%) had active disease in adulthood. All had SD/FR NS in childhood.[55] As such, proper counseling at the time of discharge from the pediatric clinic is recommended.

SUMMARY

NS is diagnosed by the presence of significant proteinuria in an edematous child. A good clinical assessment with a few laboratory tests helps rule out secondary causes for NS. All patients with INS should be treated with 2 to 3 months of corticosteroid therapy. Most patients go into remission but have relapse(s) that may need additional immunosuppression, including administration of steroid-sparing agents. The risk of a relapse can be decreased by a short 5-day course of steroid therapy during URI. Complications associated with the disease or medication side effects are not uncommon. Some patients continue to have relapses in adult life.

CLINICS CARE POINTS

- Intravenous albumin and furosemide should be used only in patients with severe edema not amenable to salt and water restriction or oral diuretic administration.
- The duration of initial corticosteroid therapy for more than 12 weeks is not necessary.
- No live vaccine should be administered during high-dose steroid therapy.
- An alternate-day, low-dose ($\leq$0.5 mg/kg) steroid for 6 months or longer can be used to sustain a remission.
- A short 5- to 7-day course of daily steroids at the onset of URI lowers the risk of a relapse.
- The commonest indication for kidney biopsy is the lack of response to initial corticosteroid therapy.
- Treatment with a non-steroidal immunosuppressant should be considered in patients with frequent relapses/steroid dependence or steroid toxicity.

DISCLOSURE

The authors have nothing to disclose.

REFERENCES

1. Nephrotic syndrome in children: prediction of histopathology from clinical and laboratory characteristics at time of diagnosis. A report of the International Study of Kidney Disease in Children. Kidney Int 1978;13(2):159–65.
2. Cameron JS. Five hundred years of the nephrotic syndrome: 1484-1984. Ulster Med J 1985;54(Suppl):S5–19.
3. Pal A, Kaskel F. History of Nephrotic Syndrome and Evolution of its Treatment. Front Pediatr 2016;4:56.
4. Hahn D, Hodson EM, Willis NS, et al. Corticosteroid therapy for nephrotic syndrome in children. Cochrane Database Syst Rev 2015;3:CD001533.
5. Veltkamp F, Rensma LR, Bouts AHM, et al. Incidence and Relapse of Idiopathic Nephrotic Syndrome: Meta-analysis. Pediatrics 2021;148(1).
6. Eddy AA, Symons JM. Nephrotic syndrome in childhood. Lancet 2003;362(9384): 629–39.
7. Moncrieff MW, White RH, Glasgow EF, et al. The familial nephrotic syndrome. II. A clinicopathological study. Clin Nephrol 1973;1(4):220–9.
8. Mattoo TK. Pediatric Nephrology in the Arabian Peninsula. In: Holliday MABT, Avner ED, editors. Pediatric nephrology. 3rd edition. Baltimore: Williams and Wilkins; 1993. p. 1436–9.
9. Haraldsson B, Nystrom J, Deen WM. Properties of the glomerular barrier and mechanisms of proteinuria. Physiol Rev 2008;88(2):451–87.
10. Barisoni L, Schnaper HW, Kopp JB. A proposed taxonomy for the podocytopathies: a reassessment of the primary nephrotic diseases. Clin J Am Soc Nephrol 2007;2(3):529–42.
11. Shalhoub RJ. Pathogenesis of lipoid nephrosis: a disorder of T-cell function. Lancet 1974;2(7880):556–60.
12. Gilbert RD, Hulse E, Rigden S. Rituximab therapy for steroid-dependent minimal change nephrotic syndrome. Pediatr Nephrol 2006;21(11):1698–700.
13. Nasr SH, Satoskar A, Markowitz GS, et al. Proliferative glomerulonephritis with monoclonal IgG deposits. J Am Soc Nephrol 2009;20(9):2055–64.
14. Sinha A, Bhatia D, Gulati A, et al. Efficacy and safety of rituximab in children with difficult-to-treat nephrotic syndrome. Nephrol Dial Transplant 2015;30(1):96–106.
15. Watts AJB, Keller KH, Lerner G, et al. Discovery of Autoantibodies Targeting Nephrin in Minimal Change Disease Supports a Novel Autoimmune Etiology. J Am Soc Nephrol 2022;33(1):238–52.
16. Ray EC, Rondon-Berrios H, Boyd CR, et al. Sodium retention and volume expansion in nephrotic syndrome: implications for hypertension. Adv Chronic Kidney Dis 2015;22(3):179–84.
17. Kallash M, Mahan JD. Mechanisms and management of edema in pediatric nephrotic syndrome. Pediatr Nephrol 2021;36(7):1719–30.
18. The primary nephrotic syndrome in children. Identification of patients with minimal change nephrotic syndrome from initial response to prednisone. A report of the International Study of Kidney Disease in Children. J Pediatr 1981;98(4): 561–4.
19. Bhimma R, Coovadia HM, Adhikari M. Nephrotic syndrome in South African children: changing perspectives over 20 years. Pediatr Nephrol 1997;11(4):429–34.
20. Nandlal L, Naicker T, Bhimma R. Nephrotic Syndrome in South African Children: Changing Perspectives in the New Millennium. Kidney Int Rep 2019;4(4):522–34.
21. Gershen RS, Brody AS, Duffy LC, et al. Prognostic value of sonography in childhood nephrotic syndrome. Pediatr Nephrol 1994;8(1):76–8.

22. Park E. Genetic Basis of Steroid Resistant Nephrotic Syndrome. Child Kidney Dis 2019;23(2):86–92.

23. Sadowski CE, Lovric S, Ashraf S, et al. A single-gene cause in 29.5% of cases of steroid-resistant nephrotic syndrome. J Am Soc Nephrol 2015;26(6):1279–89.

24. Tune BM, Mendoza SA. Treatment of the idiopathic nephrotic syndrome: regimens and outcomes in children and adults. J Am Soc Nephrol 1997;8(5):824–32.

25. Tamura H, Kuraoka S, Hidaka Y, et al. A Case of Nephrotic Syndrome that Resolved with Influenza B Infection. Case Rep Nephrol Dial 2021;11(1):103–9.

26. Nephrotic syndrome in children: a randomized trial comparing two prednisone regimens in steroid-responsive patients who relapse early. Report of the international study of kidney disease in children. J Pediatr 1979;95(2):239–43.

27. Hodson EM, Willis NS, Craig JC. Corticosteroid therapy for nephrotic syndrome in children. Cochrane Database Syst Rev 2007;4:CD001533.

28. Yoshikawa N, Nakanishi K, Sako M, et al. A multicenter randomized trial indicates initial prednisolone treatment for childhood nephrotic syndrome for two months is not inferior to six-month treatment. Kidney Int 2015;87(1):225–32.

29. Sinha A, Saha A, Kumar M, et al. Extending initial prednisolone treatment in a randomized control trial from 3 to 6 months did not significantly influence the course of illness in children with steroid-sensitive nephrotic syndrome. Kidney Int 2015;87(1):217–24.

30. Teeninga N, Kist-van Holthe JE, van Rijswijk N, et al. Extending prednisolone treatment does not reduce relapses in childhood nephrotic syndrome. J Am Soc Nephrol 2013;24(1):149–59.

31. Webb NJA, Woolley RL, Lambe T, et al. Long term tapering versus standard prednisolone treatment for first episode of childhood nephrotic syndrome: phase III randomised controlled trial and economic evaluation. BMJ 2019;365:l1800.

32. Hahn D, Samuel SM, Willis NS, et al. Corticosteroid therapy for nephrotic syndrome in children. Cochrane Database Syst Rev 2020;2015(3):CD001533.

33. Rovin BH, Adler SG, Barratt J, et al. Executive summary of the KDIGO 2021 Guideline for the Management of Glomerular Diseases. Kidney Int 2021;100(4):753–79.

34. Mocan H, Erduran E, Karaguzel G. High dose methylprednisolone therapy in nephrotic syndrome. Indian J Pediatr 1999;66(2):171–4.

35. Hoyer PF, Brodeh J. Initial treatment of idiopathic nephrotic syndrome in children: prednisone versus prednisone plus cyclosporine A: a prospective, randomized trial. J Am Soc Nephrol 2006;17(4):1151–7.

36. Zhang B, Liu T, Wang W, et al. A prospective randomly controlled clinical trial on azithromycin therapy for induction treatment of children with nephrotic syndrome. Eur J Pediatr 2014;173(4):509–15.

37. Imbasciati E, Gusmano R, Edefonti A, et al. Controlled trial of methylprednisolone pulses and low dose oral prednisone for the minimal change nephrotic syndrome. Br Med J (Clin Res Ed 1985;291(6505):1305–8.

38. Dossier C, Delbet JD, Boyer O, et al. Five-year outcome of children with idiopathic nephrotic syndrome: the NEPHROVIR population-based cohort study. Pediatr Nephrol 2019;34(4):671–8.

39. Saadeh SA, Baracco R, Jain A, et al. Weight or body surface area dosing of steroids in nephrotic syndrome: is there an outcome difference? Pediatr Nephrol 2011;26(12):2167–71.

40. Raman V, Krishnamurthy S, Harichandrakumar KT. Body weight-based prednisolone versus body surface area-based prednisolone regimen for induction of

remission in children with nephrotic syndrome: a randomized, open-label, equivalence clinical trial. Pediatr Nephrol 2016;31(4):595–604.

41. Basu B, Bhattacharyya S, Barua S, et al. Efficacy of body weight vs body surface area-based prednisolone regimen in nephrotic syndrome. Clin Exp Nephrol 2020; 24(7):622–9.

42. Kapur G, Valentini RP, Imam AA, et al. Serum osmolal gap in patients with idiopathic nephrotic syndrome and severe edema. Pediatrics 2007;119(6):e1404–7.

43. Kapur G, Valentini RP, Imam AA, et al. Treatment of severe edema in children with nephrotic syndrome with diuretics alone–a prospective study. Clin J Am Soc Nephrol 2009;4(5):907–13.

44. Kimberlin QW, Barnett ED, Lynfield R, et al. Immunizations and other considerations in immunocompromised children. Red Book: 2021–2024 Report of the Committee on Infectious Diseases. American Academy of Pediatrics; 2021.

45. Elzouki AY, Jaiswal OP. Long-term, small dose prednisone therapy in frequently relapsing nephrotic syndrome of childhood. Effect on remission, statural growth, obesity, and infection rate. Clin Pediatr (Phila) 1988;27(8):387–92.

46. Srivastava RN, Vasudev AS, Bagga A, et al. Long-term, low-dose prednisolone therapy in frequently relapsing nephrotic syndrome. Pediatr Nephrol 1992;6(3): 247–50.

47. Yadav M, Sinha A, Khandelwal P, et al. Efficacy of low-dose daily versus alternate-day prednisolone in frequently relapsing nephrotic syndrome: an open-label randomized controlled trial. Pediatr Nephrol 2019;34(5):829–35.

48. Mattoo TK, Mahmoud MA. Increased maintenance corticosteroids during upper respiratory infection decrease the risk of relapse in nephrotic syndrome. Nephron 2000;85(4):343–5.

49. Gulati A, Sinha A, Sreenivas V, et al. Daily corticosteroids reduce infection-associated relapses in frequently relapsing nephrotic syndrome: a randomized controlled trial. Clin J Am Soc Nephrol 2011;6(1):63–9.

50. Abeyagunawardena AS, Trompeter RS. Increasing the dose of prednisolone during viral infections reduces the risk of relapse in nephrotic syndrome: a randomised controlled trial. Arch Dis Child 2008;93(3):226–8.

51. Abeyagunawardena AS, Thalgahagoda RS, Dissanayake PV, et al. Short courses of daily prednisolone during upper respiratory tract infections reduce relapse frequency in childhood nephrotic syndrome. Pediatr Nephrol 2017;32(8):1377–82.

52. Soliday E, Grey S, Lande MB. Behavioral effects of corticosteroids in steroid-sensitive nephrotic syndrome. Pediatrics 1999;104(4):e51.

53. Sanjad SA, al-Abbad A, al-Shorafa S. Management of hyperlipidemia in children with refractory nephrotic syndrome: the effect of statin therapy. J Pediatr 1997; 130(3):470–4.

54. Fakhouri F, Bocquet N, Taupin P, et al. Steroid-sensitive nephrotic syndrome: from childhood to adulthood. Am J Kidney Dis 2003;41(3):550–7.

55. Korsgaard T, Andersen RF, Joshi S, et al. Childhood onset steroid-sensitive nephrotic syndrome continues into adulthood. Pediatr Nephrol 2019;34(4):641–8.

56. Mattoo TK, Giangreco AB, Afzal M, et al. Cystic lymphangiectasia of the kidneys in an infant with nephrotic syndrome. Pediatr Nephrol 1990;4(3):228–32.

57. Mattoo TK, Akhtar M. Familial glomerulopathy with proximal tubular dysfunction: a new syndrome? Pediatr Nephrol 1990;4(3):223–7.

58. Stone H, Magella B, Bennett MR. The Search for Biomarkers to Aid in Diagnosis, Differentiation, and Prognosis of Childhood Idiopathic Nephrotic Syndrome. Front Pediatr 2019;7:404.

59. Koenig JC, Rutsch F, Bockmeyer C, et al. Nephrotic syndrome and thrombotic microangiopathy caused by cobalamin C deficiency. Pediatr Nephrol 2015;30(7): 1203–6.

60. Samuel S, Bitzan M, Zappitelli M, et al. Canadian Society of Nephrology Commentary on the 2012 KDIGO clinical practice guideline for glomerulonephritis: management of nephrotic syndrome in children. Am J Kidney Dis 2014;63(3): 354–62.

61. Schijvens AM, van der Weerd L, van Wijk JAE, et al. Practice variations in the management of childhood nephrotic syndrome in the Netherlands. Eur J Pediatr 2021;180(6):1885–94.

62. Lilien M, Van de Walle J. Nefrotisch syndroom. Werkboek Kindernefrologie 2010; 2:124–31.

63. Boyer O, Baudouin V, Berard E, et al. [Idiopathic nephrotic syndrome]. Arch Pediatr 2017;24(12):1338–43.

64. Ehren R, Benz MR, Brinkkotter PT, et al. Pediatric idiopathic steroid-sensitive nephrotic syndrome: diagnosis and therapy -short version of the updated German best practice guideline (S2e) - AWMF register no. 166-001, 6/2020. Pediatr Nephrol 2021;36(10):2971–85.

65. Sinha A, Bagga A, Banerjee S, et al. Steroid Sensitive Nephrotic Syndrome: Revised Guidelines. Indian Pediatr 2021;58(5):461–81.

66. Pasini A, Benetti E, Conti G, et al. The Italian Society for Pediatric Nephrology (SINePe) consensus document on the management of nephrotic syndrome in children: Part I - Diagnosis and treatment of the first episode and the first relapse. Ital J Pediatr 2017;43(1):41.

67. Trautmann A, Vivarelli M, Samuel S, et al. IPNA clinical practice recommendations for the diagnosis and management of children with steroid-resistant nephrotic syndrome. Pediatr Nephrol 2020;35(8):1529–61.

68. Abukwaik W, Poulik JM, Mattoo TK. Calcineurin inhibitors and renal biopsy in children with idiopathic nephrotic syndrome. Clin Nephrol 2021;96(4):226–32.

69. Basu B, Sander A, Roy B, et al. Efficacy of Rituximab vs Tacrolimus in Pediatric Corticosteroid-Dependent Nephrotic Syndrome: A Randomized Clinical Trial. JAMA Pediatr 2018;172(8):757–64.

Urinary Tract Infection in Children

Per Brandström, MD, PhD[a,b,*], Sverker Hansson, MD, PhD[a,b]

KEYWORDS

- Urinary tract infection • Urine sampling • Biomarkers • Urine culture
- Kidney damage • Guidelines

KEY POINTS

- Clean-catch urine, if possible, can be used for analysis and urine culture in most infants.
- Risk factors can be used to direct investigations and follow-up of children at risk of recurrent urinary tract infection (UTI) and kidney function deterioration.
- Long-term outcome is excellent for most children with UTI.
- Severe scarring can result in hypertension and reduced kidney function later in life.

INTRODUCTION

Urinary tract infection (UTI) is common in children and affects 1.7% of boys and 8.4% of girls before the age of 7 years.[1,2] As shown in **Fig. 1**, UTI is more prevalent in boys in the first 4 to 6 months of life, but after that girls are more often affected.[3] Clinical manifestations vary from life-threatening septicemic infection to asymptomatic bacteriuria (ABU). For practical reasons, UTI can be divided into three categories: acute pyelonephritis affecting the kidney, cystitis restricted to the lower urinary tract, and ABU.

The main concern in the management of children with UTI is the preservation and protection of kidney function and kidney growth. Most published guidelines are focused on the first few years of life, when urine sampling is more challenging and symptoms often nonspecific. There is also a greater risk for more severe clinical course with septicemia in the younger children, which motivates a more intense management.[4] Kidney damage and abnormalities of the kidneys and urinary tract are usually identified during the first few years of life after the first febrile UTI or, as is happening increasingly, by prenatal ultrasound examination.

[a] Department of Pediatrics, Clinical Science Institute, Sahlgrenska Academy, University of Gothenburg, Gothenburg 416 85, Sweden; [b] Pediatric Uro-Nephrologic Center, Queen Silvia Children's Hospital, Sahlgrenska University Hospital, Gothenburg 416 85, Sweden
* Corresponding author. Pediatric Uro-Nephrologic Center, Queen Silvia Children's Hospital, Sahlgrenska University Hospital, Gothenburg 416 85, Sweden.
E-mail address: per.brandstrom@gu.se

Pediatr Clin N Am 69 (2022) 1099–1114
https://doi.org/10.1016/j.pcl.2022.07.003
0031-3955/22/© 2022 Elsevier Inc. All rights reserved.

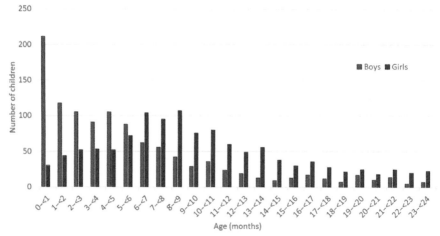

Fig. 1. First time UTI in 1111 boys and 1198 girls during the first 2 years of life. The incidence of UTI is highest the first year of life.[3]

URINARY TRACT INFECTION DIAGNOSIS

In older children, the presenting symptoms include flank pain with fever, urgency and frequent voiding, incontinence, and dysuria. In young infants, the symptoms are often vague with fever, inadequate feeding, or failure to thrive. In such cases, urinalysis is warranted and the urine specimen should be sent for culture in selected cases. Alternatively, algorithms including factors that make a UTI more likely can be used to guide clinicians when to suspect a UTI, making diagnostic procedures and urine sampling more meaningful.[5–8] As most children with kidney anomalies usually present with a UTI, the diagnostic workup and the criteria for a UTI must be thorough and accurate.

URINE SAMPLING

A representative urine sample is crucial for diagnosing a child with a suspected UTI. In nontoilet trained children, noninvasive sampling (midstream urine, adhesive bags, or nappy pads) has a high prevalence of contamination in urine cultures. Of the invasive techniques used, suprapubic aspiration (SPA) has the lowest contamination rate, followed by catheterization.[9,10] There are national or regional differences in sampling preference. Some authors have found catheterization to be less invasive and not as painful compared with SPA,[11,12] whereas in a recent study the opposite was noticed.[13] In toilet-trained children with voluntary bladder control, midstream voided urine is usually sufficient. This also happens to be the dominating sampling technique in infants in many countries,[14–18] especially with the introduction of adjuvant techniques to help enhance the possibility of getting a urine sample within a reasonable time.[19]

URINE BIOMARKERS

Leukocyturia identified with a leukocyte esterase test or by microscopy is a strong indication of bacteriuria, with a sensitivity of 83% and a specificity of 78%,[5] but can be found in children with any febrile illness.[20] Leukocyturia may be absent especially in UTIs with low bacterial count or those caused by non-*Escherichia coli* pathogens.[21,22] Urine nitrite has a low sensitivity of 23% in infants, higher in older children, but a high specificity of 99%.[23] In infant UTI, the nitrite test is mostly negative because of short bladder urine incubation time, causative bacteria that do not produce nitrite, or insufficient dietary nitrate intake.

Other urine biomarkers for the diagnosis of UTI in children have been explored.[22] Several studies have found neutrophil gelatinase-associated lipocalin (NGAL) and interleukin 8 (IL-8) to have high sensitivity and specificity in differentiating UTI from other febrile illnesses in children.[24] With the increased availability of these biomarkers, the diagnostic delay while waiting for culture results is likely to be shortened and the number of children exposed to unnecessary antibiotic treatment would also decrease. In infants with fever and low NGAL, other causes of fever should be sought.[22,24]

URINE CULTURE

The growth of a single strain of a uropathogen bacteria is indicative of a UTI, whereas multiple strains in most cases indicate contamination of the urine sample. For many years significant growth in urine was defined as $\geq$100,000 colony forming units per milliliter, a criterion originally set to exclude contaminated samples in studies of women with symptomatic UTI.[25] Infants, with short voiding intervals, can have lower bacterial counts in symptomatic UTI, especially when caused by bacteria other than E. coli.[21,26] There are divergent opinions in different guidelines on how to define significant bacterial count in children. Many recognize that uncontaminated samples from SPA should normally be sterile and that bacteria should less frequently contaminate catheterized urine samples. Hence, as shown in **Table 1**, many guidelines propose different cutoff levels for significant bacterial growth depending on the urine sampling technique.

There are new techniques being launched to identify pathogenic bacteria in the urine. These include polymerase chain reaction (PCR) for detecting 16S RNA and new generation sequencing of bacterial DNA, where genes for resistance and virulence factors also can be detected. Although promising, these techniques have to be further evaluated and refined before they can replace the current routine of urine culture.[27]

TREATMENT

When UTI is suspected, empirical antibiotic treatment should be started as soon as possible, typically before the diagnosis has been confirmed by the urine sent for culture. Oral antibiotic treatment is as effective as intravenous administration. Initial intravenous treatment can safely be switched to oral.[28] It is equally safe to start with oral treatment in nontoxic children who tolerate oral medication.[29–31] However, for children below 2 months of age the scientific data are sparse and, pending further studies, initial intravenous treatment is usually recommended, see table.

The choice of empirical treatment relies on antibiotic resistance profiles in the community and depends on the availability of drugs suitable for children. The prevalence of bacteria with multidrug resistance and extended spectrum betalactamase production poses an increasing problem.[32] Such infections also have a more complicated clinical course with a potential delay in starting appropriate antibiotic treatment, increased length of inpatient stay, and other complications.[33]

The increasing resistance, and the lack of access to drugs in a formulation and taste suitable for children, has made the treatment of childhood UTI more challenging.[34] For many years, cotrimoxazole with high bioavailability and good penetrance to parenchymal tissue was the treatment of choice in many countries. Now, owing to increasing resistance, it can only be recommended after urine culture has shown the bacteria to be sensitive.[35,36] Third-generation cephalosporins are usually

Table 1
Comparison between guidelines for UTI in children

Guidelines		Diagnostic Procedure/Test			Treatment			Imaging		
	Age	Urine Collection in Non-toilet Trained	Significant Bacteriuria	Blood Test Recommended	Route of Administration in Febrile UTI	Length of Treatment (Days) in Febrile UTI	Prophylactic Antibiotics Recommended	RBUS	VCUG	DMSA
UK/NICE[14]	0–16 years	1. MSU 2. Pad 3. Cath/SPA	Not defined	CRP *should not* be used for differentiating upper/lower UTI	<3 months: refer to hospital <1 month: iv <3 months and toxic: iv >3 months oral	10	No	<6 months: all children >6 months if atypical or recurrence	<6 months if atypical or recurrence 6–36 months: Consider if [atypical or recurrence] + risk factor[b]	<3 years if atypical or recurrence >3 years if recurrence
USA/AAP[a,5,8]	2–24 months	Cath/SPA MSU for screening	Cath/SPA $\geq 5 \times 10^4$	No recommendations given	Iv if toxic/unable to retain oral fluid Otherwise oral	7–14	No	All children	If abnormal RBUS or complicated UTI. Consider if recurrence	Not recommended
Italy[a,16]	2–36 months	Hospital- toxic: Cath/SPA Not toxic: MSU Bag for screening	Cath/SPA $\geq 10^4$ MSU $\geq 5 \times 10^4$	<3 months and hospitalized: CRP, PCT, FBC, creat	Iv if toxic/unable to retain oral fluid <3 months: iv Otherwise oral	10	Not routine. Consider if: VUR grade 4–5 >3 febrile UTIs/1 year	All children	If abnormal RBUS, recurrence or non-E. coli infection	If VUR grade 4–5
Canada[69]	>2 months	Cath/SPA MSU for screening	SPA all growth Cath $\geq 5 \times 10^4$ MSU $\geq 10^5$	Creat if "complicated" UTI	Iv if toxic/unable to retain oral fluid Otherwise oral	7–10	Not routine. VUR grade 4–5 and anomalies: discuss with urologist	<2 years all children	If abnormal RBUS <2 years if recurrence	Only if UTI diagnosis is in doubt (acute scan)
ESPU/EAU[70,71]	0–18 years	Cath/SPA/MSU Bag for screening	SPA all growth Cath $\geq 10^3$ MSU $\geq 10^5$ (10^4 if sympt)	< 1 year: CRP/PCT, FBC, creat, electrolytes	<2 months: iv Iv if toxic/unable to retain oral fluid Otherwise oral	7–14 (toilet trained, uncomplicated 7)	Consider if < 1 year and in non-toilet trained girls	All children with febrile UTI	<1 year: all children >1 year: non-E. coli UTI, recurrent febrile UTI Alternative: DMSA (top-down model)	Alternative to VCUG (top-down) within 1–2 months from infection

Country	Age	Urine sampling	Culture threshold	Blood tests	Antibiotic route	Duration (days)	VCUG	Ultrasound (RBUS)	DMSA	Comments
Spain[15]	0–18 years	Cath/SPA/MSU Bag for screening	SPA all growth, Cath $\geq 10^3$, MSU $\geq 10^5$ (10^4 if sympt)	Optional: If < 3 months blood culture	Iv if toxic/unable to retain oral fluid <3 months: iv Otherwise oral	7–10	No Consider if obstructive uropathy	<6 months: all children >6 months if atypical or recurrence		If atypical or recurrence. If UTI diagnosis is in doubt
Sweden[17]	0–18 years	1. SPA if < 1 year 2. MSU (x2) 3. Cath	Not defined	CRP, creat, blood culture if iv	Iv if toxic/unable to retain oral fluid Otherwise oral	10	VUR $\geq$ grade 3 Recurrent UTI	<2 years: all children >2 years: febrile UTI or recurrent cystitis (boys one, girls three)	<2 years if dilatation on RBUS or DMSA pathology >2 years if [recurrent febrile UTI or abnormal RBUS] + DMSA pathology	<2 years if abnormal RBUS, risk factor[c] or recurrence >2 years if abnormal RBUS or febrile recurrence
Asia[72]	not defined	Cath/SPA Bag for screening	SPA all growth, Cath $\geq 5 \times 10^4$, MSU $\geq 10^5$	Consider PCT or CRP	<3 months: refer to hospital <3 months and toxic: iv >3 months oral	7–14	VUR $\geq$ grade 3 Recurrent UTI Urinary tract obstruction	All children with febrile UTI	If abnormal RBUS and or abnormal DMSA If febrile recurrence	Severe acute pyelonephritis Hypodysplasia on RBUS If UTI diagnosis is in doubt (acute scan)
Switzerland[18]	0–16 years	1. Cath/SPA/2. MSU Bag for screening	SPA all growth, Cath $\geq 10^3$, MSU $\geq 10^5$	Consider: CRP/PCT <3 months: FBC, electrolytes, creatinine	<2 months: iv Iv if toxic/unable to retain oral fluid Otherwise oral	7–10	Consider in: VUR grade 4–5 Complex CAKUT or underlying bladder dysfunction	All children with febrile UTI	Risk factors[d] Abnormal RBUS Recurrent pyelonephritis (2 or more episodes)	Consider after interdisciplinary discussion

Abbreviations: CAKUT, congenital anomalies of the kidneys and urinary tract; cath, catheter; creat, creatinine; CRP, C-reactive protein; DMSA, ^{99m}Tc–dimercapto succinic acid scintigraphy; FBC, full blood count; iv, intravenous; MSU, mid-stream urine; PCT, procalcitonin; RBUS, renal and bladder ultrasonography; SPA, suprapubic aspiration; UTI, urinary tract infection; VCUG, voiding urethra-cystography; VUR, vesicoureteral reflux.

[a] Guideline only considers febrile UTIs.

[b] UK risk factors: dilatation on ultrasound, poor urine flow, non-*E. coli* and family history of VUR.

[c] Swedish risk factors: dilatation on ultrasound, serum CRP $\geq$ 70 mg/L, non-*E. coli* and increased serum creatinine.

[d] Swiss risk factors: abnormal ultrasound, poor urine flow, oliguria, urinary retention, non-*E. coli*, treatment failure >48 h, abnormal creatinine or electrolytes.

effective.[36] Other alternatives include amoxicillin/clavulanate and pivmecillinam. Quinolones, with their widespread use in the adult population, are discouraged in children because of safety concerns and their use should be saved for selected cases with multidrug resistance.

There is consensus in most guidelines on treating febrile UTIs for 10 days, with a span from 7 days to up to 14 days when treating the more severely ill child with a suspected or manifest septicemia (see **Table 1**). For cystitis in children above 2 to 3 years of age, where kidney involvement can be ruled out, most guidelines recommend 5 days of antibiotics, with some studies supporting an even shorter 3 days course.[37,38]

There have been attempts to decrease the risk of kidney scarring by adding steroids to the treatment of UTI, but the results have been disappointing[39,40]

ASYMPTOMATIC BACTERIURIA

Bacteriuria without clinical symptoms is referred to as ABU. It can be found in all age groups. In infants, the duration of ABU is usually limited to 1 to 3 months.[41] In older children, ABU is typically seen in girls with bladder dysfunction causing infrequent or incomplete bladder emptying, and can last longer, sometime years. ABU is also frequently found in children with neurogenic bladders with incomplete emptying or those requiring indwelling foreign materials such as catheters or vesicostomy tubes. ABU may be considered as a kind of partnership between the bacteria and the host, protecting against symptomatic UTI in susceptible individuals, and is best left untreated. Shorter courses of antibiotics may do more harm than good, with new episodes of bacteriuria after treatment in 50 to 80% and a risk of acute pyelonephritis in approximately 15% of cases.[42–45]

ANTIBIOTIC PROPHYLAXIS

Prophylactic treatment with low-dose antibiotics to prevent recurrent UTI has been common practice for children with VUR, especially dilated VUR, and other forms of dilating anomalies, or in children with recurrent UTI. The use of prophylactic antibiotics has declined substantially after proof of only moderate or no effect on the rate of recurrent UTI in several studies,[46–48] with the exception of young girls with dilated VUR.[49] The increasing bacterial resistance and the low adherence to medication have also contributed to the decreasing use of prophylaxis. However, in selected patients carefully followed, prophylaxis can protect them from recurrent UTI. The prevention of recurrent urinary tract infection in children with vesicoureteric reflux and normal renal tracts (PRIVENT) and randomized intervention for children with vesicoureteral reflux (RIVUR) studies were not able to establish whether prophylaxis protects against kidney damage or deteriorating kidney function, whereas the Swedish Reflux Trial found a significant reduction in kidney scarring in the prophylaxis group compared with surveillance only and to endoscopic subureteric injection therapy.[47,48,50] The number of recurrences is reduced by prophylactic antibiotics. In a compliant patient, de novo antibiotic resistance caused by its prolonged administration may lead to UTI recurrences by a resistant pathogen.

[51] The effectiveness of prophylaxis is dependent on family compliance and a regular contact with the family to support medication adherence is essential.[52,53]

EVALUATION AFTER URINARY TRACT INFECTION

The evaluation after a UTI aims to detect underlying congenital abnormalities of the kidneys and urinary tract, kidney damage, and bladder dysfunction, with the risk of recurrent UTI and future deterioration of kidney function. Congenital kidney anomalies in children are often diagnosed during evaluation for UTI, especially in countries where prenatal ultrasound in the last trimester is not regularly performed. Congenital kidney damage is more common in boys, whereas in girls, kidney damage is usually acquired from recurrent UTI.[54,55] The extent of kidney damage is closely associated with UTI recurrence and to higher grades of dilated VUR.[50,56,57]

ULTRASOUND

Ultrasound is the primary investigation to be considered after a first-time UTI in infants and after a febrile UTI in older children. It can identify obstruction, dilatation, and major abnormalities in the size and location of the kidneys, but cannot reliably be used to diagnose the presence or absence of kidney damage or vesicoureteral reflux.[58,59] In many countries, practitioners perform ultrasound examinations in offices whereas in other countries it is performed and interpreted by radiologists. These variations may affect the quality or interpretation of ultrasound results. It is helpful to be aware of these limitations. The following checklist can help increase the overall quality and consistency of kidney bladder ultrasound examination (**Box 1**).[60]

FURTHER IMAGING

There are two main alternative strategies for additional renal imaging after childhood UTI, either to begin with assessing for bladder dysfunction and vesicoureteral reflux (VUR), the bottom-up strategy, or to begin with the kidneys followed by the bladder and VUR assessment if there are signs of kidney involvement, the top-down approach.[61,62] The aim of the bottom-up strategy is to identify children with VUR and to manage them either with antibiotic prophylaxis until the reflux is resolved or by surgical intervention if indicated. Voiding cystourethrography (VCUG) is the gold standard for grading of VUR and to visualize posterior urethral valves in boys. One important drawback with VCUG is the need for catheterization, which is stressful for both child and parent.[63,64] It also involves radiation, and there is a small but not negligible risk of UTI caused by the catheterization during the procedure. Contrast-enhanced ultrasound and direct or indirect radionuclide techniques have been proposed as alternative ways to detect VUR, but these are less detailed in the grading of VUR. Moreover, the techniques require catheterization of the bladder and offer little benefit for the patient compared with VCUG, except for the absence of radiation in contrast-enhanced ultrasound.

The top-down model has its focus on the kidneys and the preservation of kidney function. The approach relies on the fact that VUR of any significance is associated with kidney involvement at the time of a febrile UTI.[65,66] Nuclear scintigraphy with ^{99m}Tc-dimercaptosuccinic acid (DMSA) can identify kidney involvement in the acute phase of the infection. However, to capture all acute parenchymal involvement the scintigraphy has to be done shortly after the start of treatment.[67] As soon as successful treatment is initiated, the healing process begins, and defects caused by infection start to resolve. Restricting VUR assessment by VCUG to children with manifest kidney involvement by DMSA scintigraphy or to those with dilatation of the upper urinary tract on ultrasound will reduce the number of VCUG substantially.[17,68]

URINARY TRACT INFECTION GUIDELINES

There is an ongoing effort to reduce the number of children being subjected to unnecessary, stressful, and potentially harmful investigations. Most current guidelines have

---

Box 1
Checklist for ultrasound evaluation after UTI in children

Checklist for ultrasound evaluation after UTI in children:
- Kidneys:
  - Size related to age or body size,
  - Contour
  - Echogenicity,
  - Corticomedullary differentiation
- Urinary tract:
  - Dilatation and dimensions of
    - Calyces
    - Pelvis
    - Ureters
  - Signs of duplication
- Bladder:
  - Size
  - Wall thickness
  - Diverticulae
  - Trabecules
  - Ureteroceles

---

been revised, to help identify children with kidney or urinary tract anomalies and those at a high risk of kidney damage. The risk factors for such patients are based on the presence of fever, infections with non-*E. coli* bacteria, and abnormalities on ultrasound examination, particularly dilatation of the urinary tract. Some guidelines also include inflammatory markers such as C-reactive protein (CRP), procalcitonin (PCT), and the white-blood-cell count. Recurrent UTI, the severity of clinical presentation, and a very young age, especially the first few months of life also prompt further investigations in most guidelines. The main features of selected guidelines from different parts of the world are summarized in **Table 1**.[5,8,14–18,69–72]

BLADDER AND BOWEL DYSFUNCTION

The importance of functional bladder irregularities for UTI recurrences, especially incomplete or infrequent emptying, and its association with bowel elimination dysfunction is now widely appreciated. Children with functional disorders of the bowel and/or bladder, including bladder instability, constipation, and infrequent voiding, have an increased UTI frequency.[73] Constipation should be assessed and treated in children of all ages. Assessment of incomplete bladder emptying should be done in children suspected of having bladder–bowel dysfunction. This may include completion of a validated questionnaire, voiding diary, and uroflowmetry. . Based on this evaluation the family can receive proper and individualized recommendations on bladder and bowel habits, with emphasis on regular, timely, and complete bladder and bowel emptying. Additional urotherapeutic measures, such as bio feedback, is recommended in selected patients.

The assessment of bladder function can also be done in children before they are toilet trained,[74] and severe cases of incomplete emptying or obstructive bladder outflow can be treated with catheterization or diversion of urine flow. In most cases, however, we wait for the child to achieve bladder control before we can do a complete evaluation of micturition and bladder emptying. This is also required for a successful noninvasive intervention.[75]

RISK FACTORS FOR URINARY TRACT INFECTION AND KIDNEY DAMAGE

It is important to identify children at risk of recurrent UTI and kidney damage. High-grade VUR is associated with an increased risk of kidney scarring[56,76] as are urinary tract obstruction and bladder and bowel dysfunction.[77,78] We and some other centers consider increased inflammatory markers such as and CRP >70 mg/L or PCT >0.5–1 mg/L as indicative of kidney involvement with a potential for kidney damage.[68,79]

Treatment delay increases the risk for acute kidney damage and probably permanent scarring. However, different studies show conflicting results, and it has been hard to establish a specific timeframe to minimize this risk.[80–82] In our practice we aim to diagnose a UTI and initiate empiric antibiotic treatment within 24 h of the onset of symptoms.

Non-*E. coli* UTI is a risk factor for kidney damage. It is more often seen in association with anomalies of the kidneys and urinary tract, especially in children with urinary tract obstruction, or with insufficient bladder emptying and significant residual urine.

The innate immune system plays an important role in defense against UTI and its function is altered by polymorphisms within the system.[83,84] Toll-like receptor-4 (TLR-4), which participates in the recruitment of inflammatory cells from the bloodstream to the bladder, is activated by binding to bacterial lipopolysaccharides. In a child with defective TLR-4, the defense reaction will be weak or absent and the infection may cause ABU, rather than a symptomatic UTI.[85] Other polymorphisms have been shown to increase the risk of symptomatic UTI. Mutations in the IL8-receptor CRCX7 and the INF3-receptor cause an increased inflammatory response to bacteriuria and a stronger inflammatory reaction in the kidneys with subsequent kidney scarring.[86]

Many urine proteins and peptides have been studied for their role in the clearance of bacteriuria and defense against UTI and these include uromodulin and antimicrobial peptides.[87,88] Of these, cathelicidin is found to have an antibacterial effect and its production is dependent on serum vitamin D level.[89,90] This could be the reason why low vitamin D levels have been associated with an increased risk of UTI.

LONG-TERM OUTCOME OF URINARY TRACT INFECTION

The risk of permanent kidney damage after febrile UTI during childhood has been estimated to be approximately 15%.[91] The long-term consequences of such damage have been debated for many years and include impaired kidney function, hypertension, and pregnancy-related complications. Several early studies indicated that the risk of these sequelae was high and in fact a major cause of chronic kidney disease. However, these studies were not population-based and described the outcome of selected patients. For instance, Jacobson and colleagues[92] described 30 adult patients with non-obstructive UTI with scarring and of whom 7 had hypertension and 3 had end-stage kidney failure. Smellie and colleagues[93] reported that among 226 patients with non-obstructive UTI and VUR, 15 were hypertensive, two had undergone kidney transplantation and one had died from a kidney-associated cause.

Population-based, long-term data are available from Sweden and Finland.[94–100] In the study by Wennerström and colleagues[94] 1221 children were followed for 16–26 years after their first symptomatic UTI in childhood. Glomerular filtration rate (GFR) was measured with ^{51}Cr-edetic acid clearance. Children with unilateral scarring had an unchanged mean GFR of 101 mL/min/1.73 m^2 at a mean age of 24.5 years as compared with 104 mL/min/1.73 m^2 at their mean age of 14 years. For seven children with bilateral scarring, GFR did not change significantly although it was significantly lower than the GFR of those with unilateral scarring (84 mL/min/1.73 m^2 vs 101 mL/min/1.73 m^2 at follow-up ($p = 0.007$)). 24-h ambulatory blood pressure measurements

(ABPM) did not reveal any difference between individuals with kidney scarring and a matched control group without scarring.[95]

In another population-based cohort from Göteborg, Sweden, Martinell and colleagues and later Gebäck and colleagues performed two long-term follow-ups of 86 women who were diagnosed with recurrent UTIs or kidney scarring during childhood.[96–99] The first follow-up was performed at a median age of 27 years and the second follow-up at 41 years. GFR was unchanged for women without scarring or with unilateral scarring between the two follow-ups.[97] During the same period, the GFR in those with bilateral scarring GFR dropped significantly from a median of 96 mL/min/1.73 m^2 to 81 mL/min/1.73 m^2 ($p = 0.01$). Using 24-h ABPM during the second follow-up, hypertension was diagnosed in 38% of women with kidney scarring and in 14% of those without ($p = 0.04$). Mean daytime and nighttime systolic BP was significantly higher.[98] Severity of hypertension correlated with the extent of kidney damage on DMSA scintigraphy. Pregnancy-related hypertension was diagnosed in 10 of 151 pregnancies, all in women with kidney scarring.[99] Women with kidney damage had significantly higher systolic blood pressure compared with women without kidney damage ($p = 0.005$). Other complications, including preeclampsia, were uncommon.

Hannula and colleagues[100] reported a follow-up study 6 to 17 years after UTI in a Finnish cohort of 1185 children. New kidney damage was uncommon except in those with high-grade VUR where it occurred in 20% of the cases. All individuals, 6 to 25 years of age at follow-up, had normal cystatin C-estimated GFR, were normotensive, and without proteinuria.

These findings from Sweden and Finland suggest that overall the risk of progressive kidney disease and hypertension is very low in patients with UTI in childhood. For those with kidney scarring, especially when bilateral, it may take 30 to 40 years or even more before the long-term consequences become manifest. For such patients monitoring of renal function and blood pressure, preferably with 24-h ABPM if available, are recommended. When considering these favorable results one must remember that these studies were performed in a well-controlled UTI population with early diagnosis of UTI, follow-up monitoring, and treatment of recurrent infections.

PERSPECTIVES FOR THE FUTURE

- Introduction of new biomarkers such as NGAL and IL8 may allow rapid and safe diagnosis of UTI from urine specimens, reducing the need for routine catheterization or SPA for an uncontaminated urine specimen in infants.
- Alternative diagnostic tools to replace urine culture are emerging where PCR tests and new generation sequencing of urine bacterial genome can provide faster results, not only identifying the causative agent but also its resistance to antibiotics.
- The growing insight into the innate immune system, its role in the defense against UTI, and the evolvement of kidney scarring, will hopefully give us new child-friendly alternative ways to identify children at risk of recurrent UTI and kidney scarring.
- More studies are needed on the commensal microbioma of the intestine and the urinary tract, how these are affected by antibiotic treatment, and their role in the natural defense against UTI and kidney damage.

CLINICS CARE POINTS

- Urinary tract infection (UTI) can be the initial manifestation of congenital anomalies of the kidney and urinary tract

- Infants with fever of unknown origin should be screened for a UTI
- Send urine for culture before starting antibiotic treatment when UTI is suspected
- Do not use bag or nappy pad urine for culture
- One of five infants with symptomatic UTI has urine bacterial counts less than 100,000 cfu/mL, regardless of sampling technique
- Non-*Escherichia coli* UTI should raise the suspicion of urinary tract anomalies
- Oral antibiotics are safe and effective for treating febrile UTI in children above 2 to 3 months of age
- Avoid antibiotic treatment in children with asymptomatic bacteriuria

DISCLOSURE

The authors have nothing to disclose.

REFERENCES

1. Hellstrom A, Hanson E, Hansson S, et al. Association between urinary symptoms at 7 years old and previous urinary tract infection. Arch Dis Child 1991; 66(2):232–4.
2. Shaikh N, Morone NE, Bost JE, et al. Prevalence of urinary tract infection in childhood: a meta-analysis. Pediatr Infect Dis J 2008;27(4):302–8.
3. Jakobsson B, Esbjorner E, Hansson S. Minimum incidence and diagnostic rate of first urinary tract infection. Pediatrics 1999;104(2 Pt 1):222–6.
4. Gomez B, Hernandez-Bou S, Garcia-Garcia JJ, et al. Bacteraemia Study Working Group from the Infectious Diseases Working Group SSoPE. Bacteremia in previously healthy children in emergency departments: clinical and microbiological characteristics and outcome. Eur J Clin Microbiol Infect Dis 2015; 34(3):453–60.
5. Roberts KB. Urinary tract infection: clinical practice guideline for the diagnosis and management of the initial UTI in febrile infants and children 2 to 24 months. Pediatrics 2011;128(3):595–610.
6. Hay AD, Birnie K, Busby J, et al. The Diagnosis of Urinary Tract infection in Young children (DUTY): a diagnostic prospective observational study to derive and validate a clinical algorithm for the diagnosis of urinary tract infection in children presenting to primary care with an acute illness. Health Technol Assess 2016;20(51):1–294.
7. Boon HA, Verbakel JY, De Burghgraeve T, et al. Clinical prediction rules for childhood UTIs: a cross-sectional study in ambulatory care. BJGP Open 2022. https://doi.org/10.3399/BJGPO.2021.0171.
8. Subcommittee On Urinary Tract I. Reaffirmation of AAP clinical practice guideline: the diagnosis and management of the initial urinary tract infection in febrile infants and young children 2-24 months of age. Pediatrics 2016;138(6): e20163026.
9. Diviney J, Jaswon MS. Urine collection methods and dipstick testing in non-toilet-trained children. Pediatr Nephrol 2021;36(7):1697–708.
10. Shortliffe LMD. The beginning of the end: the dilemma of obtaining a reliable urinary specimen in children under 2 years old. J Urol 2021;206(6):1359–60.

11. Pollack CV Jr, Pollack ES, Andrew ME. Suprapubic bladder aspiration versus urethral catheterization in ill infants: success, efficiency and complication rates. Ann Emerg Med 1994;23(2):225–30.

12. Kozer E, Rosenbloom E, Goldman D, et al. Pain in infants who are younger than 2 months during suprapubic aspiration and transurethral bladder catheterization: a randomized, controlled study. Pediatrics 2006;118(1):e51–6.

13. Mahdipour S, Saadat SNS, Badeli H, et al. Strengthening the success rate of suprapubic aspiration in infants by integrating point-of-care ultrasonography guidance: a parallel-randomized clinical trial. PLoS One 2021;16(7):e0254703.

14. National Institue for Health and Care Excellence (NICE). Urinary tract infection in under 16s: diagnosis and management: NICE clinical guidelines, 2018. PMID: 31971701.

15. Pineiro Perez R, Cilleruelo Ortega MJ, Ares Alvarez J, et al. [Recommendations on the diagnosis and treatment of urinary tract infection]. An Pediatr (Barc) 2019;90(6):400 e401–9.

16. Ammenti A, Alberici I, Brugnara M, et al. Updated Italian recommendations for the diagnosis, treatment and follow-up of the first febrile urinary tract infection in young children. Acta Paediatr 2020;109(2):236–47.

17. Brandstrom P, Linden M. How Swedish guidelines on urinary tract infections in children compare to Canadian, American and European guidelines. Acta Paediatr 2021;110(6):1759–71.

18. Buettcher M, Trueck J, Niederer-Loher A, et al. Swiss consensus recommendations on urinary tract infections in children. Eur J Pediatr 2021;180(3):663–74.

19. Labrosse M, Levy A, Autmizguine J, et al. Evaluation of a new strategy for clean-catch urine in infants. Pediatrics 2016;138(3):e20160573.

20. Turner GM, Coulthard MG. Fever can cause pyuria in children. BMJ 1995; 311(7010):924.

21. Swerkersson S, Jodal U, Ahren C, et al. Urinary tract infection in infants: the significance of low bacterial count. Pediatr Nephrol 2016;31(2):239–45.

22. Shaikh N, Liu H, Kurs-Lasky M, et al. Biomarkers for febrile urinary tract infection in children. Pediatr Nephrol 2022;37(1):171–7.

23. Coulthard MG. Using urine nitrite sticks to test for urinary tract infection in children aged < 2 years: a meta-analysis. Pediatr Nephrol 2019;34(7):1283–8.

24. Valdimarsson S, Jodal U, Barregard L, et al. Urine neutrophil gelatinase-associated lipocalin and other biomarkers in infants with urinary tract infection and in febrile controls. Pediatr Nephrol 2017;32(11):2079–87.

25. Kass EH. Asymptomatic infections of the urinary tract. Trans Assoc Am Physicians 1956;69:56–64.

26. Hansson S, Brandstrom P, Jodal U, et al. Low bacterial counts in infants with urinary tract infection. J Pediatr 1998;132(1):180–2.

27. Hill E, Hsieh M, Prokesch B. New direct-to-consumer urinary tract infection tests: are we ready? J Urol 2022;207(1):4–6.

28. Strohmeier Y, Hodson EM, Willis NS, et al. Antibiotics for acute pyelonephritis in children. Cochrane Database Syst Rev 2014;7:CD003772.

29. Hoberman A, Wald ER, Hickey RW, et al. Oral versus initial intravenous therapy for urinary tract infections in young febrile children. Pediatrics 1999;104(1 Pt 1): 79–86.

30. Montini G, Toffolo A, Zucchetta P, et al. Antibiotic treatment for pyelonephritis in children: multicentre randomised controlled non-inferiority trial. BMJ 2007; 335(7616):386.

31. Neuhaus TJ, Berger C, Buechner K, et al. Randomised trial of oral versus sequential intravenous/oral cephalosporins in children with pyelonephritis. Eur J Pediatr 2008;167(9):1037–47.

32. Mahony M, McMullan B, Brown J, et al. Multidrug-resistant organisms in urinary tract infections in children. Pediatr Nephrol 2020;35(9):1563–73.

33. Lukac PJ, Bonomo RA, Logan LK. Extended-spectrum beta-lactamase-producing Enterobacteriaceae in children: old foe, emerging threat. Clin Infect Dis 2015;60(9):1389–97.

34. Mattoo TK, Asmar BI. Annotations on emerging concerns about antibiotic-resistant urinary tract infection. Pediatrics 2020;145(2):e20193512.

35. Alberici I, Bayazit AK, Drozdz D, et al. Pathogens causing urinary tract infections in infants: a European overview by the ESCAPE study group. Eur J Pediatr 2015; 174(6):783–90.

36. Lashkar MO, Nahata MC. Antimicrobial pharmacotherapy management of urinary tract infections in pediatric patients. J Pharm Technol 2018;34(2):62–81.

37. Tran D, Muchant DG, Aronoff SC. Short-course versus conventional length antimicrobial therapy for uncomplicated lower urinary tract infections in children: a meta-analysis of 1279 patients. J Pediatr 2001;139(1):93–9.

38. Michael M, Hodson EM, Craig JC, et al. Short versus standard duration oral antibiotic therapy for acute urinary tract infection in children. Cochrane Database Syst Rev 2003;1:CD003966.

39. Shaikh N, Shope TR, Hoberman A, et al. Corticosteroids to prevent kidney scarring in children with a febrile urinary tract infection: a randomized trial. Pediatr Nephrol 2020;35(11):2113–20.

40. Rius-Gordillo N, Ferre N, Gonzalez JD, et al. Dexamethasone to prevent kidney scarring in acute pyelonephritis: a randomized clinical trial. Pediatr Nephrol 2022. https://doi.org/10.1007/s00467-021-05398-w. Epub 2022/01/19.

41. Wettergren B, Jodal U. Spontaneous clearance of asymptomatic bacteriuria in infants. Acta Paediatr Scand 1990;79(3):300–4.

42. Kunin CM. The natural history of recurrent bacteriuria in schoolgirls. N Engl J Med 1970;282(26):1443–8.

43. Lindberg U, Claesson I, Hanson LA, et al. Asymptomatic bacteriuria in schoolgirls. VIII. Clinical course during a 3-year follow-up. J Pediatr 1978;92(2):194–9.

44. The Cardiff-Oxford Bacteriuria Study Groups. Sequelae of covert bacteriuria in schoolgirls. A four-year follow-up study. Lancet 1978;1(8070):889–93.

45. Hansson S, Jodal U, Noren L, et al. Untreated bacteriuria in asymptomatic girls with renal scarring. Pediatrics 1989;84(6):964–8.

46. Montini G, Rigon L, Zucchetta P, et al. Prophylaxis after first febrile urinary tract infection in children? A multicenter, randomized, controlled, noninferiority trial. Pediatrics 2008;122(5):1064–71.

47. Craig JC, Simpson JM, Williams GJ, et al. Antibiotic prophylaxis and recurrent urinary tract infection in children. N Engl J Med 2009;361(18):1748–59.

48. Trial Investigators Rivur, Hoberman A, Greenfield SP, et al. Antimicrobial prophylaxis for children with vesicoureteral reflux. N Engl J Med 2014;370(25):2367–76.

49. Brandstrom P, Esbjorner E, Herthelius M, et al. The swedish reflux trial in children: III. urinary tract infection pattern. J Urol 2010;184(1):286–91.

50. Brandstrom P, Neveus T, Sixt R, et al. The swedish reflux trial in children: IV. Renal damage. J Urol 2010;184(1):292–7.

51. Selekman RE, Shapiro DJ, Boscardin J, et al. Uropathogen resistance and antibiotic prophylaxis: a meta-analysis. Pediatrics 2018;142(1).

52. Copp HL, Nelson CP, Shortliffe LD, et al. Compliance with antibiotic prophylaxis in children with vesicoureteral reflux: results from a national pharmacy claims database. J Urol 2010;183(5):1994–9.

53. Brandstrom P, Hansson S. Long-term, low-dose prophylaxis against urinary tract infections in young children. Pediatr Nephrol 2015;30(3):425–32.

54. Yeung CK, Godley ML, Dhillon HK, et al. The characteristics of primary vesico-ureteric reflux in male and female infants with pre-natal hydronephrosis. Br J Urol 1997;80(2):319–27.

55. Wennerstrom M, Hansson S, Jodal U, et al. Primary and acquired renal scarring in boys and girls with urinary tract infection. J Pediatr 2000;136(1):30–4.

56. Swerkersson S, Jodal U, Sixt R, et al. Relationship among vesicoureteral reflux, urinary tract infection and renal damage in children. J Urol 2007;178(2):647–51 [discussion: 650-651].

57. Shaikh N, Haralam MA, Kurs-Lasky M, et al. Association of renal scarring with number of febrile urinary tract infections in children. JAMA Pediatr 2019; 173(10):949–52.

58. Stokland E, Hellstrom M, Hansson S, et al. Reliability of ultrasonography in iden-tification of reflux nephropathy in children. BMJ 1994;309(6949):235–9.

59. Expert Panel on Pediatric I, Karmazyn BK, Alazraki AL, et al. ACR appropriate-ness criteria((R)) urinary tract infection-child. J Am Coll Radiol 2017;14(5S): S362–71.

60. Riccabona M, Avni FE, Blickman JG, et al. Imaging recommendations in paedi-atric uroradiology: minutes of the ESPR workgroup session on urinary tract infection, fetal hydronephrosis, urinary tract ultrasonography and voiding cys-tourethrography, Barcelona, Spain, June 2007. Pediatr Radiol 2008;38(2): 138–45.

61. Hansson S, Dhamey M, Sigstrom O, et al. Dimercapto-succinic acid scintig-raphy instead of voiding cystourethrography for infants with urinary tract infec-tion. J Urol 2004;172(3):1071–3 [discussion: 1073-1074].

62. Wang HS, Cahill D, Panagides J, et al. Top-down versus bottom-up approach in children presenting with urinary tract infection: comparative effectiveness anal-ysis using RIVUR and CUTIE data. J Urol 2021;206(5):1284–90.

63. Phillips D, Watson AR, Collier J. Distress and radiological investigations of the urinary tract in children. Eur J Pediatr 1996;155(8):684–7.

64. Stokland E, Andreasson S, Jacobsson B, et al. Sedation with midazolam for voiding cystourethrography in children: a randomised double-blind study. Pe-diatr Radiol 2003;33(4):247–9.

65. Preda I, Jodal U, Sixt R, et al. Normal dimercaptosuccinic acid scintigraphy makes voiding cystourethrography unnecessary after urinary tract infection. J Pediatr 2007;151(6):581–4, 584 e581.

66. Tullus K, Shaikh N. Urinary tract infections in children. Lancet 2020;395(10237): 1659–68.

67. Jakobsson B, Berg U, Svensson L. Renal scarring after acute pyelonephritis. Arch Dis Child 1994;70(2):111–5.

68. Preda I, Jodal U, Sixt R, et al. Imaging strategy for infants with urinary tract infec-tion: a new algorithm. J Urol 2011;185(3):1046–52.

69. Robinson JL, Finlay JC, Lang ME, et al. Urinary tract infections in infants and children: Diagnosis and management. Paediatr Child Health 2014;19(6): 315–25.

70. Stein R, Dogan HS, Hoebeke P, et al. Urinary tract infections in children: EAU/ESPU guidelines. Eur Urol 2015;67(3):546–58.

71. t Hoen LA, Bogaert G, Radmayr C, et al. Update of the EAU/ESPU guidelines on urinary tract infections in children. J Pediatr Urol 2021;17(2):200–7.
72. Yang SS, Tsai JD, Kanematsu A, et al. Asian guidelines for urinary tract infection in children. J Infect Chemother 2021;27(11):1543–54.
73. Koff SA, Wagner TT, Jayanthi VR. The relationship among dysfunctional elimination syndromes, primary vesicoureteral reflux and urinary tract infections in children. J Urol 1998;160(3 Pt 2):1019–22.
74. Holmdahl G, Hanson E, Hanson M, et al. Four-hour voiding observation in healthy infants. J Urol 1996;156(5):1809–12.
75. Clothier JC, Wright AJ. Dysfunctional voiding: the importance of non-invasive urodynamics in diagnosis and treatment. Pediatr Nephrol 2018;33(3):381–94.
76. Swerkersson S, Jodal U, Sixt R, et al. Urinary tract infection in small children: the evolution of renal damage over time. Pediatr Nephrol 2017;32(10):1907–13.
77. Spencer JR, Schaeffer AJ. Pediatric urinary tract infections. Urol Clin North Am 1986;13(4):661–72.
78. Keren R, Shaikh N, Pohl H, et al. Risk factors for recurrent urinary tract infection and renal scarring. Pediatrics 2015;136(1):e13–21.
79. Leroy S, Fernandez-Lopez A, Nikfar R, et al. Association of procalcitonin with acute pyelonephritis and renal scars in pediatric UTI. Pediatrics 2013;131(5):870–9.
80. Hewitt IK, Zucchetta P, Rigon L, et al. Early treatment of acute pyelonephritis in children fails to reduce renal scarring: data from the Italian Renal Infection Study Trials. Pediatrics 2008;122(3):486–90.
81. Shaikh N, Mattoo TK, Keren R, et al. Early antibiotic treatment for pediatric febrile urinary tract infection and renal scarring. JAMA Pediatr 2016;170(9):848–54.
82. Karavanaki KA, Soldatou A, Koufadaki AM, et al. Delayed treatment of the first febrile urinary tract infection in early childhood increased the risk of renal scarring. Acta Paediatr 2017;106(1):149–54.
83. Ragnarsdottir B, Lutay N, Gronberg-Hernandez J, et al. Genetics of innate immunity and UTI susceptibility. Nat Rev Urol 2011;8(8):449–68.
84. Ching C, Schwartz L, Spencer JD, et al. Innate immunity and urinary tract infection. Pediatr Nephrol 2020;35(7):1183–92.
85. Ragnarsdottir B, Svanborg C. Susceptibility to acute pyelonephritis or asymptomatic bacteriuria: host-pathogen interaction in urinary tract infections. Pediatr Nephrol 2012;27(11):2017–29.
86. Ragnarsdottir B, Fischer H, Godaly G, et al. TLR- and CXCR1-dependent innate immunity: insights into the genetics of urinary tract infections. Eur J Clin Invest 2008;38(Suppl 2):12–20.
87. Chromek M, Brauner A. Antimicrobial mechanisms of the urinary tract. J Mol Med (Berl) 2008;86(1):37–47.
88. Schwaderer AL, Wang H, Kim S, et al. Polymorphisms in alpha-Defensin-Encoding DEFA1A3 Associate with Urinary Tract Infection Risk in Children with Vesicoureteral Reflux. J Am Soc Nephrol 2016;27(10):3175–86.
89. Chromek M, Slamova Z, Bergman P, et al. The antimicrobial peptide cathelicidin protects the urinary tract against invasive bacterial infection. Nat Med 2006;12(6):636–41.
90. Chung C, Silwal P, Kim I, et al. Vitamin D-cathelicidin axis: at the crossroads between protective immunity and pathological inflammation during infection. Immune Netw 2020;20(2):e12.

91. Shaikh N, Ewing AL, Bhatnagar S, et al. Risk of renal scarring in children with a first urinary tract infection: a systematic review. Pediatrics 2010;126(6):1084–91.

92. Jacobson SH, Eklof O, Eriksson CG, et al. Development of hypertension and uraemia after pyelonephritis in childhood: 27 year follow up. BMJ 1989; 299(6701):703–6.

93. Smellie JM, Prescod NP, Shaw PJ, et al. Childhood reflux and urinary infection: a follow-up of 10-41 years in 226 adults. Pediatr Nephrol 1998;12(9):727–36.

94. Wennerstrom M, Hansson S, Hedner T, et al. Ambulatory blood pressure 16-26 years after the first urinary tract infection in childhood. J Hypertens 2000;18(4): 485–91.

95. Wennerstrom M, Hansson S, Jodal U, et al. Renal function 16 to 26 years after the first urinary tract infection in childhood. Arch Pediatr Adolesc Med 2000; 154(4):339–45.

96. Martinell J, Lidin-Janson G, Jagenburg R, et al. Girls prone to urinary infections followed into adulthood. Indices of renal disease. Pediatr Nephrol 1996;10(2): 139–42.

97. Geback C, Hansson S, Martinell J, et al. Renal function in adult women with urinary tract infection in childhood. Pediatr Nephrol 2015;30(9):1493–9.

98. Geback C, Hansson S, Himmelmann A, et al. Twenty-four-hour ambulatory blood pressure in adult women with urinary tract infection in childhood. J Hypertens 2014;32(8):1658–64 [discussion: 1664].

99. Geback C, Hansson S, Martinell J, et al. Obstetrical outcome in women with urinary tract infections in childhood. Acta Obstet Gynecol Scand 2016;95(4): 452–7.

100. Hannula A, Perhomaa M, Venhola M, et al. Long-term follow-up of patients after childhood urinary tract infection. Arch Pediatr Adolesc Med 2012;166(12): 1117–22.

Primary Vesicoureteral Reflux and Renal Scarring

Tej K. Mattoo, MD, DCH, FRCP (UK), FAAP[a],*, Dunya Mohammad, MD, FAAP[b]

KEYWORDS

- Vesicoureteral reflux (VUR) • Urinary tract infection (UTI) • CAKUT
- Bladder-bowel dysfunction (BBD) • Renal scarring • Reflux nephropathy
- Antimicrobial prophylaxis • VCUG

KEY POINTS

- VUR in most cases is diagnosed after a febrile UTI.
- Primary VUR, particularly low-grade, generally improves with time.
- High-grade VUR is a risk factor for pyelonephritis-associated renal scarring.
- Renal scarring diagnosed after febrile UTI may be congenital in origin.
- Renal scarring due to pyelonephritis can occur at all ages.

INTRODUCTION

Vesicoureteral reflux (VUR) may be primary or secondary. Primary VUR is the most common congenital anomaly of urinary tract that is diagnosed mostly after urinary tract infection (UTI) or during evaluation of antenatally diagnosed hydronephrosis or congenital anomalies of the kidney and urinary tract (CAKUT). In contrast, secondary VUR is less common in children and develops either because of a surgical procedure, such as a renal transplant, decompression of a ureterocele, or correction of vesicoureteral junction obstruction, or due to increased bladder pressure. Increased bladder pressure may occur due to anatomic obstruction caused by posterior urethral valves or urethral or meatal stenosis or a functional bladder abnormality as seen with neurogenic bladder, nonneurogenic neurogenic bladder (Hinman syndrome), and Ochoa syndrome. Transient VUR may occur in patients with bladder bowel dysfunction (BBD) or bladder infection. This article is exclusively about primary VUR and renal scarring in children.

The authors have nothing to disclose.
[a] Department of Pediatrics, Wayne State University School of Medicine, 400 Mack Avenue, Suite 1 East, Detroit, MI 48201, USA; [b] Pediatric Nephrology, University of South Alabama, 1601 Center Street, Suite 1271, Mobile, AL 36604, USA
* Corresponding author. 400 Mack Ave, Suite 1 East, Detroit, MI 48201
E-mail address: tmattoo@med.wayne.edu

INCIDENCE AND PREVALENCE

The reported prevalence of VUR varies from 1.3% of healthy children to 8% to 50% of children evaluated after UTI.[1] In newborns and infants, the incidence of VUR diagnosed after UTI is 36% to 49%.[1] Children with VUR detected after UTI are predominantly females.[2,3] VUR diagnosed during follow-up of antenatally diagnosed hydronephrosis is seen more often in males.[4,5] Of the 607 patients in the Randomized Intervention in Children with VUR (RIVUR) study 81% were white.[6]

DIAGNOSIS, GRADING, AND NATURAL HISTORY

The gold standard for diagnosing VUR is a voiding cystourethrogram (VCUG) based on which it is classified into 5 grades (**Fig. 1**). The RIVUR study revealed that there is a considerable interobserver variability in the VUR grading by a VCUG. Radiologists varied by 1 grade in about a fifth of patients and rarely by 2 or more grades.[7] Radionuclide VCUG can also be used to diagnose and follow children with VUR. However, using this modality, VUR can only be graded into mild, moderate, and severe because the resolution is not as good as with a contrast VCUG.

Primary VUR generally improves with time, and this is attributed to the lengthening of submucosal segment of the ureter with overall growth of the body. Factors associated with resolution of VUR include low grade at diagnosis, nonwhite race, and the absence of BBD.[8] According to a study that included 735 children and a follow-up period of 6 to 411 months, the median time for resolution of primary VUR was 38 months for grade I/II, 98 months for grade III, and 156 months for grade IV/V VUR.[9] The rate of resolution of VUR is higher in younger children,[10] undilated when compared with dilated[11] and unilateral when compared with bilateral VUR.

Bladder dysfunction in association with VUR has been reported in children as well as in adults. About 25% to 68% of children with VUR have bladder dysfunction, the 2 most common being detrusor overactivity and sphincter overactivity, and both are associated with a significant increase in bladder pressure.[12–14] In a study in 120 adults (age 33–50 years) with VUR diagnosed in childhood, the urine flow curve was abnormal in 40% cases; nearly half of the 44 operated patients had either an

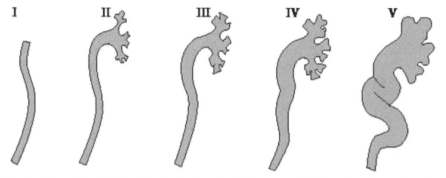

Fig. 1. International Reflux Study Grading for Vesicoureteral Reflux. Grade I: reflux into nondilated ureter. Grade II: reflux into the renal pelvis and calyces without dilatation. Grade III: mild/moderate dilatation of ureter and pelvicalyceal system. Grade IV: dilation of the renal pelvis and calyces with moderate ureteral tortuosity, blunting of fornices. Grade V: gross dilatation of the ureter, pelvis, and calyces; ureteral tortuosity; loss of papillary impressions.

interrupted or a weak flow. A high percentage of these patients also suffered from urgency and stress incontinence and annual UTIs.[15]

CLINICAL PRESENTATION

Primary VUR is often diagnosed in 1 of the 3 ways: following UTI, during follow-up for CAKUT/antenatal hydronephrosis, or while screening a sibling of a patient with VUR.

Urinary Tract Infection

UTI, particularly in younger children, is the most common presentation that leads to the diagnosis of VUR. In a large cohort of children with UTI, VUR was diagnosed in 46% of infants and 9% of preschool children.[16] Most children with VUR diagnosed after a UTI are girls; however, when considering infants younger than 6 months, no gender difference is noted.[17]

Congenital Anomalies of the Kidney and Urinary Tract/Antenatal Hydronephrosis

VUR is the most common abnormality observed in children with CAKUT.[1] About 10% to 30% of infants diagnosed with prenatal hydronephrosis have VUR[18]; the incidence is higher in boys.[4] VUR associated with antenatal hydronephrosis has a high rate of spontaneous resolution (59% by age 4 years) even in those with grades IV to V reflux.[19]

Sibling Reflux

VUR is present in about 66% of children of parents with VUR[20] and 32% of siblings of a child diagnosed with VUR.[21] A review of the natural history of VUR in siblings revealed that 52% had resolution of reflux after 18 months of follow-up, with yearly resolution rates of 28%.[22] A more "benign" course of sibling reflux diagnosed by screening[23] has led to the current approach of no routine screening for asymptomatic siblings of a diagnosed child with VUR.

RISK FACTORS FOR RENAL SCARRING

Renal scarring associated with VUR may be congenital in origin, which is also called *congenital reflux nephropathy* (RN). Renal scarring that results due to acute pyelonephritis is called acquired RN. Congenital RN is more common in boys, whereas the acquired RN is more common in girls.[24] Some other important differences between congenital and acquired RN are shown in **Table 1**.[25] In some recent randomized studies, the number of cases reported with renal scarring in children with VUR correlated with patient sex. Studies with more males reported significantly more cases of renal scarring, which is more likely to be congenital than acquired RN.[26] The reported prevalence of renal scarring after febrile UTI is about 15%[27]; it ranges from 3% after the first UTI to 29% after more than 3 febrile UTIs.[28,29] Several risk factors, including genetic predisposition, are associated with pyelonephritis-associated acquired renal scarring.

Vesicoureteral Reflux

The odds ratio of renal scarring with acute pyelonephritis in the presence of VUR is 2.8 for patients and 3.7 for renal units compared with those without VUR.[30] A systematic review revealed that the children with VUR were significantly more likely to develop pyelonephritis (relative risk [RR], 1.5; 95% confidence interval [CI], 1.1–1.9) and renal scarring (RR, 2.6; 95% CI, 1.7–3.9) compared with children with no VUR. Children with VUR grades III or higher were more likely to develop scarring than children with

Table 1
Acquired versus congenital reflux nephropathy in children

	Acquired	Congenital
Time of occurrence	Postnatal	Prenatal
History of UTI before diagnosis	Common	Uncommon
Age distribution at diagnosis	All pediatric age groups	Mostly in younger children
Gender distribution	Predominately females	Predominately males
Grade of VUR at the time of diagnosis	Variable, depending on age	Mostly high grade
Renal histology	Chronic inflammatory changes	Features of renal dysplasia

Modified from Mattoo TK.[25]

lower grades of VUR (RR, 2.1; 95% CI, 1.4–3.2).[31] Another study estimated the presence of renal damage at 6.2% for grades I to III and 47.9% for grades IV and V VUR ($P < 0.0001$).[32] In the RIVUR study, which did not include patients with grade V VUR, the proportion of new scars in renal units with grade 4 VUR was significantly higher than in units with no VUR (odds ratio, 24.2; 95% CI, 6.4–91.2).[26]

Recurrent Urinary Tract Infection

Recurrent UTI is a well-known risk factor for renal scarring. In the RIVUR study, children with a second UTI had significantly more renal scars when compared with those with a single UTI.[26] A posthoc analysis of RIVUR and CUTIE (Careful Urinary Tract Infection Evaluation) studies revealed that the odds of renal scarring after a second febrile UTI was 11.8 times and after 3 or more febrile UTIs was 13.7 times greater than after a single febrile infection.[33]

Delay in Treatment

A multivariate analysis of 158 children with febrile UTI showed that a delay of greater than 48 hours in the initiation of antibiotic treatment was associated with an increased risk of acute lesions on renal scan.[34] RIVUR study revealed that the odds ratio of new renal scarring was 74% lower among children whose treatment started within 24 hours of onset of fever, compared with those whose treatment started after 72 hours of fever.[35]

Patient Age

Recent studies have shown that young age may not be a risk factor and that older children may be at a higher risk of acquired renal scarring.[26–28] In the past, young age may have appeared as a risk factor due to the inadvertent inclusion of patients with preexisting congenital scarring. Renal scarring occurs in adult kidneys as well, as is seen in adult transplanted kidneys.[36] Also, adult pig kidneys with VUR and UTI scar as quickly as those of piglets.[37]

COMPLICATIONS OF RENAL SCARRING

In most children, renal scarring may not be clinically significant.[38] Hypertension occurs in 10% to 30% of children and young adults[39,40] and 34% to 38% of adults with renal scarring.[41,42] In a follow-up period lasting 15 years in pediatric patients with renal scarring, about 13% at age 20 to 31 years were hypertensive.[43] In a study that included 159 healthy pediatric patients (median age of 11 years) referred for evaluation of hypertension, 33 (21%) were found to have renal scars by dimercaptosuccinic acid

(DMSA) renal scan.[44] The occurrence (and severity) of hypertension does not correlate with the degree of scarring.[45] Microalbuminuria has been reported in 51% of pediatric patients (mean age 9.8 + 4.2 years) with renal scarring.[46] Overt proteinuria, which has been reported in 21% of adult patients with RN,[41] is rare in pediatric patients. Other reported complications of renal scarring are shown in **Box 1**.

In the Chronic Kidney Disease in Children Study (CKiD) study, RN was the underlying cause of chronic kidney disease (CKD) in 87 (14.8%) of 586 children aged 1 to 16 years with an estimated glomerular filtration rate (eGFR) of 30 to 90 mL/min/$1.73 m^2$.[47] According to another study, the probability of CKD for patients with bilateral severe reflux (grades III–V VUR) was 15% by 10 years after VUR diagnosis. The 4 variables that were independently associated with CKD were age at diagnosis greater than 24 months, VUR grade V, and bilateral renal damage.[48]

The complications of renal scarring are more pronounced in adults. Adult males generally present with hypertension, proteinuria, and renal failure, whereas females present mostly with UTI and pregnancy-related complications[25,49] **(Table 2)**. In a study of 21 adults (mean age 23.9 years) with gross VUR diagnosed in infancy, proteinuria and renal insufficiency was diagnosed in 3 (23%) of the 13 patients with unilateral RN and 2 (50%) of the 4 patients with bilateral RN.[50] In another study of 127 adults (mean age 41 years) with VUR diagnosed during childhood, 44 (35%) had unilateral renal scarring, 30 (24%) had bilateral renal scarring, 30 (24%) had albuminuria, and 14 (11%) had hypertension. Of the 30 patients with bilateral renal scars, 25 (83%) had an abnormal GFR.[51] The difference in sex-based outcomes in adults has previously been attributed to a delayed diagnosis in males because of an insidious onset when compared with an earlier diagnosis in females prompted by more recurrent UTI or pregnancy-related complications.[52] However, another possibility could be that the males have mostly congenital RN when compared with females who mostly have acquired RN, and the long-term outcomes of the 2 may be different.[25]

Renal Imaging

Ultrasonography
Renal ultrasonography (US) is useful in diagnosing CAKUT and complications of acute pyelonephritis such as renal abscess or pyonephrosis. A normal renal US examination

---

Box 1
Reported complications of renal scarring[25,84–87]

- Hypertension
- Microalbuminuria/proteinuria
- FSGS
- Urinary concentration defects
- Hyperkalemia and acidosis
- Urinary calculi
- Growth impairment
- Complications during pregnancy
  - Hypertension, proteinuria, edema, deterioration in renal function, preterm delivery, preeclampsia, and fetal loss
- Progressive CKD, particularly when scarring is bilateral.

Abbreviations: CKD, chronic kidney disease; FSGS, focal segmental glomerulosclerosis.

Table 2
Reflux nephropathy in adults[25]

	Males	Females
History of urinary tract infections	Uncommon	Common
Plasma creatinine at the time of diagnosis	Usually higher	Usually normal
End-stage kidney failure	More common	Less common
Proteinuria	Frequent/severe	Infrequent/less severe
Hypertension	More common	Less common

does not rule out the presence of a VUR. In the RIVUR study, only 11% of patients had an abnormal US examination as defined by the presence of hydronephrosis or ureteral duplication.[6] US findings that suggest the presence of VUR include hydronephrosis, ureteral dilatation, and renal parenchymal changes. A recent study reported a significant correlation between increased kidney echogenicity on US at the time of febrile UTI and the presence of a high-grade (grades III–V) VUR.[53]

Renal US has very low sensitivity for diagnosing acute pyelonephritis. In one study, US abnormalities for pyelonephritis were reported in 20% to 69% of patients when compared with 40% to 92% by DMSA scintigraphy.[54] It is also not a sensitive method for diagnosing renal scars. In a study of 159 patients who underwent DMSA renal scan as well as renal US for the evaluation of hypertension of unknown cause, 140 (88%) had normal result of renal US examination. Of those with abnormal renal US examination result, 12 (63%) had abnormal and 7 (37%) had normal result of DMSA renal scans. The sensitivity and specificity of renal US, to diagnose renal scars, were 36% and 94%, respectively, and the positive and the negative predictive values were 63% and 85%, respectively.[44]

Voiding cystourethrogram
Not all children with first febrile UTI need a VCUG. VCUG should be done selectively in patients with abnormal result of US examination, recurrent UTI, UTI with an atypical pathogen, significant family history, or known renal scarring. The VCUG can be obtained soon after the infection is treated. Various procedural factors that may affect a VCUG result and interobserver variability in the grading of VUR must be kept in mind when making clinical decisions.[7] Nuclear cystography has been used to reduce the radiation exposure for children during follow-up of VUR. Nuclear cystography, while being more sensitive, does not permit specific grading of VUR and does not reveal anatomic defects such as ureterocele or diverticulum. However, it is useful to determine if VUR has resolved after surgical correction.

Technetium 99^m Dimercaptosuccinic acid renal scan
DMSA is currently the gold standard for diagnosing acute pyelonephritis and renal scarring. DMSA is not recommended in the standard management of acute pyelonephritis. A delay in performing the DMSA scan to 4 to 6 months postpyelonephritis allows the acute inflammatory reaction to subside, at which point any persistent cortical defects are assumed to represent permanent renal scarring.[55] A DMSA renal scan does not help differentiate between congenital and acquired RN because they look very similar, unless there is a baseline (prepyelonephritis) DMSA scan, which is not possible in routine clinical setting. The RIVUR study revealed a significant interobserver variability in the reporting of abnormal DMSA renal scans,[56] which should be

kept in mind when making clinical decisions. Technetium 99^{m}-glucoheptonate, which is less sensitive for the detection of renal scars, may be used if DMSA is not available.

MEDICAL MANAGEMENT

The 2 main treatment modalities that have been used for VUR are long-term antimicrobial prophylaxis and surgical correction. The third option that has come up recently is surveillance only, particularly in those with low-grade VUR.

Antimicrobial Prophylaxis

The RIVUR trial revealed that trimethoprim-sulfamethoxazole (TMP/SMZ) prophylaxis reduced the risk of UTI recurrence by 50%. Similar results were reported by another placebo-controlled double-blind (PRIVENT study) trial.[57] Combined results from the RIVUR and CUTIE studies revealed that toilet-trained children with VUR and BBD exhibit the greatest benefit from antimicrobial prophylaxis.[58] However, many other randomized studies have shown either no[59–63] or a female-restricted beneficial effect with prophylaxis.[64] Systematic reviews and meta-analyses have also reported mixed results, some concluding that prophylaxis is effective,[65,66] whereas others reporting it as ineffective for the prevention of UTI recurrence.[67,68] These variations in results have been attributed to significant differences in study designs, including patient inclusion and exclusion criteria.[69]

Antimicrobial prophylaxis should be used judiciously because of the potential side effects, drug resistance in particular. In cases with febrile UTI and VUR, the American Urological Association recommends continuous antimicrobial prophylaxis in children younger than 1 year and a selective approach in older children based on patient age, severity of VUR, recurrence of UTI, presence of BBD, and renal cortical anomalies.[70] The European Association of Urology/European Society of Pediatric Urology and the Swedish and the Italian Society of Pediatric Nephrology also recommend a more selective approach based on a combination of patient age, severity of VUR, and the presence of renal scarring.[71–73] Other factors that should be considered before initiating long-term antimicrobial prophylaxis include status of toilet training, anticipated compliance with medication, parental choice, and the medication expense.[74]

Secondary analysis of the RIVUR study revealed that patients who took TMP/SMZ less than 70% of the time were 2.5 times more likely to have a recurrent UTI and were at highest risk for renal scarring when compared with more adherent patients.[75] The RIVUR study also revealed that long-term prophylaxis with TMP/SMZ was not associated with an increased risk of skin and soft tissue infections, pharyngitis or sinopulmonary infections,[76] or excessive weight gain.[77] Another RIVUR study reported no abnormalities in blood chemistry, renal function, or complete blood cell count results in children receiving long-term TMP/SMZ prophylaxis for a duration of 2 years.[78]

Depending on the local antimicrobial sensitivity profile of *Escherischia coli,* the recommendations on antimicrobial selection for prophylaxis may vary from place to place (**Table 3**). The prophylactic dose of antimicrobials is one-fourth to one-half of the therapeutic dose for acute infection, and the commonly used antimicrobial agents used in the United States and their dosages are shown in **Table 4**. During the first 2 months of life, it is advisable to avoid TMP-SMZ because it may cause hyperbilirubinemia and neurotoxicity. In toilet-trained children, prophylactic medication is generally administered at bedtime, although this recommendation is not evidence-based. The duration of prophylaxis depends on multiple factors and may range from a few days until a VCUG can be obtained in cases with recently diagnosed UTI to a couple of years for children with known VUR managed conservatively.

Bladder Bowel Dysfunction

VUR may be associated with BBD, the symptoms of which include daytime wetness, urgency, frequency, infrequency, recurrent UTI, dysuria, abdominal pain, constipation, and/or fecal incontinence. In the RIVUR study, using the dysfunctional voiding scoring system,[79] BBD was identified in 56% of 126 toilet-trained children (younger than 6 years) with grade I to IV VUR.[6] BBD increases the risk of febrile UTI in children with VUR on antimicrobial prophylaxis (44% with BBD and 3% without BBD), and it delays VUR resolution (31% with BBD and 61% without BBD at 24 months).[30] BBD can also adversely affect the results of ureteric reimplantation.[80]

Management of BBD includes treatment of constipation by dietary measures, behavioral therapy, and laxatives. Timed, frequent, and complete voiding every 2 to 3 hours is a crucial part of management. Pelvic floor exercises, biofeedback, and/or anticholinergic medication or alpha-blockers may be required to improve bladder function. Conservative medical treatment coupled with computer game-assisted pelvic floor muscle retraining decreases the incidence of breakthrough UTI and facilitates VUR resolution. Continuous intermittent catheterization may be necessary in extreme cases, as seen in Hinman syndrome.

Hypertension and/or Proteinuria

Appropriate management of hypertension and/or proteinuria is important to slow down the progression of renal disease. Angiotensin-converting enzyme inhibitors (ACEIs) or angiotensin II receptor blockers are preferred because of their renoprotective effect. Studies have revealed that ACEIs, besides lowering the blood pressure, reduce proteinuria due to RN. In a study by Lama and colleagues,[81] 15.5% of children with VUR and RN had microalbuminuria. Treatment with an ACEI (captopril) for 2 years was associated with decreased microalbuminuria. Of note, GFR, serum creatinine

Table 3
Antimicrobial agents recommended for prophylaxis in some countries

Antimicrobial Agent	EAU/ESPU[71] 2015	NICE[88] 2018	Swiss[89] 2021	ISPN[90] 2011	Asian[91] 2021	Italian[92] 2019
Trimethoprim[a]	✔	✔	✔			
Trimethoprim_sulfamethoxazole[b]	✔		✔	✔	✔	
Nitrofurantoin[c]	✔	✔	✔	✔	✔	✔
Cephalexin		✔		✔	✔	
Amoxicillin		✔	✔			
Cefaclor	✔					
Cefixime	✔					
Ceftibuten[c]	✔					✔
Cefuroxime axetil	✔					
Cefadroxil				✔		
Amoxicillin-clavulanic acid[a]						✔

Abbreviations: EAU/ESPU, European Association of Urology/European Society of Pediatric Urology; NICE, National Institute of Health and Care Excellence, United Kingdom; ISPN, Indian Society of Pediatric Nephrology.
[a] Not recommended less than 6 weeks.
[b] Not recommended less than 2 months.
[c] Not recommended less than 3 months.

Table 4 Dosage of antimicrobial agents used for prophylaxis[93]	
Antimicrobial Agent	**Dose**
TMP-sulfamethoxazole	2 mg TMP/kg/d
Nitrofurantoin	1–2 mg/kg/dose
Cephalexin	10 mg/kg/dose
Amoxicillin (infants < 2 months)	10 mg/kg/dose

Abbreviation: TMP, trimethoprim.

level, and blood pressure remained stable. However, it is not known whether this anti-proteinuric effect slows down the progressive loss of renal function. In patients with a unilateral poorly functioning scarred kidney, surgical removal of the affected kidney may normalize blood pressure.

SURGICAL MANAGEMENT

Surgical correction of VUR is usually reserved for patients with high-grade VUR, recurrent UTI despite antimicrobial prophylaxis, noncompliance or intolerance to prophylactic antibiotics, and/or the worsening of renal scars.[82] The gold standard for the surgical management of VUR is the Cohen cross-trigonal reimplantation.[83] Laparoscopic reimplantation techniques (with or without robotic assistance) have increased in recent years but utilization remains limited to specialized centers. Endoscopic

Table 5 Surgical techniques for vesicoureteral reflux[94]			
Technique	**Success Rates (%)**	**Pros**	**Cons**
Open reimplantation	95	• High success rates • Limited requirement for follow-up VCU • Reduction in hospital stays	• Surgical incision • Hospitalization required • Catheters needed during postoperative management • Need for pain control
Endoscopic injection Dextranomer and hyaluronidase (Deflux)	70–80	• Reasonable success rates • Outpatient management • Minimal pain	• Expensive • Lower success rates • Need for repeated procedures • Need for follow-up VCU
Laparoscopic or robotic reimplantation	70–90	• Reasonable success rates • Small incisions • Less discomfort	• Lower success rates • Requires hospitalization • Need for follow-up VCU • Long procedure • Expensive equipment • Significant surgical learning curve

treatment involves subureteral or intraureteral injection of a bulking agent most commonly dextranomer/hyaluronic acid (Deflux). The decision for timing and type of intervention is based on the patient age, severity of VUR, presence of renal scarring, and the parental wishes. The success rate of each procedure and their pros and cons are elaborated in **Table 5**.

SUMMARY

A high-grade VUR is a risk factor for recurrent UTI and renal scarring. Depending on the age of the patient, severity of VUR, presence of renal scarring, and the clinical course, the management options include surveillance only, antimicrobial prophylaxis, or surgical intervention. Treatment of BBD, if present, is essential for preventing recurrent UTI and help resolution of VUR. Prevention of renal scars and preservation of renal function in those with renal scars remains the most important treatment objective. Patients with renal scarring should be monitored for hypertension, and those with significant scarring, particularly bilateral, should be monitored for proteinuria and chronic kidney disease.

CLINICS CARE POINTS

- A renal US examination helps diagnose several congenital anomalies of kidney and urinary tract but is not sensitive enough to rule out the presence of a VUR.
- Prompt antibiotic administration lowers the risk of renal scarring caused by pyelonephritis and VUR.
- Prophylactic antibiotic can be used in children with high-grade VUR and other risk factors for recurrent UTI or renal scarring.
- Treatment of constipation helps improve bladder function and reduce the risk of UTI recurrence.
- Very few patients with VUR need surgical correction.
- Children with renal scarring should be monitored for hypertension, and those with significant scarring, particularly bilateral, should be monitored for chronic kidney disease.
- The complications of renal scarring are more pronounced in adults.

REFERENCES

1. Williams G, Fletcher JT, Alexander SI, et al. Vesicoureteral reflux. J Am Soc Nephrol 2008;19(5):847–62.
2. Dwoskin JY, Perlmutter AD. Vesicoureteral reflux in children: a computerized review. J Urol 1973;109(5):888–90.
3. Wennerstrom M, Hansson S, Jodal U, et al. Disappearance of vesicoureteral reflux in children. Arch Pediatr Adolesc Med 1998;152(9):879–83.
4. Marra G, Barbieri G, Dell'Agnola CA, et al. Congenital renal damage associated with primary vesicoureteral reflux detected prenatally in male infants. J Pediatr 1994;124(5 Pt 1):726–30.
5. Chand DH, Rhoades T, Poe SA, et al. Incidence and severity of vesicoureteral reflux in children related to age, gender, race and diagnosis. J Urol 2003;170(4 Pt 2):1548–50.
6. Hoberman A, Greenfield SP, Mattoo TK, et al. Antimicrobial prophylaxis for children with vesicoureteral reflux. N Engl J Med 2014;370(25):2367–76.

7. Schaeffer AJ, Greenfield SP, Ivanova A, et al. Reliability of grading of vesicoureteral reflux and other findings on voiding cystourethrography. J Pediatr Urol 2017; 13(2):192–8.
8. Silva JM, Diniz JS, Lima EM, et al. Predictive factors of resolution of primary vesico-ureteric reflux: a multivariate analysis. BJU Int 2006;97(5):1063–8.
9. Silva JM, Santos Diniz JS, Marino VS, et al. Clinical course of 735 children and adolescents with primary vesicoureteral reflux. Pediatr Nephrol 2006;21(7): 981–8.
10. Arant BS Jr. Medical management of mild and moderate vesicoureteral reflux: followup studies of infants and young children. A preliminary report of the Southwest Pediatric Nephrology Study Group. J Urol 1992;148(5 Pt 2):1683–7.
11. Schwab CW Jr, Wu HY, Selman H, et al. Spontaneous resolution of vesicoureteral reflux: a 15-year perspective. J Urol 2002;168(6):2594–9.
12. Koff SA. Relationship between dysfunctional voiding and reflux. J Urol 1992; 148(5 Pt 2):1703–5.
13. Sillen U. Bladder dysfunction in children with vesico-ureteric reflux. Acta Paediatr Suppl 1999;88(431):40–7.
14. Jansson UB, Hanson M, Hanson E, et al. Voiding pattern in healthy children 0 to 3 years old: a longitudinal study. J Urol 2000;164(6):2050–4.
15. Roihuvuo-Leskinen HM, Koskimaki JE, Tammela TL, et al. Urine flow curve shapes in adults with earlier vesicoureteral reflux. Eur Urol 2008;54(1):188–94.
16. Siegel SR, Siegel B, Sokoloff BZ, et al. Urinary infection in infants and preschool children. Five-year follow-up. Am J Dis Child 1980;134(4):369–72.
17. Chen JJ, Pugach J, West D, et al. Infant vesicoureteral reflux: a comparison between patients presenting with a prenatal diagnosis and those presenting with a urinary tract infection. Urology 2003;61(2):442–6 [discussion: 6-7].
18. Zerin JM, Ritchey ML, Chang AC. Incidental vesicoureteral reflux in neonates with antenatally detected hydronephrosis and other renal abnormalities. Radiology 1993;187(1):157–60.
19. Upadhyay J, McLorie GA, Bolduc S, et al. Natural history of neonatal reflux associated with prenatal hydronephrosis: long-term results of a prospective study. J Urol 2003;169(5):1837–41 [discussion :41, author reply: 41].
20. Noe HN, Wyatt RJ, Peeden JN Jr, et al. The transmission of vesicoureteral reflux from parent to child. J Urol 1992;148(6):1869–71.
21. Jerkins GR, Noe HN. Familial vesicoureteral reflux: a prospective study. J Urol 1982;128(4):774–8.
22. Connolly LP, Treves ST, Zurakowski D, et al. Natural history of vesicoureteral reflux in siblings. J Urol 1996;156(5):1805–7.
23. Parekh DJ, Pope JCt, Adams MC, et al. Outcome of sibling vesicoureteral reflux. J Urol 2002;167(1):283–4.
24. Wennerstrom M, Hansson S, Jodal U, et al. Primary and acquired renal scarring in boys and girls with urinary tract infection. J Pediatr 2000;136(1):30–4.
25. Mattoo TK. Vesicoureteral reflux and reflux nephropathy. Adv Chronic Kidney Dis 2011;18(5):348–54.
26. Mattoo TK, Chesney RW, Greenfield SP, et al. Renal scarring in the randomized intervention for children with vesicoureteral reflux (RIVUR) trial. Clin J Am Soc Nephrol 2016;11(1):54–61.
27. Snodgrass WT, Shah A, Yang M, et al. Prevalence and risk factors for renal scars in children with febrile UTI and/or VUR: a cross-sectional observational study of 565 consecutive patients. J Pediatr Urol 2013;9(6 Pt A):856–63.

28. Shaikh N, Craig JC, Rovers MM, et al. Identification of Children and Adolescents at Risk for Renal Scarring After a First Urinary Tract Infection: A Meta-analysis With Individual Patient Data. JAMA Pediatr 2014;168(10):893–900.

29. Roberts KB. Urinary tract infections and renal damage: focusing on what matters. JAMA Pediatr 2014;168(10):884–5.

30. Peters CA, Skoog SJ, Arant BS, et al. Summary of the AUA guideline on management of primary vesicoureteral reflux in children. J Urol 2010;184(3):1134–44.

31. Shaikh N, Ewing AL, Bhatnagar S, et al. Risk of renal scarring in children with a first urinary tract infection: a systematic review. Pediatrics 2010;126(6):1084–91.

32. Skoog SJ, Peters CA, Arant BS, et al. pediatric vesicoureteral reflux guidelines panel summary report: clinical practice guidelines for screening siblings of children with vesicoureteral reflux and neonates/infants with prenatal hydronephrosis. J Urol 2010;184(3):1145–51.

33. Shaikh N, Haralam MA, Kurs-Lasky M, et al. Association of renal scarring with number of febrile urinary tract infections in children. JAMA Pediatr 2019; 173(10):949–52.

34. Fernandez-Menendez JM, Malaga S, Matesanz JL, et al. Risk factors in the development of early technetium-99m dimercaptosuccinic acid renal scintigraphy lesions during first urinary tract infection in children. Acta Paediatr (Oslo, Norway : 1992) 2003;92(1):21–6.

35. Shaikh N, Mattoo TK, Keren R, et al. Early Antibiotic Treatment for Pediatric Febrile Urinary Tract Infection and Renal Scarring. JAMA Pediatr 2016;170(9): 848–54.

36. Howie AJ, Buist LJ, Coulthard MG. Reflux nephropathy in transplants. Pediatr Nephrol (Berlin, Germany) 2002;17(7):485–90.

37. Coulthard MG, Flecknell P, Orr H, et al. Renal scarring caused by vesicoureteric reflux and urinary infection: a study in pigs. Pediatr Nephrol (Berlin, Germany) 2002;17(7):481–4.

38. Wennerstrom M, Hansson S, Hedner T, et al. Ambulatory blood pressure 16-26 years after the first urinary tract infection in childhood. J Hypertens 2000;18(4): 485–91.

39. Faust WC, Diaz M, Pohl HG. Incidence of post-pyelonephritic renal scarring: a meta-analysis of the dimercapto-succinic acid literature. J Urol 2009;181(1): 290–7 [discussion: 7-8].

40. Smellie JM, Prescod NP, Shaw PJ, et al. Childhood reflux and urinary infection: a follow-up of 10-41 years in 226 adults. Pediatr Nephrol 1998;12(9):727–36.

41. Zhang Y, Bailey RR. A long term follow up of adults with reflux nephropathy. N Z Med J 1995;108(998):142–4.

42. Kohler J, Tencer J, Thysell H, et al. Vesicoureteral reflux diagnosed in adulthood. Incidence of urinary tract infections, hypertension, proteinuria, back pain and renal calculi. Nephrol Dial Transplant 1997;12(12):2580–7.

43. Goonasekera CD, Shah V, Wade AM, et al. 15-year follow-up of renin and blood pressure in reflux nephropathy. Lancet 1996;347(9002):640–3.

44. Ahmed M, Eggleston D, Kapur G, et al. Dimercaptosuccinic acid (DMSA) renal scan in the evaluation of hypertension in children. Pediatr Nephrol 2008;23(3): 435–8.

45. Savage JM, Koh CT, Shah V, et al. Five year prospective study of plasma renin activity and blood pressure in patients with longstanding reflux nephropathy. Arch Dis Child 1987;62(7):678–82.

46. Karlen J, Linne T, Wikstad I, et al. Incidence of microalbuminuria in children with pyelonephritic scarring. Pediatr Nephrol (Berlin, Germany) 1996;10(6):705–8.

47. Susan L, Furth AGA, Jerry-Fluker J, et al. Metabolic Abnormalities, CVD Risk Factors and GFR Decline in Children with CKD. Clin J Am Soc Nephrol (CJASN) 2011;6(9):2132–40.
48. Silva JM, Diniz JS, Silva AC, et al. Predictive factors of chronic kidney disease in severe vesicoureteral reflux. Pediatr Nephrol 2006;21(9):1285–92.
49. Bailey RR, Lynn KL, Robson RA. End-stage reflux nephropathy. Ren Fail 1994; 16(1):27–35.
50. Bailey RR, Lynn KL, Smith AH. Long-term followup of infants with gross vesicoureteral reflux. J Urol 1992;148(5 Pt 2):1709–11.
51. Lahdes-Vasama T, Niskanen K, Ronnholm K. Outcome of kidneys in patients treated for vesicoureteral reflux (VUR) during childhood. Nephrol Dial Transpl 2006;21(9):2491–7.
52. Williams DG. Reflux nephropathy. Q J Med 1990;77(284):1205–7.
53. Mohammad D, Farooqi A, Mattoo TK. Kidney Echogenicity and Vesicoureteral Reflux in Children with Febrile Urinary Tract Infection. J Pediatr 2021;242:201–5.
54. Lavocat MP, Granjon D, Allard D, et al. Imaging of pyelonephritis. Pediatr Radiol 1997;27(2):159–65.
55. Ditchfield MR, Summerville D, Grimwood K, et al. Time course of transient cortical scintigraphic defects associated with acute pyelonephritis. Pediatr Radiol 2002; 32(12):849–52.
56. Mattoo TK, Skoog SJ, Gravens-Mueller L, et al. Interobserver variability for interpretation of DMSA scans in the RIVUR trial. J Pediatr Urol 2017;13(6):616 e1–e6.
57. Craig JC, Simpson JM, Williams GJ, et al. Antibiotic prophylaxis and recurrent urinary tract infection in children. N Engl J Med 2009;361(18):1748–59.
58. Shaikh N, Hoberman A, Keren R, et al. Recurrent Urinary Tract Infections in Children With Bladder and Bowel Dysfunction. Pediatrics 2016;137(1):1–7.
59. Pennesi M, Travan L, Peratoner L, et al. Is antibiotic prophylaxis in children with vesicoureteral reflux effective in preventing pyelonephritis and renal scars? A randomized, controlled trial. Pediatrics 2008;121(6):e1489–94.
60. Garin EH, Olavarria F, Garcia Nieto V, et al. Clinical significance of primary vesicoureteral reflux and urinary antibiotic prophylaxis after acute pyelonephritis: a multicenter, randomized, controlled study. Pediatrics 2006;117(3):626–32.
61. Roussey-Kesler G, Gadjos V, Idres N, et al. Antibiotic prophylaxis for the prevention of recurrent urinary tract infection in children with low grade vesicoureteral reflux: results from a prospective randomized study. J Urol 2008;179(2):674–9 [discussion: 9].
62. Hari P, Hari S, Sinha A, et al. Antibiotic prophylaxis in the management of vesicoureteric reflux: a randomized double-blind placebo-controlled trial. Pediatr Nephrol 2015;30(3):479–86.
63. Montini G, Rigon L, Zucchetta P, et al. Prophylaxis after first febrile urinary tract infection in children? A multicenter, randomized, controlled, noninferiority trial. Pediatrics 2008;122(5):1064–71.
64. Brandstrom P, Esbjorner E, Herthelius M, et al. The Swedish reflux trial in children: III. Urinary tract infection pattern. J Urol 2010;184(1):286–91.
65. Wang ZT, Wehbi E, Alam Y, et al. A Reanalysis of the RIVUR Trial Using a Risk Classification System. J Urol 2018;199(6):1608–14.
66. Wang HH, Gbadegesin RA, Foreman JW, et al. Efficacy of Antibiotic Prophylaxis in Children with Vesicoureteral Reflux: Systematic Review and Meta-Analysis. J Urol 2014.
67. Williams G, Hodson EM, Craig JC. Interventions for primary vesicoureteric reflux. Cochrane Database Syst Rev 2019;2:CD001532.

68. Williams G, Craig JC. Long-term antibiotics for preventing recurrent urinary tract infection in children. Cochrane Database Syst Rev 2019;4:CD001534.
69. Mattoo TK, Carpenter MA, Moxey-Mims M, et al. The RIVUR trial: a factual interpretation of our data. Pediatr Nephrol 2015.
70. Peters C, Skoog SJ, Arant BS, et al. Management and Screening of Primary Vesicoureteral Reflux in Children (2010, amended 2017). 2017. Available at: https://www.auanet.org/guidelines/vesicoureteral-reflux-guideline. Accessed August, 25 2020.
71. Stein R, Dogan HS, Hoebeke P, et al. Urinary tract infections in children: EAU/ESPU guidelines. Eur Urol 2015;67(3):546–58.
72. Ammenti A, Cataldi L, Chimenz R, et al. Febrile urinary tract infections in young children: recommendations for the diagnosis, treatment and follow-up. Acta Paediatr 2012;101(5):451–7.
73. Jodal U, Lindberg U. Guidelines for management of children with urinary tract infection and vesico-ureteric reflux. Recommendations from a Swedish state-of-the-art conference. Swedish Medical Research Council. Acta Paediatr Suppl 1999;88(431):87–9.
74. Mattoo TK, Shaikh N, Nelson CP. Contemporary Management of Urinary Tract Infection in Children. Pediatrics 2021;147(2). e2020012138.
75. Gaither TW, Copp HL. Antimicrobial prophylaxis for urinary tract infections: implications for adherence assessment. J Pediatr Urol 2019.
76. Desai S, Fisher B. Impact of Trimethoprim-sulfamethoxazole Urinary Tract Infection Prophylaxis on Non-UTI Infections. Pediatr Infect Dis J 2019;38(4):396–7.
77. Edmonson MB, Eickhoff JC. Weight Gain and Obesity in Infants and Young Children Exposed to Prolonged Antibiotic Prophylaxis. JAMA Pediatr 2017;171(2):150–6.
78. Nadkarni MD, Mattoo TK, Gravens-Mueller L, et al. Laboratory Findings After Urinary Tract Infection and Antimicrobial Prophylaxis in Children With Vesicoureteral Reflux. Clin Pediatr (Phila) 2020;59(3):259–65.
79. Farhat W, Bagli DJ, Capolicchio G, et al. The dysfunctional voiding scoring system: quantitative standardization of dysfunctional voiding symptoms in children. J Urol 2000;164(3 Pt 2):1011–5.
80. Koff SA, Wagner TT, Jayanthi VR. The relationship among dysfunctional elimination syndromes, primary vesicoureteral reflux and urinary tract infections in children. J Urol 1998;160(3 Pt 2):1019–22.
81. Lama G, Salsano ME, Pedulla M, et al. Angiotensin converting enzyme inhibitors and reflux nephropathy: 2-year follow-up. Pediatr Nephrol 1997;11(6):714–8.
82. Diamond DA, Mattoo TK. Endoscopic treatment of primary vesicoureteral reflux. N Engl J Med 2012;366(13):1218–26.
83. Kennelly MJ, Bloom DA, Ritchey ML, et al. Outcome analysis of bilateral Cohen cross-trigonal ureteroneocystostomy. Urology 1995;46(3):393–5.
84. Kincaid-Smith P. Glomerular lesions in atrophic pyelonephritis and reflux nephropathy. Kidney Int Suppl 1975;4:S81–3.
85. Bailey RR, Swainson CP, Lynn KL, et al. Glomerular lesions in the 'normal' kidney in patients with unilateral reflux nephropathy. Contrib Nephrol 1984;39:126–31.
86. Das SK, Menon PS, Bagga A, et al. Physical growth in children with reflux nephropathy with normal or mildly impaired renal function. Indian J Pediatr 2010;77(6):684–6.
87. Polito C, Marte A, Zamparelli M, et al. Catch-up growth in children with vesicoureteric reflux. Pediatr Nephrol 1997;11(2):164–8.

88. National Institute for Health and Clinical Excellence (NICE) guidelines for urinary tract infection in children. 2018. Available at: https://www.nice.org.uk/guidance/cg54/evidence/full-guideline-pdf-196566877. Accessed February 5 202220.
89. Buettcher M, Trueck J, Niederer-Loher A, et al. Swiss consensus recommendations on urinary tract infections in children. Eur J Pediatr 2021;180(3):663–74.
90. Indian Society of Pediatric N, Vijayakumar M, Kanitkar M, et al. Revised statement on management of urinary tract infections. Indian Pediatr 2011;48(9):709–17.
91. Yang SS, Tsai JD, Kanematsu A, et al. Asian guidelines for urinary tract infection in children. J Infect Chemother 2021;27(11):1543–54.
92. Ammenti A, Alberici I, Brugnara M, et al. Updated Italian recommendations for the diagnosis, treatment and follow-up of the first febrile urinary tract infection in young children. Acta Paediatr 2019.
93. Saadeh SA, Mattoo TK. Managing urinary tract infections. Pediatr Nephrol 2011; 26(11):1967–76.
94. Mathews R, Mattoo TK. Primary vesicoureteral reflux and reflux nephropathy. In: Jürgen Floege RJJ, John F, editors. Comprehensive clinical Nephrology. 6th ed. St. Louis, Missouri: Elsevier Saunders; 2018. p. 738–47.

Antenatally Diagnosed Kidney Anomalies

Caoimhe S. Costigan, BSc, BM BS, MRCP[a],
Norman D. Rosenblum, MD, FRCPC, FCAHS[a,b,c,d],*

KEYWORDS

- CAKUT • Antenatal • Congenital anomalies of the kidney and urinary tract
- Development • Kidney malformations • Pediatric nephrology

KEY POINTS

- Renal anomalies account for up to 30% of all antenatally diagnosed congenital anomalies.
- The prevalence of all types of renal and urinary tract anomalies is estimated to be between 0.3 and 17 per 1000 births.
- Antenatal hydronephrosis is the most commonly detected abnormality, affecting between 1% and 4.5% of all pregnancies.
- Extrarenal malformations are described in up to 30% of cases with renal anomalies.
- Congenital renal anomalies are being detected with increased frequency and represent a spectrum of conditions with different clinical management priorities.

SECTION 1: BACKGROUND

Introduction

Congenital anomalies of the kidney and urinary tract (CAKUT) encompass a broad spectrum of developmental conditions that together account for the majority of childhood chronic kidney diseases.[1–8] These disorders include renal agenesis, hypoplasia and dysplasia, multicystic dysplasia, duplication anomalies, ureteropelvic junction obstruction (UPJO), ureterovesical junction obstruction (UVJO), megaureter, posterior urethral valves (PUV), and vesicoureteral reflux (VUR). Although not considered within the spectrum of CAKUT, hereditary cystic kidney disease can phenotypically resemble CAKUT. The detection of kidney anomalies is increasing as a result of improved antenatal care and widespread access to more sensitive screening ultrasonography. Most

[a] Division of Nephrology, The Hospital for Sick Children, 555 University Avenue, Toronto, Ontario M5G1X8, Canada; [b] Developmental & Stem Cell Biology Program, Research Institute, The Hospital for Sick Children, Toronto, ON, Canada; [c] Department of Paediatrics, Physiology, and Laboratory Medicine and Pathobiology, University of Toronto; [d] Peter Gilgan Centre for Research and Learning, 686 Bay Street, 16th Floor, Room 16.9706, Toronto, ON M5G 0A4, Canada
* Corresponding author.
E-mail address: norman.rosenblum@sickkids.ca

paediatricians will encounter children with congenital kidney anomalies across a wide spectrum of disorders.

In this article, the authors focus predominantly on antenatally diagnosed kidney anomalies in the CAKUT spectrum and also discuss cystic kidney diseases to be considered in the context of CAKUT. The authors review relevant aspects of kidney development and embryology and provide an outline for classification of CAKUT and a framework for investigation and key aspects of management, including the evidence informing current guidelines relating to management of children with kidney anomalies.

Epidemiology

Both the kidneys and ureters arise from a common structure, the intermediate mesoderm.[9] Lower tract abnormalities involving the ureters and bladder are identified in about 50% of patients with renal malformations, including VUR (25%), UPJO (11%), and UVJO (11%).[10,11]

The fetal kidney and bladder can be detected by maternal ultrasound between gestational week 12 and week 15. In the presence of at least one functional kidney, the bladder should be urine filled, and a distinction between the kidney cortex and medulla should be possible by week 20.[12,13] The sensitivity of antenatal ultrasound for detecting kidney abnormalities may be as high as 82% but this depends on timing of the ultrasound.[14]

Kidney formation occurs in concert with the development of many other major organ systems. Extrarenal malformations are described in up to 30% of cases of renal anomalies and more than 200 multiorgan syndromes that involve renal or urinary tract manifestations are described.[6,15,16] The epidemiology of some renal anomalies is outlined in **Table 1**.

Classification

Renal anomalies are classified based on their sonographic appearance and can be broadly defined as abnormalities in kidney size, shape, position, or number as outlined in **Table 2**.

Renal agenesis describes failure of renal development, which can be either unilateral or bilateral. Bilateral renal agenesis is associated with oligohydramnios, consequent pulmonary hypoplasia, and perinatal demise. With unilateral renal agenesis (URA)

Table 1 Epidemiology of renal anomalies	
Condition	**Incidence**
Antenatal hydronephrosis	1%–4.5% of pregnancies[8,12]
Bilateral renal agenesis	1:3000–10, 000 births[17]
Unilateral renal agenesis	1:1000 autopsies[17]
Unilateral hypoplasia/dysplasia	1:3000–5000 births[17]
Bilateral dysplasia	1: 10, 000[17]
MCDK	1:3,640[17]
Renal ectopia	1:10,000 births &1:1,000 autopsies[18]
Renal fusion anomalies	1:600[19]
ARPKD	1:20,000[20,21]
ADPKD	1:1,000[22]

| Table 2 | | | |
| Classification of renal anomalies | | | |
Abnormal Size	Abnormal Shape	Abnormal Location	Abnormal Number
Renal hypoplasia	Cystic renal disease	Renal ectopia	Renal agenesis
Renal dysplasia	Renal fusion	Renal fusion	Renal duplication

and normal functioning other kidney, there are no expected deleterious effects on amniotic fluid volume or lung development. URA is associated with urinary tract anomalies on the contralateral side in 32% of patients; VUR (24%); PUJO (6%); megaureter (7%); and duplex kidney (3%).[23]

Hypoplasia describes kidneys that are small based on the ultrasonographic assessment of renal length—typically defined as greater than 2 standard deviations less than the normal mean for age and height.[24] Such kidneys have normal morphology but the number of nephrons is reduced. Reference tables exist defining mean length by gestational age for antenatal ultrasound and by height and age postnatally.[24,25]

Dysplasia, sometimes also called "cystic dysplasia," describes kidneys that contain abnormal renal tissue or structures. Dysplasia may manifest on ultrasound as hyperechogenicity, loss of normal corticomedullary differentiation, with or without the presence of cysts. Distinguishing hypoplasia and dysplasia can be difficult on a practical level, as the dysplastic kidney may also be small, but small kidneys are not necessarily dysplastic.

Congenital cystic kidney disease can broadly be categorized into hereditary and nonhereditary disorders. Hereditary cystic kidney disease includes both autosomal dominant and recessive polycystic kidney disease (ADPKD and ARPKD) as well as some syndromic presentations such as nephronophthisis and glomerulocystic kidney diseases. Many of these hereditary forms of cystic kidney disease can be difficult to distinguish from classic CAKUT antenatally.

A *multicystic dysplastic kidney (MCDK)* is technically a cystic subtype of renal dysplasia in which the kidney is devoid of normal tissue and composed of large noncommunicating cysts. There is classically no functional renal tissue. The natural history of MCDK is involution over time.[26]

An *ectopic kidney* is usually a unilateral phenomenon, most commonly with one kidney failing to ascend out of the pelvis, remaining on the ipsilateral side as a pelvic kidney. Ectopic kidneys can also be found on the contralateral side and in locations other than the pelvis (such as the thorax); this is uncommon.[27,28]

Horseshoe kidney, a fusion abnormality, is the commonest with an incidence as 1 in 500 in the general population and higher in certain groups such as children with Turner and Down syndrome.[29] In horseshoe kidney, both kidneys fail to migrate normally, and fusion is usually of the lower poles; a horseshoe kidney is typically found in the pelvis. Crossed fused ectopia describes an ectopic kidney that fuses with the contralateral kidney, generally at its lower pole, and can be found anywhere from the normal position of the contralateral kidney to the pelvis.

A *duplex system* is common. Duplication abnormalities can be either complete or incomplete, distinguished by the entry of the ureter into the bladder. In complete duplication 2 ureters develop that enter the bladder separately. In incomplete subtypes the pelvis and ureters can be bifid but the urethral orifice at the bladder is singular. There are many varieties of duplication abnormalities. The upper pole ureter may insert ectopically into the vagina or posterior urethra, may be associated with a ureterocele that can cause obstruction, or be associated with dysplastic tissue.[30] The lower pole ureter usually has a normal insertion at the bladder but may be associated with VUR.[31]

SECTION 2: CAUSE
Embryology and Molecular Control Mechanisms

The cause of CAKUT is multifactorial, representing a complex interplay between genetic, epigenetic, and environmental factors. Kidney development in humans commences at the end of the fourth gestational week and is complete by 34 to 36 weeks' of gestation.[9] A basic understanding of the embryological processes involved in kidney development is a useful foundation for appreciating the various components involved in pathogenesis of such conditions.[9] **Fig. 1** is a simplified overview of the key stages in kidney development.

Genetics

CAKUT has been recognized as having a defined monogenetic cause in up to 20% of cases with more than 40 monogenic causes identified, some of which are outlined in **Table 3**.[15,32] In addition to single gene mutations, copy number variants (structural variation of the genome resulting from duplications or deletions) are recognized to have a role in CAKUT.[33,34]

Environmental Factors

Some environmental factors that have been suggested to be involved in the pathogenesis in CAKUT are outlined in **Table 4**.

SECTION 3: CLINICAL APPROACH
An Antenatal Approach

The kidneys and bladder can be detected on transvaginal ultrasound by the 12th gestational week. Reference data exist to assess renal size from 15 weeks' gestation. Small kidneys usually suggest some form of hypodysplasia, whereas large kidneys can be seen in some cystic kidney diseases (eg, ARPKD, TCF2 mutations) and in overgrowth syndromes such as Beckwith-Wiedemann, Simpson-Golabi-Behmel, and Sotos syndrome. Parenchymal abnormalities such as increased echogenicity, cortical thinning, and cysts, although nonspecific, can indicate dysplasia or hereditary cystic disease.[35] HNF1ß (*TCF2*) mutations have been reported to be the main cause of echogenic kidneys in the fetus.[36] Amniotic fluid volume is an important indicator of fetal

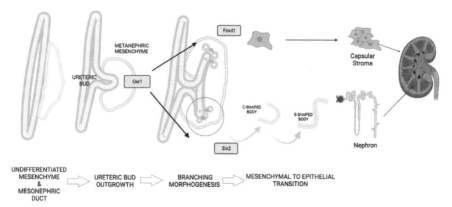

Fig. 1. An overview of kidney development. Created with BioRender.com

Table 3
Monogenic forms of congenital anomalies of the kidney and urinary tract

Gene	Protein	Inheritance Pattern
ACE	Angiotensin-I-converting enzyme	AR
AGT	Angiotensinogen	AR
AGTR1	Angiotensin II receptor, type 1	AR
BMP4	Bone morphogenic protein 4	AD
CHRM3	Muscarinic acetylcholine receptor M3	AR
CHD1L	Chromodomain helicase DNA binding protein 1	AD
CRKL	CRK-like proto-oncogene, adaptor protein	AD
DSTYK	Dual serine/threonine & tyrosine protein kinase	AD
EYA1	Eyes absent homolog 1	AD
FRAS1	ECM protein FRAS1	AR
FREM1	FRAS1-related ECM protein 1	AR
FREM2	FRAS1-related ECM protein 1	AR
GATA3	GATA binding protein 3	AD
GLI3	GLI family zinc finger 3	AD
GPC3	Glypican 3	XLR
GRIP1	Glutamate receptor interacting protein 1	AR
HNF1B	HNF homeobox B	AD
HPSE2	Heparanase B	AR
ITGA8	Integrin-alpha 8	AR
LRIG2	Leucine-rich repeats and Ig-like domains	AR
MUC1	Mucin 1	AD
NRIP1	Nuclear receptor interacting protein 1	AD
PAX2	Paired box gene 2	AD
PBX1	PBX homeobox 1	AD
REN	Renin	AR
RET	Proto-oncogene tyrosine-protein kinase receptor Ret	AD
ROBO2	Roundabout, axon guidance receptor, homolog 2	AD
SALL1	Sal-like protein 1	AD
SIX1	SIX homeobox 1	AD
SIX2	SIX homeobox 2	AD
SIX5	SIX homeobox 5	AD
SLIT2	Slit homolog 2	AD
SOX17	Transcription factor SIX-17	AD
SRGAP1	SLIT-ROBO Rho GTPase activating protein 1	AD
TBX18	T-box transcription factor	AD
TNXB	Tenascin XB	AD
TRAP1	Heat shock protein 75	AR
UPK3A	Uroplakin 3A	AD
UMOD	Uromodulin	AD
WNT4	Protein Wnt-4	AD
KAL1	Anosmin-1	XLR

Abbreviation: Ig, immunoglobulin.

Table 4
Environmental factors in congenital anomalies of the kidney and urinary tract

	Environmental Factors
Maternal Factors	Diabetes mellitus
	Overweight/Obesity
	Vitamin A deficiency
	Folic acid deficiency
Nephrotoxic Medication	ACE inhibitors, ARBs
	NSAIDs
	Folate antagonists
	Maternal use or administration to preterm neonate
Other	Alcohol consumption
	Cocaine use
	Fertility treatment

Abbreviations: ACE, angiotensin-converting enzyme; ARB, angiotensin receptor blocker; NSAIDs, nonsteroidal antiinflammatory drugs.

urine production; oligo- or anhydramnios are major risk factors for pulmonary hypoplasia. Antenatal genetic testing is often performed when an abnormality of a second affected organ system is identified. **Table 5** outlines some kidney conditions that do not fall under CAKUT and may be detected antenatally.

A Postnatal Approach

As with any clinical assessment, the initial steps in an infant with a kidney or urinary tract abnormality is a detailed history and clinical examination.

Antenatal history of relevant environmental exposures is important to illicit. Family history is important, as it may influence a decision to pursue genetic investigation. In the context of antenatal hydronephrosis (AH), a description of the urinary stream is pertinent, as a poor stream is associated with lower tract obstruction, such as PUV.

Physical examination is focused on identifying associated abnormalities or syndromic features. Palpable kidneys are usually easily identifiable in children with ARPKD but may also be present in severe hydronephrosis or MCDK. A distended bladder after voiding could indicate lower tract obstruction. Because of their related embryonic origin, genital abnormalities can co-exist with CAKUT. Evidence of anorectal or cloacal abnormalities should also be sought. Some syndromes associated with CAKUT are outlined in **Table 6**.

INVESTIGATION

A variety of imaging modalities are available to investigate renal abnormalities—knowing which to choose and when can be challenging.

Kidney bladder ultrasound: ultrasound is the primary mode of imaging used. Ultrasound is minimally invasive, low-cost, and can provide information on kidney size, position, and parenchymal features—echogenicity, echotexture, corticomedullary differentiation, cysts, and assessment of the collecting system and bladder—which is comparable over serial assessments (**Box 1**).

The purpose of an *early* (within 24 hours of life) postnatal ultrasound is to confirm the antenatal findings and to determine the need for urgent intervention, which is usually surgical.

Indications include the following:

- Oligohydramnios

Table 5
Non-CAKUT antenatally detectable kidney anomalies

Condition	Gene	Kidney Phenotype	Extrarenal Manifestations	Possible Antenatal Findings
ARPKD	PKHD1 DZIP1L	Enlarged kidneys with microcysts (collecting duct origin) Hypertension Progressive CKD	Congenital hepatic fibrosis, biliary dysgenesis, caroli disease	Markedly enlarged echogenic kidneys Poor CMD +/− cysts +/− oligohydramnios Can have normal antenatal appearance
ADPKD	PKD1 PKD2	Larger cysts Often presents in adolescence/adulthood Progressive CKD	Mitral valve prolapse Arachnoid cysts Congenital hepatic fibrosis	Often have normal antenatal appearance Can be enlarged (often mildly) Echogenic Poor CMD +/− cysts
Nephronophthisis (NPHP) • Infantile • Juvenile • Adolescent	NPHP 2 &3 NPHP 1 NPHP 3	Impaired urinary concentrating ability Chronic tubulointerstitial nephropathy Progressive CKD Hypertension in infantile form	More in infantile form Skeletal, cardiac, liver, eye	Hyperechogenicity +/− cysts Poor CMD Can be normal, large, or small Both oligo- or polyhydramnios possible Can have normal antenatal appearance

(continued on next page)

Table 5
(continued)

Condition	Gene	Kidney Phenotype	Extrarenal Manifestations	Possible Antenatal Findings
Syndromes associated with NPHP				
Meckel Gruber syndrome	NPHP6, NPHP8, & MKS	NPHP	Occipital encephalocele Postaxial polydactyly	Hyperechogenicity +/− cysts
Joubert syndrome	Multiple possible loci	NPHP	Cerebellar vermis hypoplasia (molar tooth sign) Polydactyly, hypotonia, hepatic fibrosis, retinal dystrophy, ocular coloboma	Poor CMD Can be normal, large or small Both oligo- or polyhydramnios possible Can have normal antenatal appearance
Sensenbrenner syndrome	IFT122, WDR35, IFT43, & WDR19	NPHP	Craniosynostosis, short limbs, brachydactyly, narrow thorax, and facial anomalies	
Senior-Loken syndrome	NPHP5 & NPHP6	NPHP	Retinitis Pigmentosa/Leber congenital amaurosis	
Overgrowth Syndromes with Kidney phenotypes				
Beckwith-Wiedemann syndrome	11p15.5 region	Medullary dysplasia/sponge kidney, cystic change, nephromegaly	Omphalocele, macroglossia, macrosomia, tumors	Large kidneys ± increased echogenicity ± cysts
Sotos syndrome	NSD1	Nephromegaly VUR, duplication defects, single kidney, PUJO, urethral abnormalities	Characteristic facial appearance, learning disability, and overgrowth	
Simpson-Golabi-Behmel syndrome	GPC3	Medullary dysplasia	Overgrowth, coarse facies, congenital heart defects	

Abbreviations: CKD, cystic kidney disease; CMD, corticomedullary differentiation.

Table 6
Syndromic forms of congenital anomalies of the kidney and urinary tract

Syndrome	Genetics	Kidney Phenotype	Other
Branchio-oto-renal (BOR) syndrome	EYA1, SIX1, SIX5, SALL1	Unilateral or bilateral agenesis/dysplasia, hypoplasia, collecting system anomalies	Major features: hearing loss, branchial defects, ear pits, and renal anomalies Minor features: preauricular pits, lacrimal duct stenosis, congenital cataracts Classic BOR defined as 3 major features Highly variable phenotype Inheritance is AD with incomplete penetrance and variable expressivity
VACTERL Syndrome	TRAP1	Unilateral or bilateral renal agenesis, horseshoe kidney, cystic kidneys, dysplastic kidneys, urinary tract, and genital defects	Defined as at least 3 of the following: vertebral anomalies, anal atresia, cardiac defects, tracheoesophageal defects, renal malformations, and limb anomalies 50%–80% have renal anomalies Fanconi anemia is an important differential
Renal-Coloboma syndrome (RCS)	PAX2	Hypoplasia, vesicoureteral reflux, MCDK, UPJO	Optic phenotype is variable—most optic disc pit with mild visual impairment Can also include hearing loss, Arnold Chiari malformation, seizures, joint laxity
Renal cysts and diabetes (RCAD) syndrome	TCF2 (HNF1β)	Dysplasia, hypoplasia, bilateral cortical cysts	Glucose intolerance/diabetes mellitus (60%), hyperuricemia, elevation of liver enzymes, hypomagnesemia, abnormalities of the genital tract, and exocrine pancreatic abnormalities
CHARGE	CHD7	Horseshoe kidney, renal agenesis, VUR, and renal cysts	Choanal atresia, malformations of the heart, ear & ocular anomalies, cranial nerve dysfunction, dysmorphism Renal anomalies in 10%–40%

Abbreviations: CHARGE, Colobomas, Heart defects, choanal Atresia, Retarded growth and development, Genital hypoplasia, and Ear anomalies; VACTERL, vertebral anomalies, anal atresia, cardiac defects, tracheo-esophageal defects, renal malformations, and limb anomalies..

Box 1 Ultrasound pearls[37]	
Echogenicity	Refers to relative "brightness" on ultrasound
	Normal cortical echogenicity is less than the liver or spleen and more than the medulla
	Infants, particularly premature infants, have relatively echogenic kidneys
Corticomedullary differentiation	Normal kidneys demonstrate a distinction between the cortex, which is relatively echogenic (bright), and the more hypoechoic medulla
	Loss of this distinction can be a feature of dysplasia.

- Progressive AH
- Significant hydronephrosis in a single kidney (SK)
- Abnormal bladder
- Bilateral hydroureteronephrosis (particularly male infants)

In abnormalities that do not require urgent assessment, there is benefit in delaying sonographic assessment by at least 48 to 72 hours, particularly in breastfed infants, to allow for normal urine flow to be established.[38] Assessment of AH, performed too early, in an underhydrated infant with suboptimal urine output, may underestimate the degree of dilatation. The specific timing of the initial postnatal ultrasound is guided by the clinical severity of hydronephrosis in the third trimester. Mild to moderate degrees of severity require less urgent postnatal assessment (eg, within 1–2 months of life), whereas severe hydronephrosis will need earlier imaging.

Voiding cystourethrogram (VCUG): a VCUG is often considered in suspected VUR. The VCUG can also provide information on bladder size, shape, and emptying capacity. An early VCUG is performed when there is strong suspicion of bladder outlet obstruction such as PUV; suspicious findings include bilateral hydroureteronephrosis (moderate to severe), a large, thick-walled or trabeculated bladder and/or a "keyhole" appearance. A dilated and elongated posterior urethra during the voiding phase of the VCUG study provides the presumptive diagnosis of PUV, which is confirmed on cystoscopy.

Renal scans: functional renal imaging involves the administration of a radionucleotide tracer and analysis of its uptake and excretion. Different radiotracers with different mechanisms of uptake and clearance are used for different indications.[37]

A ^{99m}Tc-MAG3 or a diethylenetriamine pentacetic acid renogram can assess both differential renal function and urinary drainage. Various protocols including administration of intravenous fluids and diuretics exist to augment urine output during the test—hence the name "diuretic renogram." As it is glomerular filtration rate (GFR) dependent, a "MAG3" is not as effective as a^{99m}Tc-DMSA at determining split renal function in very young infants with a naturally lower GFR. A ^{99m}Tc-DMSA scan be used to identify functional renal tissue in children with MCDK or suspected ectopic renal tissues, as well as providing information on bilateral function in children with dysplasia, hypoplasia, or scarring.

INVESTIGATION
Genetic Testing

Defining patients who are most likely to benefit from genetic testing is an evolving subject. CAKUT presents in heterogenous ways with significant overlap between phenotypes, making a tailored approach difficult at the moment.

Establishing a genetic diagnosis can lead to more precise management and prognostication. It may allow patients to circumvent invasive diagnostics or potentially toxic medications and provide an opportunity for genetic counseling and more precise advice regarding recurrence risk. Recurrence risk is becoming increasingly relevant, as medical and surgical advances allow children with CAKUT to reach adulthood and reproductive age.

Both cost and ethical implications of genetic investigation must be considered. The risk of actionable incidental findings exists, particularly as advanced gene sequencing technologies become more accessible; this may lead to insurance or employment discrimination and has the potential to invoke psychological distress.

A recent review of genomic diagnostics for CAKUT has recommended considering genetic testing in children with syndromic or severe CAKUT, and including children with a clearly relevant family history also seems reasonable.[39] The relatively low cost of microarray testing makes it a reasonable first line for suspected syndromic forms of CAKUT.

AN APPROACH TO MANAGEMENT OF SPECIFIC ANOMALIES
Single Kidney

An apparent SK can be the result of URA, aplasia, spontaneous involution of an MCDK, or an unidentified ectopic kidney. Renal ultrasound is usually sufficient to identify an empty renal fossa; however, functional imaging such as a DMSA scan may distinguish URA from other possibilities with more certainty.[40]

The most reassuring finding with URA is the presence of a normal-appearing contralateral kidney displaying compensatory hypertrophy—renal length is greater than 95th percentile.[41] URA is associated with abnormalities of the contralateral kidney in almost one-third of cases, of which VUR is most common, occurring in 24%.[23] The presence of associated CAKUT and the absence of compensatory hypertrophy are independent risk factors for renal injury in children with solitary kidney.[42]

Although previously thought to be a relatively benign entity with compensatory hypertrophy preserving renal function, there is some more recent evidence that questions this assumption and strengthens the rationale for monitoring these children for the development of renal injury, specifically hypertension, microalbuminuria, or reduced GFR.[42,43]

The proposed mechanism of renal injury is based on the hyperfiltration hypothesis. The increased burden of glomerular filtration on the remaining nephron mass leads to hyperfiltration, precipitating glomerular hypertension and ultimately leading to sclerosis and loss of function, which further compounds the issue in a vicious cycle of diminishing nephron mass.

The goal of management in children with an SK is nephroprotection (prevention of further loss of nephron mass) and early identification of signs of glomerular hypertension. These include albuminuria and elevated blood pressure, both of which can perpetuate glomerular injury if left untreated. Our general approach is regular surveillance—blood pressure, urinalysis, and kidney function—which continues for life. The intention is detection in sufficient time to intervene and prevent further decline in kidney function.[44] Surveillance of growth of the contralateral kidney with ultrasound is also recommended. Despite the relatively high incidence of VUR in this population, neither routine VCUG nor antibiotic prophylaxis is recommended routinely.[44]

General nephroprotective measures such as avoiding nephrotoxic medication, for example, nonsteroidal antiinflammatory drugs, and urinary tract infection (UTI) prevention strategies are advised; these might include addressing dysfunctional voiding routines, avoidance of constipation, and ensuring adequate hydration.

Lifestyle advise to avoid obesity and excessive salt intake should be recommended, as these factors increase the risk of hypertension in an already at-risk cohort. Previous practice was to advise avoidance of contact sports due to a concern for direct traumatic injury to the single functioning kidney; however, recent evidence suggests this is not necessary.[45]

Cystic Kidney Disease

Postnatal management of suspected hereditary cystic kidney disease highly depends on the condition involved with the trajectory and priorities for children with ARPKD are quite different from those with nephronophthisis. Generally, infants suspected of having cystic kidney disease antenatally will be followed-up with postnatal ultrasound. Genetic investigations may be warranted depending on the clinical scenario, and ultrasound of the parents' kidneys is sometimes requested.

Multicystic Dysplastic Kidney

Historically the diagnosis of MCDK raised concerns for an increased risk of hypertension, and malignancy, often prompting surgical nephrectomy. However, a more conservative approach to management is now favored. Multiple studies have demonstrated that the natural history of MCDK is to involute over time, with the proportion of involution being 33% by 2 years of age, 47% by 5 years, and 59% by 10 years.[46] The risk of both malignancy and hypertension has been demonstrated to be very low.[47]

Ultrasound is sufficient to make a diagnosis of MCDK; confirmatory functional imaging is not routine. Contralateral VUR is reported in up to 21% of children with MCDK; this is usually low grade and self-resolving—VCUG is again not routinely recommended.[46,48]

In the authors' center, patients with a congenital SK and MCDK who demonstrate no other renal-urinary tract abnormalities and size of the normal kidney greater than 50th centile for length are followed-up at age 6 months and at 2, 5, 10, and 15 years with ultrasound, blood pressure, and urinalysis as well as a serum creatinine at age 5 and 15 years.[49]

Hypoplasia and Dysplasia

The clinical trajectory of children with renal hypoplasia depends on the degree of hypoplasia, whether it is unilateral or bilateral, and the presence of abnormal/dysplastic tissue. All children with suspicion on antenatal imaging should have postnatal follow-up to clarify the findings.

Children with unilateral hypoplasia are likely to do well; however, they should undergo intermittent surveillance to ensure adequate renal growth. Children with bilateral hypoplasia or those with evidence dysplasia should be offered renoprotective advise and be monitored for evolving renal injury—hypertension, proteinuria, and declining GFR.

Fusion Anomalies, Ectopia, and Duplication

Renal ectopia is often asymptomatic and detected either antenatally or on routine postnatal ultrasound performed for another indication. There is a high incidence of lower tract abnormalities associated with renal ectopia. VUR is present in 30% of children with simple unilateral ectopia and 20% with crossed ectopia.[18] The known association with VUR should prompt earlier referral for consideration of a VCUG in the context of other evidence of VUR such as dilatation on ultrasound or a history of UTI.

The most common fusion abnormality, the horseshoe kidney, is associated with urological abnormalities in up to 52% of children in one study; this may include VUR, PUJO, or ectopic ureter.[50] Kidney stones also have a higher incidence with horseshoe kidney (25%) in a recent review. The same report described the incidence of end-stage kidney disease was 2.6/10,000, which is higher than control individuals.[51] This risk of chronic kidney disease should prompt these children to be surveyed in a similar manner to those with SK.

Typically, unless abnormalities such as hydronephrosis are detected, or there are recurrent UTIs, duplication abnormalities do not require routine investigations or follow-up.

Antenatal Hydronephrosis

AH is one of the most common antenatal findings (1%–5%) and can represent a spectrum of conditions (**Box 2**). AH is not synonymous with obstruction, and in many cases it is a transient and self-resolving phenomenon.[52]

Measurement of the anteroposterior diameter (APD) of the renal pelvis is the simplest and probably most well-established method to classify AH.

It is widely accepted that increasing APD correlates with increasing risk of underlying pathology; however, the timing of the measurement is also relevant.[52–54] A renal pelvic diameter greater than 15 mm has a high likelihood of being associated with a clinically significant underlying pathology that may require surgical intervention.[52] Other clinically significant findings include bilateral involvement, abnormalities of the renal parenchyma, abnormalities of the bladder, or reduction in the amniotic fluid volume.[53]

It is important to consider hydronephrosis as a dynamic state—high-grade dilation can resolve, and low-grade can deteriorate. Most published guidelines recommend that all infants with AH have a postnatal ultrasound; this should be deferred until the infant is well hydrated, generally more than 72 hours, and should be completed within 1 to 4 weeks of birth, depending on the individual situation.[55] Late worsening or recurrent hydronephrosis is a well-recognized entity informing the suggestion that a single early postnatal ultrasound is inadequate to out-rule obstruction.[56] A repeat ultrasound at 4 to 6 weeks of life is generally recommended.[53]

Children with moderate to severe hydronephrosis should have further investigation, typically a VCUG and/or a MAG3 renogram. Mild to moderate AH does not warrant routine VCUG, given the invasive nature of this test, low risk of UTI, and the ambiguity regarding management of low-grade VUR, if identified.[57]

The role of continuous antibiotic prophylaxis (CAP) is also controversial in children with AH. The incidence of UTI in patients with low-grade hydronephrosis was reported as 2% to 5% in one study, climbing to 15% to 29% in children with higher grades of dilatation (SFU grade >3–4).[58] Similar results were found in a large systematic

---

Box 2
Causes of antenatal hydronephrosis

Most common
  Transient hydronephrosis
  UPJ obstruction
  VUR

Less common
  UVJ obstruction
  Posterior urethral valves/urethral abnormality
  Ureterocele/ectopic ureter

Uncommon
  Prune-Belly syndrome
  Cystic kidney disease

review—children with high-grade hydronephrosis were 4 times more likely to develop UTI than those with low-grade hydronephrosis. Both this and another more recent systematic review have suggested that CAP seems to be of benefit in the high-grade hydronephrosis group.[59,60] CAP is not warranted in mild hydronephrosis.[61] All parents of infants with hydronephrosis should be counseled on UTI awareness, as well as the possibility of late recurrence hydronephrosis, from UPJO, for example, which can present with flank or abdominal pain.

SUMMARY

Renal and urinary tract anomalies are the most common congenital anomaly and are being detected antenatally with increased frequency due to advancing sonographic technologies. Pediatricians will undoubtedly encounter children with these complex problems, and a broad understanding of the classification, investigation, and basis of management is important to appropriately direct their care.

CLINICS CARE POINTS

- Newborn male infants with moderate/severe bilateral hydrouteronephrosis should have an early postnatal ultrasound and VCUG to assess for bladder outlet obstruction, for example, posterior urethral valves.

- In general, non -urgent postnatal ultrasounds should be delayed for at least 72 hours, to allow for establishment of urinary flow and reduce the risk of underestimating hydronephrosis.

- Infants with mild antenatal hydronephrosis do not require routine VCUG or continuous antibiotic prophylaxis; however, parents should be counseled about UTI awareness.

- Despite the high prevalence of VUR in many forms of CAKUT, a VCUG is not indicated in all patients, as VUR alone is not viewed as a risk to kidney health. Rather, a VCUG is restricted to patients who present with a UTI or hydronephrosis.

- Infants and children with unilateral CAKUT and a normal-appearing contralateral kidney and no evidence of hydronephrosis on renal ultrasound do not require further initial evaluation. Intermittent follow-up is directed to determine normal growth of the contralateral kidney, absence of proteinuria, normal blood pressure, and a normal serum creatinine.

DISCLOSURE

No conflicts of interest to declare.

REFERENCES

1. Ardissino G, Daccò V, Testa S, et al. Epidemiology of Chronic Renal Failure in Children: Data From the ItalKid Project. Pediatrics 2003;111(4):e382–7. https://doi.org/10.1542/peds.111.4.e382.
2. Harambat J, van Stralen KJ, Kim JJ, et al. Epidemiology of chronic kidney disease in children. Pediatr Nephrol Berl Ger 2012;27(3):363–73. https://doi.org/10.1007/s00467-011-1939-1.
3. Dillon E, Walton SM. The antenatal diagnosis of fetal abnormalities: a 10 year audit of influencing factors. Br J Radiol 1997;70(832):341–6. https://doi.org/10.1259/bjr.70.832.9166068.
4. Queisser-Luft A, Stolz G, Wiesel A, et al. Malformations in newborn: results based on 30,940 infants and fetuses from the Mainz congenital birth defect monitoring system (1990-1998). Arch Gynecol Obstet 2002;266(3):163–7.

5. Melo BF, Aguiar MB, Bouzada MCF, et al. Early risk factors for neonatal mortality in CAKUT: analysis of 524 affected newborns. Pediatr Nephrol Berl Ger 2012; 27(6):965–72.
6. Wiesel A, Queisser-Luft A, Clementi M, et al, EUROSCAN Study Group. Prenatal detection of congenital renal malformations by fetal ultrasonographic examination: an analysis of 709,030 births in 12 European countries. Eur J Med Genet 2005;48(2):131–44.
7. Dudley JA, Haworth JM, McGraw ME, et al. Clinical relevance and implications of antenatal hydronephrosis. Arch Dis Child Fetal Neonatal Ed 1997;76(1):F31–4.
8. Ismaili K, Hall M, Donner C, et al. Results of systematic screening for minor degrees of fetal renal pelvis dilatation in an unselected population. Am J Obstet Gynecol 2003;188(1):242–6.
9. Potter EL. Normal and abnormal development of the kidney. Chicago: Year Book Medical Publishers; 1972.
10. Jain S, Chen F. Developmental pathology of congenital kidney and urinary tract anomalies. Clin Kidney J 2019;12(3):382–99.
11. Piscione TD, Rosenblum ND. The malformed kidney: disruption of glomerular and tubular development. Clin Genet 1999;56(5):341–56.
12. Dugoff L. Ultrasound diagnosis of structural abnormalities in the first trimester. Prenat Diagn 2002;22(4):316–20.
13. Cohen HL, Kravets F, Zucconi W, et al. Congenital abnormalities of the genitourinary system. Semin Roentgenol 2004;39(2):282–303.
14. Vanderheyden T, Kumar S, Fisk NM. Fetal renal impairment. Semin Neonatol SN 2003;8(4):279–89.
15. Sanna-Cherchi S, Westland R, Ghiggeri GM, et al. Genetic basis of human congenital anomalies of the kidney and urinary tract. J Clin Invest 2018; 128(1):4–15.
16. van der Ven AT, Vivante A, Hildebrandt F. Novel Insights into the Pathogenesis of Monogenic Congenital Anomalies of the Kidney and Urinary Tract. J Am Soc Nephrol JASN 2018;29(1):36–50.
17. Winyard P, Chitty L. Dysplastic and polycystic kidneys: diagnosis, associations and management. Prenat Diagn 2001;21(11):924–35.
18. Guarino N, Tadini B, Camardi P, et al. The incidence of associated urological abnormalities in children with renal ectopia. J Urol 2004;172(4 Pt 2):1757–9 [discussion: 1759].
19. Weizer AZ, Silverstein AD, Auge BK, et al. Determining the incidence of horseshoe kidney from radiographic data at a single institution. J Urol 2003;170(5): 1722–6.
20. Guay-Woodford LM, Bissler JJ, Braun MC, et al. Consensus expert recommendations for the diagnosis and management of autosomal recessive polycystic kidney disease: report of an international conference. J Pediatr 2014;165(3):611–7.
21. Zerres K, Rudnik-Schöneborn S, Senderek J, et al. Autosomal recessive polycystic kidney disease (ARPKD). J Nephrol 2003;16(3):453–8.
22. Torres VE, Harris PC. Autosomal dominant polycystic kidney disease: the last 3 years. Kidney Int 2009;76(2):149–68.
23. Westland R, Schreuder MF, Ket JCF, et al. Unilateral renal agenesis: a systematic review on associated anomalies and renal injury. Nephrol Dial Transpl 2013;28(7): 1844–55.
24. Cain JE, Di Giovanni V, Smeeton J, et al. Genetics of Renal Hypoplasia: Insights Into the Mechanisms Controlling Nephron Endowment. Pediatr Res 2010; 68(2):91–8.

25. Cohen HL, Cooper J, Eisenberg P, et al. Normal length of fetal kidneys: sonographic study in 397 obstetric patients. AJR Am J Roentgenol 1991;157(3): 545–8.

26. Damen-Elias HaM, De Jong TPVM, Stigter RH, et al. Congenital renal tract anomalies: outcome and follow-up of 402 cases detected antenatally between 1986 and 2001. Ultrasound Obstet Gynecol Off J Int Soc Ultrasound Obstet Gynecol 2005;25(2):134–43.

27. Murphy JJ, Altit G, Zerhouni S. The intrathoracic kidney: should we fix it? J Pediatr Surg 2012;47(5):970–3.

28. N'Guessen G, Stephens FD, Pick J. Congenital superior ectopic (thoracic) kidney. Urology 1984;24(3):219–28.

29. Glodny B, Petersen J, Hofmann KJ, et al. Kidney fusion anomalies revisited: clinical and radiological analysis of 209 cases of crossed fused ectopia and horseshoe kidney. BJU Int 2009;103(2):224–35.

30. Schwarz RD, Stephens FD, Cussen LJ. The pathogenesis of renal dysplasia. II. The significance of lateral and medial ectopy of the ureteric orifice. Invest Urol 1981;19(2):97–100.

31. Zissin R, Apter S, Yaffe D, et al. Renal duplication with associated complications in adults: CT findings in 26 cases. Clin Radiol 2001;56(1):58–63.

32. Kohl S, Habbig S, Weber LT, et al. Molecular causes of congenital anomalies of the kidney and urinary tract (CAKUT). Mol Cell Pediatr 2021;8(1):2.

33. Verbitsky M, Westland R, Perez A, et al. The copy number variation landscape of congenital anomalies of the kidney and urinary tract. Nat Genet 2019;51(1): 117–27.

34. Sanna-Cherchi S, Kiryluk K, Burgess KE, et al. Copy-number disorders are a common cause of congenital kidney malformations. Am J Hum Genet 2012; 91(6):987–97.

35. Tsatsaris V, Gagnadoux MF, Aubry MC, et al. Prenatal diagnosis of bilateral isolated fetal hyperechogenic kidneys. Is it possible to predict long term outcome? BJOG Int J Obstet Gynaecol 2002;109(12):1388–93.

36. Decramer S, Parant O, Beaufils S, et al. Anomalies of the TCF2 gene are the main cause of fetal bilateral hyperechogenic kidneys. J Am Soc Nephrol JASN 2007; 18(3):923–33.

37. Viteri B, Calle-Toro JS, Furth S, et al. State-of-the-Art Renal Imaging in Children. Pediatrics 2020;145(2):e20190829.

38. Bueva A, Guignard JP. Renal function in preterm neonates. Pediatr Res 1994; 36(5):572–7.

39. Westland R, Renkema KY, Knoers NVAM. Clinical integration of genome diagnostics for congenital anomalies of the kidney and urinary tract. Clin J Am Soc Nephrol 2021;16(1):128–37.

40. Grabnar J, Rus RR. Is renal scintigraphy really a necessity in the routine diagnosis of congenital solitary kidney? Pediatr Surg Int 2019;35(6):729–35.

41. van Vuuren SH, van der Doef R, Cohen-Overbeek TE, et al. Compensatory enlargement of a solitary functioning kidney during fetal development. Ultrasound Obstet Gynecol 2012;40(6):665–8.

42. Westland R, Kurvers RAJ, van Wijk JAE, et al. Risk factors for renal injury in children with a solitary functioning kidney. Pediatrics 2013;131(2):e478–85.

43. Kim S, Chang Y, Lee YR, et al. Solitary kidney and risk of chronic kidney disease. Eur J Epidemiol 2019;34(9):879–88.

44. Groen in 't Woud S, Westland R, et al. Clinical management of children with a congenital solitary functioning kidney: overview and recommendations. Eur Urol Open Sci 2021;25:11–20.
45. Psooy K, Franc-Guimond J, Kiddoo D, et al. Canadian Urological Association Best Practice Report: Sports and the solitary kidney — What primary caregivers of a young child with a single kidney should know (2019 update). Can Urol Assoc J 2019;13(10):315–7.
46. Aslam M, Watson AR. Unilateral multicystic dysplastic kidney: long term outcomes. Arch Dis Child 2006;91(10):820–3.
47. Chang A, Sivananthan D, Nataraja RM, et al. Evidence-based treatment of multicystic dysplastic kidney: a systematic review. J Pediatr Urol 2018;14(6):510–9.
48. Kuwertz-Broeking E, Brinkmann OA, Von Lengerke HJ, et al. Unilateral multicystic dysplastic kidney: experience in children. BJU Int 2004;93(3):388–92.
49. Jawa NA, Rosenblum ND, Radhakrishnan S, et al. Reducing unnecessary imaging in children with multicystic dysplastic kidney or solitary kidney. Pediatrics 2021;148(2). e2020035550.
50. Cascio S, Sweeney B, Granata C, et al. Vesicoureteral reflux and ureteropelvic junction obstruction in children with horseshoe kidney: treatment and outcome. J Urol 2002;167(6):2566–8.
51. Kang M, Kim YC, Lee H, et al. Renal outcomes in adult patients with horseshoe kidney. Nephrol Dial 2021;36(3):498–503.
52. Lee RS, Cendron M, Kinnamon DD, et al. Antenatal hydronephrosis as a predictor of postnatal outcome: a meta-analysis. Pediatrics 2006;118(2):586–93.
53. Nguyen HT, Herndon CDA, Cooper C, et al. The Society for Fetal Urology consensus statement on the evaluation and management of antenatal hydronephrosis. J Pediatr Urol 2010;6(3):212–31.
54. Capolicchio JP, Braga LH, Szymanski KM. Canadian Urological Association/Pediatric Urologists of Canada guideline on the investigation and management of antenatally detected hydronephrosis. Can Urol Assoc J 2018;12(4):85–92.
55. Dejter SW, Gibbons MD. The fate of infant kidneys with fetal hydronephrosis but initially normal postnatal sonography. J Urol 1989;142(2 Pt 2):661–2. https://doi.org/10.1016/s0022-5347(17)38846-8 [discussion: 667-668].
56. Matsui F, Shimada K, Matsumoto F, et al. Late recurrence of symptomatic hydronephrosis in patients with prenatally detected hydronephrosis and spontaneous improvement. J Urol 2008;180(1):322–5. https://doi.org/10.1016/j.juro.2008.03.065 [discussion: 325].
57. Szymanski KM, Al-Said AN, Pippi Salle JL, et al. Do infants with mild prenatal hydronephrosis benefit from screening for vesicoureteral reflux? J Urol 2012;188(2):576–81.
58. Montini G, Rigon L, Zucchetta P, et al. Prophylaxis after first febrile urinary tract infection in children? A multicenter, randomized, controlled, noninferiority trial. Pediatrics 2008;122(5):1064–71.
59. Braga LH, Mijovic H, Farrokhyar F, et al. Antibiotic prophylaxis for urinary tract infections in antenatal hydronephrosis. Pediatrics 2013;131(1):e251–61.
60. Easterbrook B, Capolicchio JP, Braga LH. Antibiotic prophylaxis for prevention of urinary tract infections in prenatal hydronephrosis: An updated systematic review. Can Urol Assoc J J Assoc Urol Can 2017;11(1–2Suppl1):S3–11.
61. Yalçınkaya F, Özçakar ZB. Management of antenatal hydronephrosis. Pediatr Nephrol Berl Ger 2020;35(12):2231–9.

Diagnosis and Management of Nephrolithiasis in Children

Larisa Kovacevic, MD*

KEYWORDS

- Nephrolithiasis • Hypercalciuria • Hyperuricosuria • Hypocitraturia • Cystinuria
- Hyperoxaluria • Lithotripsy • Nephrolithotomy

KEY POINTS

- Nephrolithiasis is a common condition in pediatric population; a predisposing cause for stone formation is found in approximately two-thirds of affected children.
- Hypercalciuria and hypocitraturia are the commonest causes of kidney stones in children.
- Initial evaluation should include a detailed history and physical examination, laboratory investigation, stone fragment analysis, and radiological imaging of the urinary tract.
- Stones up to 5 mm have a high likelihood of spontaneous passage in children of all ages. Depending on size and location of the stone, a surgical intervention may be necessary.
- All patients with nephrolithiasis should be advised increased fluid intake, dietary salt restriction, and an increased intake of vegetables and fruits.

INTRODUCTION

Kidney stone disease or nephrolithiasis is a common condition in the pediatric population and its prevalence and incidence have increased in the last decade.[1–4] Changes in epidemiology, etiology, and stone composition that have been noted in pediatric nephrolithiasis are partly related to the modern lifestyle.[5,6] New trends for nephrolithiasis in children are notable. These include a marked increase in the annual incidence of nephrolithiasis, particularly among children between 12 and 17 years of age, females, and African Americans; a change in the most common cause of nephrolithiasis from infectious to metabolic causes; hypocitraturia replacing hypercalciuria as the main metabolic risk factor in older children; and changes in stone composition from ammonium and urate to calcium.[7–9]

In contrast with adults, pediatric patients have a heterogeneous clinical presentation; a high frequency of an underlying etiology (anatomic and genetic in younger

Department of Pediatric Urology, Michigan State University and Central Michigan University, Stone Clinic, Children's Hospital of Michigan, 3901 Beaubien Boulevard, Detroit 48201, MI, USA
* Corresponding author.
E-mail address: lkovacev@dmc.org

Pediatr Clin N Am 69 (2022) 1149–1164
https://doi.org/10.1016/j.pcl.2022.07.008
0031-3955/22/© 2022 Elsevier Inc. All rights reserved.

pediatric.theclinics.com

and metabolic in older children); a great variability of risk factors in relation to age, gender, and race; and a high rate of recurrence posing the risk for chronicity.[10–13] Moreover, nephrolithiasis has a significant morbidity owing to its association with various conditions such as cardiovascular disease, diabetes mellitus, the metabolic syndrome, atherosclerosis, low bone mineral density, and chronic kidney disease.[14–20] Without adequate treatment nephrolithiasis may lead to obstruction, urinary tract infections, and recurrent pain. Therefore, the optimal management of pediatric nephrolithiasis is important to prevent recurrence and associated complications, and preserve kidney function.

Epidemiology

A 4% to 16% annual increase in the incidence of pediatric nephrolithiasis has been noted over the past 2 decades.[1–3] However, the prevalence, incidence, and risk of nephrolithiasis vary with gender, age, race, climate, geographic location, dietary habits, and socioeconomic factors. Boys are more affected in the first decade of life and girls in the second decade.[21] This difference is due to the main risk factor for stones in these age groups, namely, obstructive urinary malformations in boys and urinary tract infections in postpubertal, sexually active girls. Children aged 14 to 18 years have a 10.2-fold greater risk for nephrolithiasis and hospitalization as compared with children 0 to 13 years of age.[7] Nephrolithiasis is more common in non-Hispanic White children as compared with Hispanic children and is least common in African American children.[22–24] A higher incidence of kidney stones has been reported in children living in Western countries (5%–10% of that in adults), in rural communities, and in those living in hot and dry climate.

Pathogenesis

The mechanism of stone formation is explained by 3 theories: (1) the free particle theory, (2) the fixed particle theory, and (3) the vascular theory of Randall's plaque formation. The initiation and growth of calculus requires high urinary solute concentration (supersaturation) and low urinary volume. Further growth and aggregation are favored by ionic strength, urinary pH, and the concentration of promoters (calcium, oxalate, sodium, urate, and cystine) and inhibitors of crystallization (citrate, magnesium, pyrophosphate, glycosaminoglycans, Tamm-Horsfall protein, and osteopontin).

The free particle theory[25] is particularly important for stone formation in cystinuria, where high urinary levels of cystine initiate intratubular nucleation. Adherence to the epithelial renal tubular cells is required to allow for crystal growth (the fixed particle theory),[26] a process especially important in patients with brushite and apatite stones. Injured renal tubular cells by either toxins, infection, or medications (eg, calcineurin inhibitors and gentamycin) favor crystal attachment. The expected urine washout of crystal aggregates is impaired by stasis caused by congenital anomalies of the urinary tract.

In Randall's hypothesis, apatite plaques or other sources of uroepithelial damage such as infection and foreign bodies represent a nidus for calcium oxalate stone formation.[27] Randall's plaque originates from the basal membrane of the thin loops of Henle, expands through the interstitium, and protrudes into the papillary vasculature causing injury and repair in an atherosclerosis like fashion.[28] This theory, which accounts for stones that seem to be embedded in the papillary wall, is supported by the physiology of turbulent flow, high osmolality, and hypoxia in the renal papilla.[29]

Etiology

A predisposing cause for stone formation is found in approximately two-thirds of affected children. These include metabolic ($\leq$95% cases), anatomic ($\leq$32% cases), and urinary tract infections ($\leq$24% cases), alone or in combination.[30,31] The composition of stones varies with calcium oxalate being the most common.[30,32]

Metabolic risk factors

A detailed list of metabolic risk factors for nephrolithiasis in children in presented in **Table 1**. The more common causes are discussed here.

Hypercalciuria is the most common metabolic abnormality in children with kidney stones. It is found in 50% to 97% of those with identifiable underlying metabolic disease. Hypercalciuria is mostly idiopathic and polygenic, caused by disturbances in the kidney (decreased calcium reabsorption in the renal tubules, ie, renal hypercalciuria), intestinal tract (increased calcium intestinal absorption, ie, absorptive hypercalciuria), and bone (increased calcium bone resorption, ie, resorptive hypercalciuria).

Hyperoxaluria is found in approximately 10% to 20% of children with nephrolithiasis. The most common is idiopathic hyperoxaluria, which is mostly seen in association with hypercalciuria and causes calcium oxalate stones.

Hyperuricosuria is seen in 2% to 8% of children with nephrolithiasis. Pure uric acid stones in children are rare. These occur owing to an overproduction of uric acid owing

Table 1	
Metabolic causes of nephrolithiasis	
Condition	**Metabolic Causes**
Hypercalciuria	Idiopathic
	Inherited
	Polygenic (renal, absorptive, resorptive);
	Monogenic (Dent and Bartter diseases)
	Hypercalcemia: vitamin D excess, hyperparathyroidism, sarcoidosis,
	malignancy, William syndrome
	Primary distal renal tubular acidosis
	Metabolic acidosis
	Loop diuretics, glucocorticoids, ketogenic diet
	Immobilization
	Excessive sodium intake
	Medullary sponge kidney
Hyperoxaluria	Idiopathic
	Primary hyperoxaluria types I, II, and III
	Secondary hyperoxaluria
	Excessive oxalate ingestion (ethylene glycol, ascorbic acid, and
	methoxyflurane);
	Fat malabsorption (cystic fibrosis, celiac disease, Inflammatory bowel
	disease, short bowel syndrome, pancreatitis);
	Medication (orlistat)
Hypocitraturia	Idiopathic
	Chronic metabolic acidosis (chronic diarrhea, distal tubular acidosis,
	medication: topiramate, acetazolamide)
	Hypokalemia
	Ketogenic diet
Hyperuricosuria	Idiopathic
	Dietary: excessive purine intake, ketogenic diet
	Metabolic syndrome
	Overproduction of uric acid: tumor lysis syndrome, malignant
	proliferative disorders
	Genetic disorders: Lesch–Nyhan syndrome, glycogen storage disease
Cystinuria	Cystinuria: types I, II, and III

to tumor lysis syndrome, lymphoproliferative and myeloproliferative disorders, and genetic disorders (Lesch–Nyhan syndrome and glycogen storage disorders).

Cystinuria is found in approximately 5% of children with renal calculi. It is an autosomal-recessive disorder of renal tubular transport caused by mutations in 2 genes, SLC3A1 and SLC7A9. Cystinuria is characterized by excessive excretion of the dibasic amino acids cystine, ornithine, lysine, and arginine. The hexagonal cystine crystals are pathognomonic, but are seen only in 20% to 25% of cases. Recurrent nephrolithiasis is common.

Hypocitraturia in children is increasing and now seems to be one of the leading causes of pediatric renal stones in older children.[9] Citrate combines with calcium in the tubular lumen to form a soluble complex resulting in less free calcium available to combine with oxalate. Citrate also inhibits crystal aggregation and growth.

Anatomic risk factors
Congenital and structural abnormalities of kidney and the urinary tract are associated with urinary stasis, which facilitates stone formation. The most common conditions are medullary sponge disease, autosomal dominant polycystic kidney disease, ureteropelvic junction obstruction, ureterocele, horseshoe kidney, bladder exstrophy, neuropathic bladder, and surgically reconstructed or augmented bladders.

Urinary tract infection as a risk factor
Urinary tract infection occurs in approximately one-fourth of children with nephrolithiasis, and it may either be the cause or the result of stone disease. It is commonly seen in boys younger than 5 years of age with obstructive uropathy. Urease produced by bacteria such as Proteus, Klebsiella, Pseudomonas, and enterococci breaks down urea to form ammonium and bicarbonate. This creates a favorable milieu for struvite stones (magnesium ammonium phosphate), which can further grow into the renal calyces, and produce staghorn calculi.

Other risk factors for nephrolithiasis include (1) prematurity and low birth weight and the use of diuretics and nephrotoxic drugs, (2) chronic bowel disease owing to malabsorption and increased intestinal absorption of oxalate, (3) neurological diseases owing to immobilization and poor water intake, and (4) administration of commonly used medications such as antibiotics (cephalosporins, fluoroquinolones and broad-spectrum penicillins) diuretics, and anticonvulsants.

CLINICAL PRESENTATION

The presenting symptoms of nephrolithiasis differ in children as compared with adults and depend on the child's age. Typical renal colic and gross hematuria are more often seen in older children and adolescents, who have higher rates of ureteral stones and spontaneous passage. Younger children may present with irritability, vomiting, nonspecific abdominal pain, microhematuria, and urinary tract infection. Gross or microscopic hematuria is seen in approximately one-half of the children with nephrolithiasis and dysuria and frequency is seen in approximately 10% of cases. Urinary retention and pain may occur with obstruction. Other presentations include failure to thrive, hypertension, and kidney failure; enuresis, penile edema, and anorexia have been reported rarely.

Initial Evaluation of a Child with Nephrolithiasis

A comprehensive diagnostic evaluation should be performed in every child who presents with nephrolithiasis because it will guide treatment and will allow a better prevention strategy.[33–35] This workup consists of a detailed history and physical examination; laboratory investigation such as serum chemistry, urine microscopy, and solute excretion rates; stone fragment analysis when available; and radiological imaging of the urinary tract as elaborated in **Fig. 1**.

Spot urines for calcium, citrate, uric acid, and oxalate can be used for the initial screening for a metabolic abnormality. The normal values for age, gender, body weight, and body surface area are presented in **Table 2**. Spot urines are particularly important in children who are not toilet trained and in those in whom a 24-hour urine collection may not be possible. Whenever possible, a timed 24-hour urine collection should be obtained to confirm the results of initial screening by spot urine. A timed collection provides information on urine volume and saturation, as well as urinary excretion of calcium, phosphorus, oxalate, citrate, uric acid, sodium, potassium, and magnesium. In view of a day-to-day variation in diet and fluid intake, two 24-hour urine collections are preferred. Urine creatinine should be checked to verify the completeness of urine collection; a concentration of greater than 15 mg/kg/d is desired. The timed collection should be performed without altering the child's usual fluid or dietary intake or activity, in the absence of a urinary tract infection, and at least 1 month after the spontaneous passage of stone or surgical intervention. Patients should be asked to complete a diet diary at the same time as 24-hour urine collection. The diary should include the type and amount of each consumed food and drink.

Stone analysis is an important step in the evaluation of nephrolithiasis. The composition of all recovered stone fragments should be analyzed by either infrared spectroscopy or x-ray diffraction, and components exceeding 5% should be reported. This should be done with each passage of stone because the composition may differ from time to time. Most kidney stones are calcium based.[15]

Radiologic Imaging

Initial diagnostic imaging is aimed at detecting the stone, estimating the stone size and its likelihood of passing, identifying whether it is obstructing urinary flow that may need

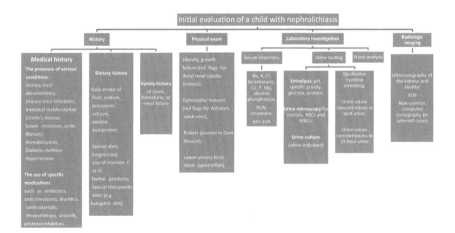

Fig. 1. Evaluation of nephrolithiasis. BUN, blood urea nitrogen; Ca, calcium; Cl, chloride; K, potassium; KUB, kidney, ureter, and bladder radiograph; Mg, magnesium; Na, sodium; P, phosphorus; RBCs, red blood cells; WBCs, white blood cells.

Table 2
Normal values for urinary metabolite excretion

	Age	Random in mg/mg (mmol/mmol)	Timed (All Ages)
Calcium	0–6 months	<0.8[a]	<4 mg/kg per 24 hours
	7–12 months	<0.6[a]	(<0.1 mmol/kg per 24 hours)
	>2 years	<0.2[a]	
Oxalate	0–6 months	<0.26[a]	<40 mg/1.73 m^2 per 24 hours
	7–24 months	<0.11[a]	(<0.5 mmol/1.73 m^2 per
	2–5 years	<0.08[a]	24 hours)
	5–14 years	<0.06[a]	
	>16 years	<0.32[a]	
Cystine	> 6 months	<0.075[a]	<60 mg/1.73 m^2 per 24 hours
			(<250 μmol/1.73 m^2 per
			24 hours)
Uric acid	<1 year	<2.2 (<1.5)	<815 mg/1.73 m^2 per 24 hours
	1–3 years	<1.9 (<1.3)	(<486 mmol/1.73 m^2 per
	3–5 years	<1.5 (<1.0)	24 hours)
	5–10 years	<0.9 (<0.6)	
	>10 years	<0.6 (<0.4)	
Citrate[b]	0–5 years	>0.2–0.42 (>0.12–0.25)	>310 mg/1.73 m2 per 24 hours
	>5 years	>0.14–0.25 (>0.08–0.15)	(>1.6 mmol/1.73 m^2 per
			24 hours) in girls;
			>365 mg/1.73 m2 per 24 hours
			(>1.9 mmol/1.73 m^2 per
			24 hours) in boys
Magnesium	> 2 years	>0.13[a]	>0.8 mg/kg (>0.04 mmol/kg)

[a] Same value for mg/mg and mmol/mmol.
[b] A range for normal random citrate values is presented in the table to account for regional variations.

surgical intervention, and diagnosing any structural abnormality of the urinary tract that might cause local urinary stasis.

Ultrasound examination is the mainstay of initial radiological imaging[36–39] Simultaneous plain abdominal radiograph showing the kidney, ureter, and bladder should be performed to identify ureteral stones and to appreciate the calcium content of the stone. A computed tomography scan without contrast is used sparingly during the initial evaluation of nephrolithiasis in children owing to its high risk of radiation (**Table 3**). Low radiation dose, noncontrast computed tomography scan protocols have been developed for pediatric patients and are mainly indicated when the patient is symptomatic and a stone is suspected but not seen by ultrasound examination.

Acute Management

The immediate treatment goals during an acute stone episode include management of pain, nausea and vomiting, hydration, and associated infection, if present. Pain control can be achieved with oral nonsteroidal anti-inflammatory medications (if renal function and hydration are adequate) or with oral or intravenous narcotics (eg morphine 0.3 mg/ kg by mouth every 3–4 hours or 0.05 mg/kg intravenously every 2–4 hours). The preferred antiemetic agent is ondansetron because of its minimal side effects; metoclopramide hydrochloride or prochlorperazine are also acceptable options.

With adequate pain control, uncomplicated unilateral stones causing only minimal or partial obstruction can be managed conservatively for several weeks before

Table 3
Radiologic imaging of the kidneys and the urinary tract

Ultrasound Examination (Sensitivity 77%–90%)	Plain Abdominal Radiography (Kidney, Ureter, and Bladder) (Sensitivity 45%–58%)	Noncontrast Computed Tomography Scan (Sensitivity 90%–100%)
Advantages		
Easy to perform, no pain, no radiation, low cost, no need for anesthesia	Detects large enough ureteral stones not seen on ultrasound examination	Detects small and radiolucent stones
Shows stones of all compositions	Detects calcium (radiodense), struvite and cystine stones (intermediate radiodensity)	Provides anatomic details of the kidneys and urinary tract.
Reveals the anatomy of the kidneys and the urinary tract, detects hydronephrosis		
Can be repeated as many times as needed		
Disadvantages		
Operator dependent	Misses radiolucent stones: uric acid, xanthine, and indinavir	Risk of malignancy with radiation
Overestimates stone size		Potential need for sedation
Can miss ureteral calculi, papillary or calyceal stones, and small calculi (<5 mm)	Risk of malignancy with radiation	High cost
Stone visualization can be affected by the body habitus and bowel gas		

surgical intervention is considered. Stones up to 5 mm in size have a high likelihood of spontaneous passage in children of all ages. Medical expulsive therapy for smaller ureteral stones has been used, especially in older children, with some success. The most commonly used agent is tamsulosin, which causes relaxation of ureteral smooth muscle with inhibition of ureteral spasm and dilatation of the ureter. Alternatively, alpha blockers or calcium channel blockers can be used to facilitate the passage of ureteral stones that are less than 10 mm in size.[39–43] During an acute episode, all patients with a stone should be asked to filter urine through a sieve to capture stones for analysis.

The indications for hospitalization include the following:

- An urgent need for upper tract decompression (nephrostomy tube or a lower urinary tract stent).
- Severe vomiting requiring intravenous hydration.
- Severe pain requiring intravenous analgesia.
- Urosepsis or acute pyelonephritis requiring intravenous antibiotic therapy.

METABOLIC WORKUP AND EVALUATION FOR RISK OF RECURRENT UROLITHIASIS

After the initial presentation and acute management, children with nephrolithiasis should be evaluated for risk factors that might predispose to recurrence of stone formation.[34,35] This step is particularly important in pediatrics because of a high risk of recurrence that reaches up to 50% within 3 years from the first episode of nephrolithiasis.[44] The rate of recurrence is higher in patients with an identifiable metabolic abnormality and in those with a family history of stones in first-degree relatives.[45] Additionally, recurrent stone formers have a 2 times higher risk of developing chronic kidney disease and end-stage kidney failure compared with nonstone formers.[1] Ideally, a combined stone clinic should provide nephrology and urology expertise, genetic testing, dietary services, and access to appropriate metabolic laboratory investigation.

Basic metabolic panel testing and 24-hour urine analysis should be repeated. Blood levels of parathyroid hormone and 1,25-dihydroxyvitamin D are additional tests required in some patients with calcium-based stones and when abnormal blood levels of calcium and/or phosphorus are identified. Primary hyperparathyroidism is rare in children, but evidence for suppression of parathyroid hormone offers a clue to states of vitamin D excess. Moreover, a workup for uric acid stones up should include serum uric acid levels and enzyme assays to check if hyperuricosuria is due to enzyme deficiencies.[46] The measurement of blood level oxalate is important in hyperoxaluria to identify the primary types of the disease.

Genetic testing should be considered in following patients:

- Young age at presentation and strong family history of stone disease, as well as consanguineous marriages.
- Failure to thrive with developmental delay, dysmorphic features, vision and hearing impairment, or presence of rickets.
- Recurrent stones in spite of treatment.
- Presence of rare tubulopathies.
- Stone composition (cysteine, uric acid, dihydroadenine, xanthine).

Early recognition of the monogenic forms of nephrolithiasis such as primary hyperoxalurias, cystinuria, distal renal tubular acidosis, Dent's disease, Bartter syndrome, and adenine phosphoribosyl transferase deficiency will allow timely treatment and prevention of various complications including irreversible kidney damage.

Follow-up Imaging and Surveillance

Repeat metabolic assessment and renal ultrasound examinations are needed to diagnose stone recurrence or increasing size of an existing stone. The frequency of these tests depends on the presence and severity of the metabolic abnormality, the number of stones and recurrence rate. A child with a single stone and no evidence of an underlying metabolic abnormality will require less frequent monitoring than a child with multiple stones or a significant metabolic problem associated with recurrent nephrolithiasis such as primary hyperoxaluria or cystinuria. Compliance with high fluid intake should be monitored by measuring urine specific gravity. Children receiving drug therapy should be closely monitored for adverse effects.

In an asymptomatic child, a repeat ultrasound examination is usually performed 6 months after the initial episode. If the ultrasound examination shows no stone recurrence or change in residual stone size, the study can be performed yearly. A metabolic workup is repeated 4 to 6 weeks after therapy has been initiated. If the metabolic abnormality was corrected, repeat studies should be done at 6 months, and then yearly. Reevaluation is needed if metabolic abnormalities persist.

Treatment

Treatment of nephrolithiasis includes dietary modification and pharmacological intervention.

Dietary Modification

A general dietary recommendation in all children with nephrolithiasis, regardless of etiology, include high fluid consumption, salt restriction, and increased intake of vegetables and fruits, as well as a high-fiber diet (**Table 4**).[47,48] Aggressive fluid intake that is evenly distributed throughout the day is aimed to prevent tubular precipitation of various salts. Adequate hydration can be estimated from the urine specific gravity and/or urine osmolality. Water is preferable to help avoid the side effects of sugary drinks. Furthermore, fructose found in sweet beverages may increase the urinary excretion of calcium and oxalate and thus enhance the risk of stone formation or its enlargement. Fruits and vegetables represent a good source of potassium, which facilitates urinary citrate excretion, and a good source of phytates, which increase the solubility of calcium salt. A high-fiber diet facilitates the binding of intestinal calcium.

Excessive salt intake causes increased excretion of urinary calcium and sodium restriction is advised in all stone formers. Patients should be advised to avoid adding salt or sodium-rich seasoning to food either during preparation or during consumption. Processed and canned food should also be avoided.

Restriction of calcium and protein intake is not recommended in children because they are necessary for growth and bone health. Additionally, calcium binds to free oxalate in the digestive tract and prevents hyperoxaluria. Avoiding high oxalate food, such as chocolate, spinach, nuts, and cola, is particularly helpful in children with secondary hyperoxaluria.[31] Patients with hyperuricosuria should be advised low intake of purine-containing foods such as red meat.

Targeted Therapy

Targeted pharmacological therapy based on the identified metabolic risk factor(s) is presented in **Table 5**. Urinary alkalinization with oral potassium citrate to achieve a pH of greater than 7.0 is useful in patients with distal renal tubular acidosis or hypercalciuria, hyperoxaluria, hyperuricosuria, hypocitraturia, and cystinuria because it increases the solubility of these solutes.[49–51] The recommended dose is 0.5 to 2.0 mmol/kg/d in divided doses, which effectively and safely decreases urinary calcium without significant adverse effects. Potassium citrate therapy should be taken after a meal or with a snack and with a big glass of water to prevent stomach pain, which could cause poor therapy adherence. Urinary pH should be closely monitored, because a higher pH may decrease the solubility of phosphate leading to calcium phosphate urolithiasis. Additionally, serum K and bicarbonate should be measured periodically. Another treatment option for urinary alkalinization is high lemon extract intake (the lemon protocol), but there are no studies to prove its efficiency in pediatrics

Table 4
General dietary recommendations in pediatric nephrolithiasis

Factor	Recommendation
Fluid Intake	High at >2 L/1.73 m²/d, mainly water
Sodium intake	Low at <3 mEq/kg/d
Vegetables and fruit intake	High
Calcium intake	100% of the daily allowance
Protein intake	100% of the daily allowance
Vitamin D intake	Supplement if low
Vitamin C intake	Avoid excess

Table 5
Pharmacologic intervention in pediatric nephrolithiasis

Condition	Pharmacologic Treatment	Adverse Effects
Hypercalciuria	Hydrochlorothiazide (1 to 2 mg/kg per day, older children 25–100 mg/d)	Hypokalemia, hyponatremia, or hyperuricemia
Hyperoxaluria	Pyridoxine (5–10 mg/kg/d) for primary hyperoxaluria Magnesium (if hypomagnesuria is present) Calcium supplements[a] Treatment of secondary hyperoxaluria should be directed at the treatment of the underlying cause	Numbness and tingling, drowsiness, decreased sensation, sensory nerve damage, nausea, loss of appetite, decreased folic acid Diarrhea, muscle weakness, fatigue Constipation, bloating
Hyperuricosuria	Allopurinol (4–10 mg/kg/d, older children 300 mg/d)[b]	Nausea, diarrhea, stomach upset, skin rash, changes in liver function test
Cystinuria	Tiopronin (5 mg/kg/dose 3 times a day) D-Penicillamine (30 mg/kg/d divided in 4 doses) Captopril (0.5–1.5 mg/kg/d divided in 4 doses)	Skin and mucosal eruption Arthralgias Zinc and copper deficiency Lupus like drug reaction, myasthenia gravis like reaction, pemphigus Hematological: aplastic anemia, neutropenia, thrombocytopenia Altered taste Renal: proteinuria Vitamin B deficiency Hyperkalemia Elevated serum creatinine Cough

[a] Calcium supplements can be prescribed because calcium binds to oxalate in the intestinal tract forming calcium oxalate complex that is excreted in the feces. However, calcium should be taking during a meal because otherwise can cause hypercalciuria.
[b] Reserved for children with a known disorder of uric acid metabolism.

and it may not be well-tolerated in children, leading to noncompliance.[52.] Sodium citrate should be avoided because increased sodium intake increases the risk of stone formation.

Thiazide diuretics (eg, hydrochlorothiazide and chlorthalodine) decrease urinary calcium excretion by causing volume contraction that increases calcium absorption in the proximal tubule.[53–56] The starting dose is 0.5 to 1.0 mg/kg/d as a single dose, titrated to achieve maximum efficacy and good tolerance. Laboratory monitoring is required because it may cause hypokalemia, hyponatremia, or hyperuricemia. Long-term nonadherence to medication is reported in approximately one-third of patients and hypercalciuria recurs in 44% cases when the medication is discontinued.[56]

Children with cystinuria require aggressive hydration, low salt intake, a limited animal protein diet, and urinary alkalinization. In many cases, these measures are insufficient and a cystine-binding thiol containing medication (D-penicillamine, tiopronin, and captopril) is needed. Both D-penicillamine and tiopronin act by reducing the disulfide bond of cystine to produce 2 molecules of cysteine. Both drugs are equally effective and have similar results. Owing to potential significant adverse effects, each drug should be started at a lower dose and should be gradually increased based on urinary cystine concentration over several weeks. The targeted goal is a urinary cystine concentration of less than 1250 μmol/L.[57] Close dose monitoring for both efficacy and toxicity is required, with the goal of effectively reducing urinary cystine levels, while minimizing side effects.

Surgical Treatment

The indications for surgical management are as follows.

- Large (>5 mm), obstructing, and infected stones.
- History of sepsis with kidney stone.
- Patients with acute kidney injury owing to obstruction.
- Patients with pain refractory to analgesics.

Various minimally invasive surgery (techniques are available for stone removal from kidney and the urinary tract. These include extracorporeal shock wave lithotripsy (ESWL), ureteroscopy, percutaneous nephrolithotomy, and laparoscopic and robotic surgery (pyelolithotomy and nephrolithotomy). These procedures are increasingly being used in children because they allow faster recovery than open surgery, but run the risk of a need for repeat procedures (**Table 6**).[58–61]

The choice of surgical intervention depends on the child's age and body habitus, stone characteristics (composition, size, and location), number of calculi (single vs multiple), presence of obstruction or infection, the anatomy of the urinary tract, associated conditions (bladder dysfunction), patient or family preference, and the surgeon's experience and skills. Careful patient selection for the best choice of minimally invasive surgery ensures a better outcome for stone treatment and renal preservation as well as patient safety.

Open surgery is mainly reserved for patients with associated congenital renal anomalies requiring anatomical repair combined with stone removal (such as ureteropelvic or ureterovesical junction obstruction), for infected and staghorn stones, and for patients with previous multiple abdominal surgeries (augmented bladder with large bladder calculus).

ESWL is usually successful in children and is becoming the first-line intervention in many centers.[59,62] The likelihood of success depends on stone size (lower with larger stones), stone location (poorer with calyceal stones located in the lower pole compared with those located in the upper and mid-pole), stone composition (lower with struvite, cystine and calcium oxalate monohydrate), and the number of previous ESWL sessions. Struvite fragments in particular are friable facilitating stone fragment retention. Decreased urine output in chronic kidney disease may also compromise the stone clearance. Success rates are lower in children with an abnormal anatomy of the urinary tract or obesity.

Repeated ESWL may be needed for stones larger than 1.5 cm, and nomograms and scoring systems for prediction of outcomes after ESWL have been developed.[63–65] Younger children require an insertion of a ureteral stent. Stones larger than 1.5 to 2.0 cm are not usually amenable to ESWL and will require other surgical techniques including percutaneous nephrolithotomy, ureteroscopy or retrograde intrarenal surgery, and robotic-assisted pyelolithotomy.[66] Nephrectomy may be a consideration if renal function is markedly decreased, in association with a large stone burden and recurrent urinary tract infections. Infected stones require careful antibiotic treatment because bacteria may be released during stone fragmentation after any surgical procedure.

Table 6
Surgical management of pediatric nephrolithiasis

Indications and Advantages	Disadvantages and Specific Complications
ESWL	
First-line treatment of small renal and proximal ureteral stones <1.5 cm	Ureteric obstruction with stone fragments causing pain[1]
Noninvasive outpatient approach	Debate on the long-term effect on the kidney development
High safety, minimal morbidity	
Overall success rate range of 81%–96%	
Ureteroscopy/retrograde intrarenal surgery	
Best choice for stones located in the lower pole calices (<1.5–2.0 cm) and for mid- or distal ureteral stones (<1.0 cm)	Ureteral injury, which may be prevented by a double stent placement for 2–3 weeks before the treatment to induce passive ureteral dilatation
Shorter operative time and in-hospital stay owing to less invasive approach	
Good visualization owing to their fiber optic and video systems	
The stone can be directly extracted (using basket or grasping forceps), or can be fragmented (by laser or electrohydraulic or ultrasonic probes)	
Overall success rate range from 47% to 100%	
Percutaneous nephrolithotomy	
Best choice for kidney stones >1.5 cm and staghorn stones;	Longer operative time and in-hospital stay owing to more invasive approach;
B Overall success rate ranges from 67% to 100%	Hemorrhage (0.4%–23.9% of cases), which can be severe requiring blood transfusion
	Can be difficult in patients with obesity, hemorrhagic diathesis, and renal tumors
	Renal pelvis perforation
Laparoscopic and robotic surgery (pyelolithotomy and nephrolithotomy)	
Indicated in hard stones difficult to fragment (staghorn calculi, stone in calyceal diverticulum)	Bleeding and sepsis (lower rate)
When simultaneous reconstruction and repair is needed (concurrent ureteropelvic junction obstruction)	Renal pelvis perforation
Stones in ectopic kidney	
Failed previous endourological procedures	
Stones containing gas	
Decreased need for repeat procedures	
It can be done retroperitoneally	
Improving suturing and reconstruction	
Excellent clearance rate up to 96% owing to complete stone removal without fragmentation	

SUMMARY

The incidence of kidney stones in children is increasing, causing significant morbidity and increased health care costs. Optimal management of pediatric nephrolithiasis is important to prevent recurrence and associated complications, and preserve kidney function. A multidisciplinary management is the key to successful treatment and prevention of pediatric nephrolithiasis.

CLINICS CARE POINTS

- All children with nephrolithiasis should undergo a complete metabolic workup, the results of which would provide a targeted pharmacological treatment.
- The signs and symptoms of a possible genetic involvement should be recognized early.
- High fluid consumption, dietary salt restriction, and increased intake of vegetables and fruits should be recommended in all children with nephrolithiasis.
- Medical expulsion therapy should not be tried in children with kidney stones less than 5 mm in size.
- Observation without surgical intervention is an acceptable approach in stones up to 5 mm in an asymptomatic child.
- The need for hospitalization and the indications for surgical management should be recognized early.
- A multidisciplinary management is the best approach in pediatric nephrolithiasis.

DISCLOSURE

The author has nothing to disclose.

REFERENCES

1. Tasian GE, Ross ME, Song L, et al. Annual Incidence of Nephrolithiasis among Children and Adults in South Carolina from 1997 to 2012. Clin J Am Soc Nephrol 2016;11:488–96. Available at: https://pubmed.ncbi.nlm.nih.gov/26769765/.
2. Bonzo JR, Tasian GE. The emergence of kidney stone disease during childhood-impact on adults. Curr Urol Rep 2017;18:44–50.
3. Dwyer ME, Krambeck AE, Bergstralh EJ, et al. Temporal trends in incidence of kidney stones among children: a 25-year population based study. J Urol 2012; 188:247–52.
4. Sas DJ, Hulsey TC, Shatat IF, et al. Increasing incidence of kidney stones in children evaluated in the emergency department. J Pediatr 2010;157:132–7.
5. Bush NC, Xu L, Brown BJ, et al. Hospitalizations for pediatric stone disease in United States, 2002-2007. J Urol 2010;183:1151–6.
6. Bowen DK, Tasian GE. Pediatric stone disease. Urol Clin North Am 2018;45: 539–50.
7. Sas DJ. An update on the changing epidemiology and metabolic risk factors in pediatric kidney stone disease. Clin J Am Soc Nephrol 2011;6:2062–8.
8. Schissel BL, Johnson BK. Renal stones: evolving epidemiology and management. Pediatr Emerg Care 2011;27:676–81.
9. Kovacevic L, Wolfe-Christensen C, Edwards L, et al. From hypercalciuria to hypocitraturia–a shifting trend in pediatric urolithiasis? J Urol 2012;188:1623–7.
10. Li Y, Bayne D, Wiener S, et al. Stone formation in patients less than 20 years of age is associated with higher rates of stone recurrence: results from the Registry for Stones of the Kidney and Ureter (ReSKU). J Pediatr Urol 2020;16:373.
11. Tasian GE, Kabarriti AE, Kalmus A, et al. Kidney stone recurrence among children and adolescents. J Urol 2017;197:246–52.
12. Kovacevic L, Lu H, Kovacevic N, et al. Cystatin C, Neutrophil gelatinase-associated lipocalin, and lysozyme C: urinary biomarkers for detection of early kidney dysfunction in children with urolithiasis. Urology 2020;143:221–6.

13. Valentini RP, Lakshmanan Y. Nephrolithiasis in children. Adv Chronic Kidney Dis 2011;18:370–5.

14. Kovacevic L, Lu H, Caruso JA, et al. Urinary proteomics reveals association between pediatric nephrolithiasis and cardiovascular disease. Int Urol Nephrol 2018;50:1949–54.

15. Reiner AP, Kahn A, Eisner BH, et al. Kidney stones and subclinical atherosclerosis in young adults: the CARDIA study. J Urol 2011;185:920–5.

16. Gambaro G, Ferraro PM, Capasso G. Calcium nephrolithiasis, metabolic syndrome and the cardiovascular risk. Nephrol Dial Transpl 2012;27:3008–10.

17. Goldfarb DS. Kidney stones and the risk of coronary heart disease. Am J Kidney Dis 2013;62:1039–41.

18. Kovacevic L, Lu H, Caruso JA, et al. Marked increase in urinary excretion of apolipoproteins in children with nephrolithiasis associated with hypercalciuria. Pediatr Nephrol 2017;32:1029–33.

19. Jungers P, Joly D, Barbey F, et al. ESRD caused by nephrolithiasis: prevalence, mechanisms, and prevention. Am J Kidney Dis 2004;44:799–805.

20. Kovacevic L, Lu H, Caruso JA, et al. Renal tubular dysfunction in pediatric urolithiasis: proteomic evidence. Urology 2016;92:100–5.

21. Novak TE, Lakshmanan Y, Trock BJ, et al. Sex prevalence of pediatric kidney stone disease in the United States: an epidemiologic investigation. Urol 2009;74:104–7.

22. Stamatelou KK, Francis ME, Jones CA, et al. Time trends in reported prevalence of kidney stones in the United States: 1976-1994. Kidney Int 2003;63:1817–23.

23. Mente A, Honey RJ, McLaughlin JR, et al. Ethnic differences in relative risk of idiopathic calcium nephrolithiasis in North America. J Urol 2007;178:1992–2027.

24. Pearle MS, Calhoun EA, Curhan GC. Urologic diseases in America project: urolithiasis. J Urol 2005;173:848–57.

25. Finlayson B, Reid F. The expectation of free and fixed particles in urinary stone disease. Invest Urol 1978;15:442–8.

26. Kok DJ, Khan SR. Calcium oxalate nephrolithiasis, a free or fixed particle disease. Kidney Int 1994;46:847–54.

27. Randall A. The Origin and Growth of Renal Calculi. Ann Surg 1937;105:1009–27.

28. Evan AP, Lingeman JE, Coe FL, et al. Randall's plaque of patients with nephrolithiasis begins in basement membranes of thin loops of Henle. J Clin Invest 2003;111:607–16.

29. Kwon MS, Lim SW, Kwon HM. Hypertonic stress in the kidney: a necessary evil. Physiology (Bethesda) 2009;24:186–91.

30. Sas DJ, Becton LJ, Tutman J, et al. Clinical, demographic, and laboratory characteristics of children with nephrolithiasis. Urolithiasis 2016;44:241–6.

31. Marra G, Taroni F, Berrettini A, et al. Pediatric nephrolithiasis: a systematic approach from diagnosis to treatment. J Nephrol 2019;32:199–210.

32. Bergsland KJ, Coe FL, White MD, et al. Urine risk factors in children with calcium kidney stones and their siblings. Kidney Int 2012;81:1140–8.

33. Ellison JS, Hollingsworth JM, Langman CB, et al. Analyte variations in consecutive 24-hour urine collections in children. J Pediatr Urol 2017;13:632.

34. Bevill M, Kattula A, Cooper CS, et al. The modern metabolic stone evaluation in children. Urology 2017;101:15–20.

35. Gouru VR, Pogula VR, Vaddi SP, et al. Metabolic evaluation of children with urolithiasis. Urol Ann 2018;10:94–9.

36. Smith SL, Somers JM, Broderick N, et al. The role of the plain radiograph and renal tract ultrasound in the management of children with renal tract calculi. Clin Radiol 2000;55:708–10.
37. Vrtiska TJ, Hattery RR, King BF, et al. Role of ultrasound in medical management of patients with renal stone disease. Urol Radiol 1992;14:131–8.
38. Morrison JC, Kawal T, Van Batavia JP, et al. Use of Ultrasound in Pediatric Renal Stone Diagnosis and Surgery. Curr Urol Rep 2017;18:22.
39. Seitz C, Liatsikos E, Porpiglia F, et al. Medical therapy to facilitate the passage of stones: what is the evidence? Eur Urol 2009;56:455–71.
40. Aydogdu O, Burgu B, Gucuk A, et al. Effectiveness of doxazosin in treatment of distal ureteral stones in children. J Urol 2009;182:2880–4.
41. Pickard R, Starr K, MacLennan G, et al. Medical expulsive therapy in adults with ureteric colic: a multicentre, randomised, placebo-controlled trial. Lancet 2015; 386:341–9.
42. Velázquez N, Zapata D, Wang HH, et al. Medical expulsive therapy for pediatric urolithiasis: systematic review and meta-analysis. J Pediatr Urol 2015;11:321–7.
43. Mokhless I, Zahran AR, Youssif M, et al. Tamsulosin for the management of distal ureteral stones in children: a prospective randomized study. J Pediatr Urol 2012; 8:544–8.
44. Ranabothu S, Bernstein AP, Drzewiecki BA. Diagnosis and management of non-calcium-containing stones in the pediatric population. Int Urol Nephrol 2018;50: 1191–8.
45. Pietrow PK, Pope JCt, Adams MC, et al. Clinical outcome of pediatric stone disease. J Urol 2002;167:670–3.
46. Shekarriz B, Stoller ML. Uric acid nephrolithiasis: current concepts and controversies. J Urol 2002;168:1307–14.
47. Copelovitch L. Urolithiasis in children: medical approach. Pediatr Clin North Am 2012;59:881–96.
48. Scoffone CM, Cracco CM. Pediatric calculi: cause, prevention and medical management. Curr Opin Urol 2018;28(5):428–32.
49. Tekin A, Tekgul S, Atsu N, et al. Oral potassium citrate treatment for idiopathic hypocitruria in children with calcium urolithiasis. J Urol 2002;168(6):2572–4.
50. Phillips R, Hanchanale VS, Myatt A, et al. Citrate salts for preventing and treating calcium containing kidney stones in adults. Cochrane Database Syst Rev 2015; 10:CD010057.
51. Rodgers A, Allie-Hamdulay S, Jackson G. Therapeutic action of citrate in urolithiasis explained by chemical speciation: increase in pH is the determinant factor. Nephrol Dial Transpl 2006;21:361–9.
52. Shen J, Zhang X. Potassium citrate is better in reducing salt and increasing urine pH than oral intake of lemonade: a cross-over study. Med Sci Monit 2018;24: 1924–9.
53. Sarica K. Pediatric urolithiasis: etiology, specific pathogenesis and medical treatment. Urol Res 2006;34:96–101.
54. Voskaki I, al Qadreh A, Mengreli C, et al. Effect of hydrochlorothiazide on renal hypercalciuria. Child Nephrol Urol 1992;12(1):6–9.
55. Parvin M, Shakhssalim N, Basiri A, et al. The most important metabolic risk factors in recurrent urinary stone formers. Urol J 2011;8(2):99–106.
56. Liern M, Bohorquez M, Vallejo G. Treatment of idiopathic hypercalciuria and its impact on associated diseases. Arch Argent Pediatr 2013;111:110–4.

57. Malieckal DA, Modersitzki F, Mara K, et al. Effect of increasing doses of cystine-binding thiol drugs on cystine capacity in patients with cystinuria. Urolithiasis 2019;47:549–55.

58. Smaldone MC, Docimo SG, Ost MC. Contemporary surgical management of pediatric urolithiasis. Urol Clin North Am 2010;37:253–67.

59. Sultan S, Aba Umer S, Ahmed B, et al. Update on Surgical Management of Pediatric Urolithiasis. Front Pediatr 2019;7:252.

60. Destro F, Selvaggio GGO, Lima M, et al. Minimally Invasive Approaches in Pediatric Urolithiasis. The Experience of Two Italian Centers of Pediatric Surgery. Front Pediatr 2020;8:377.

61. Fernández Alcalde Á A, Ruiz Hernández M, Gómez Dos Santos V, et al. Comparison between percutaneous nephrolithotomy and flexible ureteroscopy for the treatment of 2 and 3cm renal lithiasis. Actas Urol Esp 2019;43:111–7.

62. D'Addessi A, Bongiovanni L, Sasso F, et al. Extracorporeal shockwave lithotripsy in pediatrics. J Endourol 2008;22:1–12.

63. Dogan HS, Altan M, Citamak B, et al. A new nomogram for prediction of outcome of pediatric shock-wave lithotripsy. J Pediatr Urol 2015;11:84.

64. Onal B, Tansu N, Demirkesen O, et al. Nomogram and scoring system for predicting stone-free status after extracorporeal shock wave lithotripsy in children with urolithiasis. BJU Int 2013;111:344–52.

65. Çitamak B, Dogan HS, Ceylan T, et al. A new simple scoring system for prediction of success and complication rates in pediatric percutaneous nephrolithotomy: stone-kidney size score. J Pediatr Urol 2019;15:67.

66. Ghani KR, Trinh QD, Jeong W, et al. Robotic nephrolithotomy and pyelolithotomy with utilization of the robotic ultrasound probe. Int Braz J Urol 2014;40:125–6.

Hypertension in Children and Young Adults

Emily Haseler, BM BCh[a,b], Manish D. Sinha, PhD[a,b],*

KEYWORDS

- Hypertension • Blood pressure • Adolescence • Pediatric • Obesity • Left ventricle
- Haemodynamics

KEY POINTS

- The prevalence of primary hypertension continues to increase across childhood populations.
- Secondary hypertension remains the predominant cause of hypertension in young children, in whom underlying kidney disease is the most common pathology.
- Hypertension-mediated organ damage occurs during childhood and prompt diagnosis and appropriate management is important.
- Out-of-office blood pressure monitoring, preferably by 24-h ambulatory blood pressure monitoring is essential for the diagnosis and management of hypertension.
- The Dietary Approach to Stop Hypertension diet, weight control, and increased physical activity are central to the management of hypertension.

INTRODUCTION

Hypertension affects over a billion adults worldwide and is one of the leading causes of premature death.[1] In younger children, most hypertension is secondary but primary hypertension (PH), particularly during adolescence, continues to steadily increase in its prevalence over the past 2 to 3 decades. PH is now the predominant form of hypertension diagnosed in adolescents, in large part due to the epidemic of obesity.[2] This article reviews the epidemiology, diagnosis, and management of hypertension in children and young adults, with a focus on aspects that have not been reviewed recently including global perspective, hemodynamic determinants, and challenges in the provision of care of childhood and adolescent hypertension.[3–5]

[a] Department of Paediatric Nephrology, Evelina London Children's Hospital, Guys & St Thomas NHS Foundation Trust, Westminster Bridge Road, 3rd Floor Beckett House, London SE1 7EH, United Kingdom; [b] Kings College London, United Kingdom
* Corresponding author. Department of Paediatric Nephrology, Evelina London Children's Hospital, Guys & St Thomas NHS Foundation Trust, Westminster Bridge Road, 3rd Floor Beckett House, London SE1 7EH, United Kingdom.
E-mail address: manish.sinha@gstt.nhs.uk

Pediatr Clin N Am 69 (2022) 1165–1180
https://doi.org/10.1016/j.pcl.2022.07.005
0031-3955/22/© 2022 Elsevier Inc. All rights reserved.

Prevalence

A recent study on the global prevalence of pediatric hypertension included a meta-analysis of 47 studies, covering five continents and data spanning 25 years from 1990 to 2014.[6] The pooled prevalence was 4.0% [95% confidence interval [CI] 3.3%–4.8%], with increasing prevalence over the reported period.[6] Prevalence of elevated blood pressure (BP) (previously known as prehypertension and in Europe known as high normal BP), was 9.7% [7.3%–12.4%]. A strength of this study was the inclusion of only studies in which office BP had been measured on three separate occasions. It is recognized that a lower prevalence of elevated BP is observed if BP is measured repeatedly on more than one visit; this is in keeping with various Clinical Practice Guidelines.[7–11] However, given the practical challenges repeated visits pose, particularly when conducting a research study, many studies report measurements performed during a single visit.

Studies from Australia, Canada, and central Europe published following the meta-analysis by Song and colleagues[6] corroborate its findings, reporting prevalence at 3.1%, 4.5%, and 6%, respectively.[6,12–14] The reported prevalence of hypertension has been affected following a change in the diagnostic threshold as per the 2017 AAP Clinical Practice Guideline.[10] Analysis of a large US cohort from the National Health and Nutrition Survey (NHANES) found that the application of these guidelines increased the prevalence from 2.7% to 5.5%.[15] Similarly, a Spanish study reported an increase in the prevalence of hypertension from 6.6% when using 2016 European Society of Hypertension (referred to as "2016 ESH") guidelines to 10.6% under the 2017 American Academy of Pediatrics (referred to as "2017 AAP") guidelines.[16] The 2017 AAP guideline change should therefore be kept in mind when interpreting data regarding the prevalence of childhood hypertension.

Hypertension in Low- and Middle-Income Countries

The majority of adults with hypertension live in low- and middle-income countries (LIMCs), with one in three estimated to be hypertensive.[17] Data regarding pediatric hypertension prevalence in LIMCs is mixed: the Middle East, South America, China, India, and Nigeria were represented in the meta-analysis by Song and colleagues, with prevalence varying from 1.1% (India, 1994) to 12.8% (Nigeria, 2017).[6,18,19] Two recent studies in Sub-Saharan Africa using repeated BP measurements found a prevalence of 3.1% in rural Uganda and 1.6% in rural Cameroon using 2016 ESH and the so-called, 2004 Fourth Report guidelines.[20,21] In contrast, a Tanzanian study observed a much higher prevalence of 10.2% following three repeated measurements.[9] It remains unclear whether the significant variation in prevalence across studies is primarily because of inherent differences in population and lifestyle factors, or methodological differences pertaining to included age range, definition of hypertension, or sampling bias. With these potential confounders, it remains difficult to compare the true prevalence of hypertension in childhood across different global regions to monitor trends and ultimately focus resources.

Genetics

Monogenic forms of hypertension remain extremely rare and have been well described elsewhere.[22] It has long been known that PH has a substantial polygenic component, with twin studies over the past 30 years in children and adults confirming significant heritability.[23] A recent meta-analysis of twin studies on familial aggregation in childhood BP, suggested that approximately 70% of the BP variability was explained by a shared environment, whereas genetics comprised a relatively modest 25%.[24]

Genome-wide association studies (GWAS) allow simultaneous comparison of hundreds of thousands of gene variants and have dramatically advanced the identification of the specific gene variants determining hypertension. In 2011, a GWAS consortium collated the known 29 genome-wide significant variants, developing the first genetic risk score for hypertension; there are now over 1000 loci of interest.[25,26] A study based on TwinsUK and UK Biobank cohorts found pulsatile and systolic components of BP showed a much higher heritability than diastolic and mean arterial pressure.[27] This is an interesting finding when paired with hemodynamic observations regarding pulsatile components of BP contributing disproportionately to hypertension in childhood. To date, the association between reported loci and BP during childhood has not been tested. Overall, although significant advances in this area are expected in the coming decades, there is currently no role in clinical practice for genetic testing in PH.

Excess Weight and Hypertension

Obesity is well established as an independent risk factor for hypertension.[8,28] In a Canadian study where BP was measured at mean ages of 12.8, 15.2, and 17 years, an increase in 1 body mass index (BMI) unit was associated with an increase of 0.7 mm Hg systolic blood pressure (SBP).[29] Prevalence of hypertension in those with overweight and obesity has been estimated between 15.3% and 40%, although studies again vary in the number of BP measurements performed and definition of hypertension.[6,8,14,30] However, the relationship between excess weight and BP is not observed in all populations. Data from Tanzania and South Africa report a low prevalence of obesity within their hypertensive cohorts.[9,31] Furthermore, an analysis of changes in BMI and BP from 1974 to 1993 in subjects of the Bogalusa Heart Study showed that the increased rate of obesity from 6% to 17% during this time was not associated with an increase in SBP and DBP.[32] These findings imply that obesity-independent processes are also important in the development of PH in childhood.

Obesity and hypertension have both independent and summative effects on left ventricular remodeling. A decrease in abdominal obesity and an increase in lean body mass are the main predictors of left ventricular hypertrophy (LVH) regression in hypertensive adolescents.[33] The main metabolic abnormalities associated with excess weight are hyperinsulinaemia and insulin resistance. This results from a pro-inflammatory state established by excess adipose tissue, in particular visceral as opposed to subcutaneous adipose tissue.[34] Hyperinsulinaemia is known to result in sympathetic nervous system (SNS) activation and several cross-sectional and epidemiological studies have observed higher heart rate (HR), stroke volume (SV), or cardiac output (CO) in those with excess weight.[30] These observations have underpinned the hyperdynamic state theory.

Hemodynamics

The predominant phenotype of hypertension in children, adolescents, and young adults is isolated systolic hypertension (ISH), characterized by a raised pulse pressure (PP), whereas hypertension diagnosed in 30–50-year-olds is predominantly isolated diastolic hypertension (IDH) and systo-diastolic hypertension (SDH), before ISH becomes the main phenotype with increasing age.[30,35,36] These changing phenotypes are thought to be driven by age-related changes in the arterial tree, a phenomenon less likely to be occurring in hypertensive children during the first two decades of life.

Support for a "hyperdynamic state" has emerged following observations that CO or its component, HR, and SV are raised in hypertensive children and young adults.[8,30,37] These data suggest that instead of a "vascular"-driven process, a "cardiac"-driven process is dominant in at least a subset of children and young adults with hypertension. Increased SNS activity is proposed as the pathophysiological link between obesity, PH, increased CO, and altered ventricular ejection dynamics.[34,38] Recent evidence suggests a presence of distinct hemodynamic phenotypes within PH, eg, males tending toward a "cardiac" phenotype and females tending toward "vascular."[39] It remains interesting to consider that the earliest hemodynamic changes may be cardiac driven and that these promote vascular remodeling which over time switches the phenotype to more of a vascular phenotype.[40] Arguments for and against the "hyperdynamic state" theory are subject to ongoing debate in the literature and the interested reader is directed to recent reviews on the subject.[41,42] **Fig. 1** summarizes important hemodynamic relationships and a proposed pathophysiological model of factors leading to hypertension in young people.[27,28,36,41]

Studies measuring detailed hemodynamic parameters in healthy weight hypertensive and obese hypertensive individuals compared with normotensive subjects are needed. Further, studies to investigate the effect of different antihypertensive medications on these emerging distinct hypertensive phenotypes may help develop a more logical approach to the management of childhood hypertension.

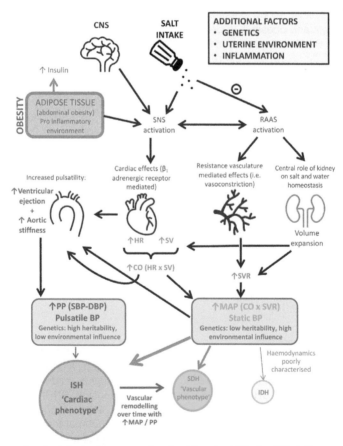

Fig. 1. Key pathophysiological processes involved in raised BP–simplified diagram. CNS, central nervous system; CO, cardiac output; HR, heart rate; HTN, hypertension; IDH, isolated diastolic hypertension; MAP, mean arterial pressure; PP, pulse pressure; RAAS, renin angiotensin aldosterone system; SDH, systo-diastolic hypertension; SNS, sympathetic nervous system; SV, stroke volume; SVR, systemic vascular resistance.

Blood Pressure Tracking

Tracking refers to the tendency for an individual with normal BP to increase with time such that it remains around the percentile of initial measurement. Robust data provide evidence of tracking of BP from childhood to adult life, with correlation coefficient estimated at 0.38 for SBP and 0.28 for DBP.[43] These data suggest that children with high BP have a high risk for future hypertension. Correlation increased with age, into adolescence, and in the presence of obesity.[43]

Intrauterine environment, including both fetal under and overnutrition, have been shown to influence BP in early life.[44] Fetal "programming" is likely to interact with childhood weight trajectory, environmental and genetic factors to influence BP trajectory, and risk of cardiovascular disease as an adult.[44] Hypertension in adulthood is more likely with sustained rather than transient high BP in childhood.[45] In the Bogalusa cohort, the presence of LVH in adulthood was associated with a trajectory of higher BP measurements beginning in childhood.[46] These observations reinforce the importance of measuring BP at regular intervals throughout childhood and adolescence.

Linking Hypertension to Cardiovascular Events in Adults

Increasing BP is on a continuum with increasing risk of adverse cardiovascular outcomes in old age: with each 20 mm Hg SBP or 10 mm Hg DBP rise above a threshold of 115/75 mm Hg, the risk of death from heart disease, stroke or other vascular disease is doubled.[47] Subgroup analysis within a recent meta-analysis of subjects aged <30 years showed that compared with "optimal BP" (BP < 120/80 mm Hg), the relative risk (RR) of any adverse cardiovascular event for Grade 1 hypertension (140–159/90–99 mm Hg) was 1.46 (1.24–1.72) and for Grade 2 hypertension was 2.22 (1.46–3.39).[48] These data support the current hypertension guidelines for young adults. For all participants 18 to 45 years, number needed to treat (NNT) for one year to prevent one cardiovascular event for those with Stage 2 hypertension was 236 and for high normal BP was 1450.[48]

Defining Hypertension in Children

BP increases physiologically throughout childhood with increasing age and height, with the largest increment during adolescence, and with greater changes in boys than girls. The diagnosis of hypertension in children has historically been based on normative values for age, height, and sex and defined as BP > 95th percentile.

- The 2017 AAP updated diagnostic criteria offered a simplified single threshold for children of ≥13 years of 130/80 mm Hg in line with the adult American Heart Association definition.[10]
- Hypertension Canada similarly in 2020 suggested a simplified threshold of 120/80 mm Hg for 6–11-year-olds and 130/85 mm Hg for ≥ 12-year-olds.[11]
- The 2016 ESH guideline specifies that the 95th centile should be used for hypertension diagnosis in all young people <16 years, and a threshold of 140/90 mm Hg in those ≥16 years to keep in line with adult ESH thresholds.[49]

Normative data for the 2016 ESH guidelines are taken from the "2004 Fourth Report." Of note, both European and Canadian datasets were derived from healthy US children from the NHANES program, but the 2017 AAP guidelines excluded overweight and obese children from this dataset. These differences between Clinical Practice Guidelines highlight the significant knowledge gaps that remain to help make firm and grounded recommendations to lower age cutoffs. The decision of what age to transition to an "adult" single cutoff remains difficult as it implies that age, sex, and height have become irrelevant.

Since the publication of the 2017 AAP and 2016 ESH guidelines, considerable research and debate has focused on which approach maximizes positive predictive value for patients at risk of cardiovascular morbidity.[50,51] Application of the 2017 AAP guidelines in longitudinal cohorts increases the prevalence of hypertension for most patients compared with the 2004 Fourth Report and 2016 ESH guidelines, especially for those with excess weight.[15,50] A recent systematic review and meta-analysis found that although the 2017 AAP guideline classified more patients as hypertensive, no difference in detection of LVH within hypertensive groups was seen.[52] Despite the differing guidelines, there is widespread consensus that both approaches are clinically valid in the absence of definitive data on cardiovascular endpoints, and that studies delineating the optimum BP threshold to lower the risk of these cardiovascular endpoints are urgently needed.[51] Overall, these issues also highlight that the relationships among age, body size, and left ventricular mass (LVM) are complex, especially during the process of growth as seen during adolescence.

Hypertension-Mediated Organ Damage

In the absence of longitudinal data linking childhood hypertension to cardiovascular events, the rationale for identifying and treating hypertension is largely based on evidence reporting markers of hypertensive-mediated organ damage (HMOD) in hypertensive young people.

Indexed left ventricular mass (LVMI) expressed as $g/m^{2.7}$ is the most widely reported HMOD marker, shown to relate to adverse cardiovascular outcomes in adults.[53] Increased prevalence of LVH has been consistently found in hypertensive compared with normotensive pediatric cohorts, but the percentile of BP above which the risk for LVH increases has been unclear.[54] A recent multicentre cohort study in the United States has improved clarity regarding this issue. Echocardiography in 360 participants stratified into low-, mid-, and high-risk BP (BP < 80th, 81st-90th, and >90th percentiles, respectively) found a stepwise increase in LVMI across BP risk groups.[55] LVH was present in 13%, 21%, and 27% of the low-, mid-, and high-risk groups, respectively.[55] Following specific analysis of increasing SBP, the 90th percentile represented the best balance between sensitivity (0.44) and specificity (0.75) to predict presence of LVH, suggesting that evaluation for LVH may be indicated if clinic SBP >90th centile.[55]

In addition to cardiac remodeling, pediatric hypertension is associated with signs of early vascular aging, in the form of structural (as assessed by carotid intima medial thickness, cIMT) and functional (as assessed by carotid-femoral PWV, PWVcf, and flow-mediated dilatation) impairment of the arterial tree.[56] Urbina and colleagues[57] reported progressive worsening of arterial stiffness measures with increasing BP levels in a large cohort of hypertensive and normotensive adolescents. Neurocognitive impairment in those with PH has been suggested, implying involvement of the wider vascular tree.[58] Microvascular components of the arterial tree are also impacted as shown in a recent study reporting a close association between macrovascular injury (increased cIMT) and retinal microcirculation injury (increased foveal avascular zone).[59] At present, no guidelines recommend specific investigation for vascular HMOD outside the research setting due to insufficient normative data.

Importantly, evidence supporting the reversibility of LVH in children was reported by Litwin and colleagues with a reduction in LVH from 47% to 31% after 12 months of antihypertensive therapy. They reported a reduction in excess weight as an independent predictor for LVH regression.[33] This is corroborated by weight loss studies in obese young people; with one study finding that a combined diet and exercise weight reduction program is more effective at reducing cIMT than dietary interventions alone, although BP outcomes were not presented.[60] These data highlight the value of early and aggressive management of hypertension in the presence of HMOD and the importance of a multifaceted approach to treatment including lifestyle modification.

Investigation and Diagnosis

Suggested pathway to diagnosis and management is covered in detail in the relevant guidelines, with evidence for rationale, and is summarized in **Fig. 2**.[10,11,49,61] Following confirmation of high office BP, the most helpful procedure is out-of-office BP measurement in the form of 24-h ambulatory BP measurement (ABPM). This is recommended to confirm the diagnosis of hypertension and has been found to be cost-effective in a hospital setting, as a normal ABPM study often negates the need for significant further investigation.[62]

Although ABPM is the gold standard, it is not feasible across all settings or patients. Purchase of ABPM equipment and training staff to use and interpret the results is expensive and difficult to implement in general pediatric settings, not to mention LIMCs. ABPM is not recommended in children under 5 due to lack of normative data and lack of feasibility, and may not be tolerated in some special populations of children over 5. In such cases, Home BP (HBP) monitoring can be a useful adjunct

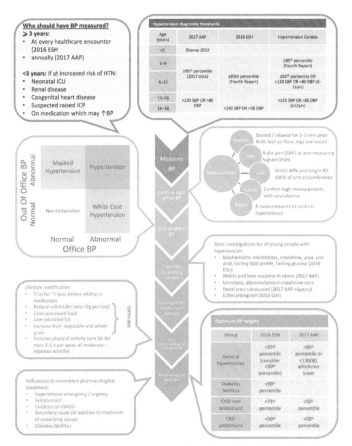

Fig. 2. Hypertension diagnosis and management: key factors. AAP, American Academy of Pediatrics guidelines 2017; BP, blood pressure; CKD, chronic kidney disease; DASH, dietary approaches to stop hypertension; DBP, diastolic BP; ESH, European Society for Hypertension guidelines 2016; HTN, hypertension; ICP, intracranial pressure; ICU, intensive care unit; SBP, systolic BP.

to gain some insight into out-of-office BP. HBP has been shown to correlate with ABPM, office BP and for SBP, signs of HMOD.[63] A validated oscillometric device can be used but these are known to overestimate BP in children. HBP monitoring using a doppler probe to detect SBP has also been shown to have a good correlation with office BP and to be feasible to teach to parents.[64] However, normative data for HBP monitoring with either automated or doppler devices do not currently exist and published experience remains limited outside single centers for HBP. Additional clinical studies are needed, although a recent systematic review on HBP concluded that until further data become available, a 7-day, morning, and evening (minimum 12) series of measurements should be used for HBP.[63]

Once the diagnosis of hypertension has been confirmed, a targeted consideration and investigation for secondary causes should be undertaken. Beyond a basic investigation panel indicated in every young person diagnosed with hypertension (see **Fig. 2**), this will vary according to the clinical situation. **Table 1** summarizes common secondary causes with investigations to consider.[65] An echocardiogram to assess for HMOD is recommended for all patients with hypertension by 2016 ESH guidelines and at the time of consideration of pharmacological therapy by 2017 AAP guidelines.[10,49]

Treatment

For PH and high normal BP in the absence of symptoms or markers of HMOD, the first-line management outlined in all major guidelines is lifestyle modification; primarily reduction in salt intake and weight loss through dietary modification and increased exercise. Focus on lifestyle modification should continue following initiation of medication, especially in the case of obesity-related hypertension where weight loss is the most important therapeutic intervention.[10,49]

A recent randomized controlled trial (RCT) showed that an intervention consisting of four 90-min exercise sessions per week for 1 year reduced the proportion of children in hypertensive BP range from 86% to 16% in a group of obese children with a mean age of 10.4 ± 1.4 years.[66] Meta-analyses of studies focusing on general and obese populations show more modest reductions of 1-2 mm Hg for both SBP and DBP from exercise programs involving three or more sessions lasting at least 60 minutes per week.[67]

Salt intake has long been associated with BP.[68,69] In adults, a decreased salt intake of 6 g/day was associated with a fall in SBP of approximately 6 mm Hg.[69] In children, a 42% reduction in salt intake was associated with a decrease in SBP of 2.47 mm Hg (4.00 to 0.94 mm Hg; $P < 0.01$).[68] There is evidence that salt intake from infancy influences BP trajectory. A 20-year follow-up of participants in a neonatal salt restriction study found a lower SBP of 3.6 mm Hg (-6.6 to -0.5) in those assigned a lower salt diet as a neonate.[70]

Given the prevalence of salt in processed foods, for families who find it difficult to reduce the proportion of processed foods in their diet, referral to a dietician or community/school-based dietary education program may be more effective than advice alone. One large 20-year prospective study found that following bi-annual dietary advice focused on increasing fruit, vegetables, and fiber and reducing saturated fat, attainment of these dietary targets was associated with a modest reduction in BP.[71] Interest has gathered around the Dietary Approaches to Stop Hypertension (DASH), a healthy eating approach specific to hypertension by promoting foods that are low in sodium, high in potassium and magnesium, and low in saturated fat. Evidence of its efficacy in children is limited mainly due to lack of data and poor adherence to the diet in the few RCTs which have been performed.[72]

Indications for commencing antihypertensive therapy and target BP are detailed in **Fig. 2**. There is very limited evidence to support which medication to use; the most

Table 1
Important secondary causes for hypertension with suggested diagnostic investigations

Category	Specific Cause	Investigations
All hypertension cases		Renal ultrasound scan Plasma electrolytes, creatinine, and urea Urinalysis Urine albumin: creatinine ratio Echocardiogram (2016 ESH)
Obesity		Fasting glucose &/or HbA1$_c$ Lipid profile Uric acid
	In selected cases only	
Parenchymal renal disease	Glomerulonephritis Focal and segmental glomerulosclerosis Pyelonephritis-related renal scarring Acute kidney injury with salt and water overload Polycystic kidney disease Chronic kidney disease Obstructive uropathy	Tc99 dimercaptosuccinic acid (DMSA) scan
Renovascular	Renal artery stenosis (*Idiopathic, Fibromuscular dysplasia, Neurofibromatosis type 1, Williams syndrome*) Mid-aortic syndrome Thrombosis of renal artery or vein Acute or post hemolytic uremic syndrome Fistulae External compression	Renin and aldosterone Doppler studies of renal arteries CT angiography MR angiogram Digital Subtraction Angiography (DSA) Selective renal vein renin measurement
Endocrine	Cortisol/glucocorticoid excess Aldosterone/mineralocorticoid excess Catecholamine excess Congenital adrenal hyperplasia Thyroid disease	Thyroid Function Tests Plasma cortisol Urinary steroid profile Plasma/urine catecholamines and metanephrines
Cardiovascular	Coarctation of aorta Takayasu arteritis	Echocardiogram Cardiac MRI
Central nervous system	Pain Convulsions Increased intracranial pressure Guillain–Barré syndrome Dysautonomia	
Malignancy	Wilms' tumor (nephroblastoma) Neuroblastoma Pheochromocytoma	Plasma/urine catecholamines and metanephrines Metaiodobenzylguanidine (MIBG) scan CT abdomen/pelvis

(continued on next page)

Table 1 (continued)		
Category	Specific Cause	Investigations
Drugs	Amphetamine or sympathomimetics	Urine toxicology screen
	Acute vitamin D intoxication, hypercalcemia	
	Calcineurin inhibitors (ciclosporin/tacrolimus)	
	Decongestants	
	Erythropoietin	
	Oral contraceptive pills	
	Steroids	
Others	Obstructive sleep apnea	Sleep study
	Bronchopulmonary dysplasia	
	Single gene defects causing hypertension (eg, Liddle's syndrome)	

Investigations are suggested for each category rather than specific causes and may not be indicated in all cases.

Adapted from Singh C, Jones H, Copeman H, Sinha MD. Fifteen-minute consultation: the child with systemic arterial hypertension. Arch Dis Child Educ Pract Ed. 2017 Feb;102(1):2-7.

recent meta-analysis in 2018 found angiotensin-converting enzyme inhibitors (ACEi) and angiotensin receptor blockers (ARB) are superior to placebo.[73] A recent interesting study adopted an n-of-1 methodology (single patient randomized crossover trials) to develop a personalized approach to antihypertensive medication choice.[74] Lisinopril was preferred and effective in 16 of the 32 patients studied, with the next most popular agents being amlodipine and hydrochorothiazide.[74]

Until further data become available, ACEi, ARB, calcium channel blocker, or thiazide diuretic could be considered as initial agents, starting at the lowest dose and titrating up every 2-4 weeks until BP is in the target range.[10,49] ACEi/ARB are most suitable as they increase insulin sensitivity and peripheral blood flow but have potential side effects and need to be avoided in sexually active girls. Calcium channel blockers are useful first-line agents but may be associated with pedal edema. Beta-blockers especially more recent agents in those with evidence of hyperdynamic circulation are helpful and all agents can be used in combination. There may be specific circumstances in which choice of medication is clear, eg, ACEi/ARB in chronic kidney disease with proteinuria, a diuretic in corticosteroid-induced hypertension. If a second agent is needed, a thiazide diuretic is useful to counter the salt and water retention caused by several other medications.

Challenges in Management

Hypertension in children and young adults is an expanding clinical problem. However many clinical settings are not resourced to measure or interpret BP and there remains heterogeneity in its management which is discordant with the published guidelines. Further, hypertension is poorly screened for and recognized, especially in obese young people.[75] Diagnosis depends on out-of-office BP monitoring, a limited resource to clinicians in primary and secondary care, and in LIMCs.[76] Diet, weight control, and increased physical activity are the most important management strategy for obesity-related hypertension and yet parity of access to multidisciplinary weight loss services is not clear. Engagement with lifestyle modification interventions is notoriously

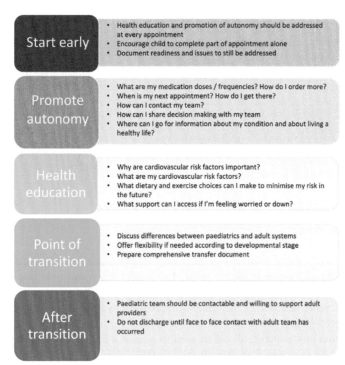

Start early
- Health education and promotion of autonomy should be addressed at every appointment
- Encourage child to complete part of appointment alone
- Document readiness and issues to still be addressed

Promote autonomy
- What are my medication doses / frequencies? How do I order more?
- When is my next appointment? How do I get there?
- How can I contact my team?
- How can I share decision making with my team
- Where can I go for information about my condition and about living a healthy life?

Health education
- Why are cardiovascular risk factors important?
- What are my cardiovascular risk factors?
- What dietary and exercise choices can I make to minimise my risk in the future?
- What support can I access if I'm feeling worried or down?

Point of transition
- Discuss differences between paediatrics and adult systems
- Offer flexibility if needed according to developmental stage
- Prepare comprehensive transfer document

After transition
- Paediatric team should be contactable and willing to support adult providers
- Do not discharge until face to face contact with adult team has occurred

Fig. 3. Transition to adult services–suggested schematic of key themes. (Based on Nagra A, McGinnity PM, Davis N, Salmon AP. Implementing transition: Ready Steady Go. Arch Dis Child Educ Pract Ed. 2015 Dec;100(6):313-20 [www.readysteadygo.net] and National Institute for Health and Care Excellence, Transition from children's to adults' services. Quality standard [QS140] Published date: 21 December 2016.)

difficult, especially as most PH patients are adolescents, a group of patients with specific needs and vulnerabilities.

Transition to Adult Services

Adolescence and transition to adult services is a particularly challenging period of clinical care for young people, their families, and clinical teams. Young people are expected to follow a developmental trajectory that culminates in self-management of their condition, but the speed and pattern of this trajectory may not align with the traditional timings of transition from pediatric to adult care.[77] In hypertension this is even more problematic; as a largely asymptomatic condition, there are high risks for young people to drop out of clinical care and/or medication compliance.[78] Children with PH are often cared for by pediatric specialists (eg, nephrologists or cardiologists) however adult hypertension care may be based on cardiology or family medicine/general practice depending on local arrangements and the severity of the condition. This adds to the complexity of the transition process and to the opportunity for interruptions in care. Regardless of the quality of BP control under pediatric care, if a young adult drops out of care during the transition to adult services, there may be significant effects on their cardiovascular risk.[48] There are no unified guidelines to aid in the planning of transition services for young people with hypertension but suggested general good practice principles are outlined in **Fig. 3**.[79,80]

SUMMARY

Hypertension in children and young adults is a growing clinical problem linked to the increasing prevalence of obesity worldwide. If BP is poorly controlled, there is likely to be a significant increase in health care-related costs due to excess adverse cardiovascular events in middle age or sooner. Improvements in care for this group of patients depend on prompt diagnosis, supported nonpharmacological interventions, and robust local frameworks for the transition from pediatric to adult services. Future research should aim to address unknowns regarding future risk of adverse cardiovascular outcomes, establish normative datasets for home BP monitoring and elucidate the hemodynamic processes distinguishing hypertension in young people. These may form the starting point for randomized controlled trials into optimum antihypertensive agents for different hypertensive phenotypes, patient ethnicities, and underlying etiologies.

CLINICS CARE POINTS

- Clinicians should have an increasing index of suspicion for primary rather than secondary hypertension with increasing age and especially in the context of excess weight."

- There is currently no role for genetic testing in paediatric hypertension unless a monogenic cause is suspected.

- Out of office BP monitoring should be used to support a diagnosis of hypertension and investigate for white coat hypertension. ABPM is preferred."

- Guidelines differ regarding diagnostic threshold, minimum investigations and treatment threshold for managing hypertension."

- Lifestyle changes remain the most important management strategy for primary hypertension and include a combination of weight management, reduction in salt intake and moderate exercise."

DISCLOSURE

The authors have nothing to disclose.

REFERENCES

1. Hypertension: fact sheet, world health organisation. Available at: https://www.who.int/health-topics/hypertension#tab=tab_1. Accessed 10th January, 2022.
2. Gupta-Malhotra M, Banker A, Shete S, et al. Essential hypertension vs. secondary hypertension among children. Am J Hypertens 2015;28(1):73–80.
3. Khoury M, Urbina EM. Hypertension in adolescents: diagnosis, treatment, and implications. Lancet Child Adolesc Health 2021;5(5):357–66.
4. Dionne JM. Evidence gaps in the identification and treatment of hypertension in children. Can J Cardiol 2020;36(9):1384–93.
5. Taylor-Zapata P, Baker-Smith CM, Burckart G, et al. Research gaps in primary pediatric hypertension. Pediatrics 2019;143(5).
6. Song P, Zhang Y, Yu J, et al. Global Prevalence of Hypertension in Children: A Systematic Review and Meta-analysis. JAMA Pediatr 2019;173(12):1154–63.
7. Sun J, Steffen LM, Ma C, et al. Definition of pediatric hypertension: are blood pressure measurements on three separate occasions necessary? Hypertens Res 2017;40(5):496–503.

8. Chiolero A, Cachat F, Burnier M, et al. Prevalence of hypertension in schoolchildren based on repeated measurements and association with overweight. J Hypertens 2007;25(11):2209–17.
9. Nsanya MK, Ayieko P, Hashim R, et al. Sustained high blood pressure and 24-h ambulatory blood pressure monitoring in Tanzanian adolescents. Sci Rep 2021; 11(1):8397.
10. Flynn JT, Kaelber DC, Baker-Smith CM, et al. Clinical practice guideline for screening and management of high blood pressure in children and adolescents. Pediatrics 2017;140(3):e20171904.
11. Rabi DM, McBrien KA, Sapir-Pichhadze R, et al. Hypertension Canada's 2020 comprehensive guidelines for the prevention, diagnosis, risk assessment, and treatment of hypertension in adults and children. Can J Cardiol 2020;36(5): 596–624.
12. Larkins NG, Teixeira-Pinto A, Kim S, et al. The population-based prevalence of hypertension and correlates of blood pressure among Australian children. Pediatr Nephrol 2019;34(6):1107–15.
13. Robinson SK, Rodd CJ, Metzger DL, et al. Prevalence of high blood pressure among Canadian Children: 2017 American Academy of Pediatrics guidelines with the Canadian Health Measures Survey. Paediatr Child Health 2021;26(3): e158–65.
14. Martin L, Oepen J, Reinehr T, et al. Ethnicity and cardiovascular risk factors: evaluation of 40,921 normal-weight, overweight or obese children and adolescents living in Central Europe. Int J Obes (Lond) 2015;39(1):45–51.
15. Sharma AK, Metzger DL, Rodd CJ. Prevalence and severity of high blood pressure among children based on the 2017 american academy of pediatrics guidelines. JAMA Pediatr 2018;172(6):557–65.
16. Lurbe E, Torró I, Álvarez J, et al. Impact of ESH and AAP hypertension guidelines for children and adolescents on office and ambulatory blood pressure-based classifications. J Hypertens 2019;37(12):2414–21.
17. Sarki AM, Nduka CU, Stranges S, et al. Prevalence of hypertension in low- and middle-income countries: a systematic review and meta-analysis. Medicine (Baltimore) 2015;94(50):e1959.
18. Ajayi IO, Soyannwo MAO, Asinobi AO, et al. Blood pressure pattern and hypertension related risk factors in an urban community in Southwest Nigeria: The Mokola hypertension initiative project, Ibadan, Nigeria. J Public Health Epidemiol 2017;9:51–64.
19. Verma M, Chhatwal J, George SM. Obesity and hypertension in children. Indian Pediatr 1994;31(9):1065–9.
20. Katamba G, Agaba DC, Migisha R, et al. Prevalence of hypertension in relation to anthropometric indices among secondary adolescents in Mbarara, Southwestern Uganda. Ital J Pediatr 2020;46(1):76.
21. Chelo D, Mah EM, Chiabi EN, et al. Prevalence and factors associated with hypertension in primary school children, in the centre region of Cameroon. Transl Pediatr 2019;8(5):391–7.
22. Aggarwal A, Rodriguez-Buritica D. Monogenic hypertension in children: a review with emphasis on genetics. Adv Chronic Kidney Dis 2017;24(6):372–9.
23. Wang X, Xu X, Su S, et al. Familial aggregation and childhood blood pressure. Curr Hypertens Rep 2015;17(1):509.
24. Huang Y, Ollikainen M, Muniandy M, et al. Identification, heritability, and relation with gene expression of novel DNA methylation loci for blood pressure. Hypertension 2020;76(1):195–205.

25. Surendran P, Feofanova EV, Lahrouchi N, et al. Discovery of rare variants associated with blood pressure regulation through meta-analysis of 1.3 million individuals. Nat Genet 2020;52(12):1314–32.

26. Ehret GB, Munroe PB, Rice KM, et al. Genetic variants in novel pathways influence blood pressure and cardiovascular disease risk. Nature 2011;478(7367): 103–9.

27. Cecelja M, Keehn L, Ye L, et al. Genetic aetiology of blood pressure relates to aortic stiffness with bi-directional causality: evidence from heritability, blood pressure polymorphisms, and Mendelian randomization. Eur Heart J 2020;41(35): 3314–22.

28. Litwin M, Kułaga Z. Obesity, metabolic syndrome, and primary hypertension. Pediatr Nephrol 2021;36(4):825–37.

29. Maximova K, O'Loughlin J, Paradis G, et al. Changes in anthropometric characteristics and blood pressure during adolescence. Epidemiology 2010;21(3): 324–31.

30. Sorof JM, Poffenbarger T, Franco K, et al. Isolated systolic hypertension, obesity, and hyperkinetic hemodynamic states in children. J Pediatr 2002;140(6):660–6.

31. Naidoo S, Kagura J, Fabian J, et al. Early Life factors and longitudinal blood pressure trajectories are associated with elevated blood pressure in early adulthood. Hypertension 2019;73(2):301–9.

32. Freedman DS, Goodman A, Contreras OA, et al. Secular trends in BMI and blood pressure among children and adolescents: the Bogalusa Heart Study. Pediatrics 2012;130(1):e159–66.

33. Litwin M, Niemirska A, Sladowska-Kozlowska J, et al. Regression of target organ damage in children and adolescents with primary hypertension. Pediatr Nephrol 2010;25(12):2489–99.

34. Brady TM. Obesity-Related Hypertension in Children. Front Pediatr 2017;5:197.

35. Franklin SS, Jacobs MJ, Wong ND, et al. Predominance of isolated systolic hypertension among middle-aged and elderly US hypertensives: analysis based on National Health and Nutrition Examination Survey (NHANES) III. Hypertension 2001;37(3):869–74.

36. Alsaeed H, Metzger DL, Blydt-Hansen TD, et al. Isolated diastolic high blood pressure: a distinct clinical phenotype in US children. Pediatr Res 2021;90(4): 903–9.

37. McEniery CM, Yasmin, Wallace S, et al. Increased stroke volume and aortic stiffness contribute to isolated systolic hypertension in young adults. Hypertension 2005;46(1):221–6.

38. Gu H, Singh C, Li Y, et al. Early ventricular contraction in children with primary hypertension relates to left ventricular mass. J Hypertens 2021;39(4):711–7.

39. Nardin C, Maki-Petaja KM, Miles KL, et al. Cardiovascular phenotype of elevated blood pressure differs markedly between young males and females: the enigma study. Hypertension 2018;72(6):1277–84.

40. Falkner B. Cardiac output versus total peripheral resistance. Hypertension 2018; 72(5):1093–4.

41. Li Y, Haseler E, Chowienczyk P, et al. Haemodynamics of hypertension in children. Curr Hypertens Rep 2020;22(8):60.

42. Litwin M, Feber J. Origins of primary hypertension in children. Hypertension 2020; 76(5):1400–9.

43. Chen X, Wang Y. Tracking of blood pressure from childhood to adulthood: a systematic review and meta-regression analysis. Circulation 2008;117(25):3171–80.

44. Sinha MD. From pregnancy to childhood and adulthood: the trajectory of hypertension. In: Lurbe EW E, editor. Hypertension in children and adolescents: new perspectives. Switzerland AG: Springer Nature; 2019. p. 1–16, chap 1. Updates in Hypertension and Cardiovascular Protection.

45. Urbina EM, Khoury PR, Bazzano L, et al. Relation of blood pressure in childhood to self-reported hypertension in adulthood. Hypertension 2019;73(6):1224–30.

46. Zhang T, Li S, Bazzano L, et al. Trajectories of childhood blood pressure and adult left ventricular hypertrophy: the bogalusa heart study. Hypertension 2018; 72(1):93–101.

47. Lewington S, Clarke R, Qizilbash N, et al. Age-specific relevance of usual blood pressure to vascular mortality: a meta-analysis of individual data for one million adults in 61 prospective studies. Lancet 2002;360(9349):1903–13.

48. Luo D, Cheng Y, Zhang H, et al. Association between high blood pressure and long term cardiovascular events in young adults: systematic review and meta-analysis. BMJ 2020;370:m3222.

49. Lurbe E, Agabiti-Rosei E, Cruickshank JK, et al. 2016 European Society of Hypertension guidelines for the management of high blood pressure in children and adolescents. J Hypertens 2016;34(10):1887–920.

50. Khoury M, Khoury PR, Dolan LM, et al. Clinical Implications of the Revised AAP Pediatric Hypertension Guidelines. Pediatrics 2018;142(2):e20180245.

51. Stabouli S, Redon J, Lurbe E. Redefining hypertension in children and adolescents: a review of the evidence considered by the European Society of Hypertension and American Academy of Pediatrics guidelines. J Hypertens 2020;38(2): 196–200.

52. Di Bonito P, Valerio G, Pacifico L, et al. Impact of the 2017 Blood Pressure Guidelines by the American Academy of Pediatrics in overweight/obese youth. J Hypertens 2019;37(4):732–8.

53. Levy D, Garrison RJ, Savage DD, et al. Prognostic implications of echocardiographically determined left ventricular mass in the framingham heart study. New Engl J Med 1990;322(22):1561–6.

54. Woroniecki RP, Kahnauth A, Panesar LE, et al. Left ventricular hypertrophy in pediatric hypertension: a mini review. Front Pediatr 2017;5:101.

55. Urbina EM, Mendizábal B, Becker RC, et al. Association of blood pressure level with left ventricular mass in adolescents. Hypertension 2019;74(3):590–6.

56. Litwin M, Feber J. Origins of primary hypertension in children: early vascular or biological aging? Hypertension 2020;76(5):1400–9.

57. Urbina EM, Khoury PR, McCoy C, et al. Cardiac and vascular consequences of pre-hypertension in youth. J Clin Hypertens (Greenwich) 2011;13(5):332–42.

58. Lande MB, Batisky DL, Kupferman JC, et al. Neurocognitive function in children with primary hypertension. J Pediatr 2017;180:148–55.e1.

59. Rogowska A, Obrycki Ł, Kułaga Z, et al. Remodeling of retinal microcirculation is associated with subclinical arterial injury in hypertensive children. Hypertension 2021;77(4):1203–11.

60. Woo KS, Chook P, Yu CW, et al. Effects of diet and exercise on obesity-related vascular dysfunction in children. Circulation 2004;109(16):1981–6.

61. Dionne JM, Abitbol CL, Flynn JT. Hypertension in infancy: diagnosis, management and outcome. Pediatr Nephrol 2012;27(1):17–32.

62. Swartz SJ, Srivaths PR, Croix B, et al. Cost-effectiveness of ambulatory blood pressure monitoring in the initial evaluation of hypertension in children. Pediatrics 2008;122(6):1177–81.

63. Stergiou G, Stambolliu E, Bountzona I, et al. Home blood pressure monitoring in children and adolescents: systematic review of evidence on clinical utility. Curr Hypertens Rep 2019;21(8):64.

64. Newton J, Singh C, Sinha MD. Measurement of SBP at home by parents using hand-held Doppler device and aneroid sphygmomanometer: a single-centre experience. J Hypertens 2021;39(5):904–10.

65. Singh C, Jones H, Copeman H, et al. Fifteen-minute consultation: the child with systemic arterial hypertension. Arch Dis Child Educ Pract Ed 2017;102(1):2–7.

66. Aguilar-Cordero MJ, Rodríguez-Blanque R, Leon-Ríos X, et al. Influence of physical activity on blood pressure in children with overweight/obesity: a randomized clinical trial. Am J Hypertens 2020;33(2):131–6.

67. Cai L, Wu Y, Wilson RF, et al. Effect of childhood obesity prevention programs on blood pressure: a systematic review and meta-analysis. Circulation 2014;129(18):1832–9.

68. He FJ, MacGregor GA. Importance of salt in determining blood pressure in children: meta-analysis of controlled trials. Hypertension 2006;48(5):861–9.

69. He FJ, Li J, Macgregor GA. Effect of longer term modest salt reduction on blood pressure: cochrane systematic review and meta-analysis of randomised trials. BMJ 2013;346:f1325.

70. Geleijnse JM, Hofman A, Witteman JC, et al. Long-term effects of neonatal sodium restriction on blood pressure. Hypertension 1997;29(4):913–7.

71. Laitinen TT, Nuotio J, Niinikoski H, et al. Attainment of targets of the 20-year infancy-onset dietary intervention and blood pressure across childhood and young adulthood. Hypertension 2020;76(5):1572–9.

72. Paula Bricarello L, Poltronieri F, Fernandes R, et al. Effects of the Dietary Approach to Stop Hypertension (DASH) diet on blood pressure, overweight and obesity in adolescents: a systematic review. Clin Nutr ESPEN 2018;28:1–11.

73. Burrello J, Erhardt EM, Saint-Hilary G, et al. Pharmacological treatment of arterial hypertension in children and adolescents: a network meta-analysis. Hypertension 2018;72(2):306–13.

74. Samuel JP, Tyson JE, Green C, et al. Treating hypertension in children with n-of-1 trials. Pediatrics 2019;143(4):e20181818.

75. Rea CJ, Brady TM, Bundy DG, et al. Pediatrician adherence to guidelines for diagnosis and management of high blood pressure. J Pediatr 2021;242(e1):12–7.

76. Peterson CG, Miyashita Y. The use of ambulatory blood pressure monitoring as standard of care in pediatrics. Front Pediatr 2017;5:153.

77. Farre A, McDonagh JE. Helping health services to meet the needs of young people with chronic conditions: towards a developmental model for transition. Healthcare (Basel) 2017;5(4):77.

78. Chung RJ, Mackie AS, Baker A, et al. Cardiovascular risk and cardiovascular health behaviours in the transition from childhood to adulthood. Can J Cardiol 2020;36(9):1448–57.

79. Nagra A, McGinnity PM, Davis N, et al. Implementing transition: ready Steady Go. Arch Dis Child Educ Pract Ed 2015;100(6):313–20.

80. National Institute for Health and Care Excellence. Transition from children's to adults' services, quality standard [QS140] 2016.

Hemolytic-Uremic Syndrome in Children

Olivia Boyer, MD, PhD[a,b], Patrick Niaudet, MD, PhD[a,*]

KEYWORDS

- Hemolytic uremic syndrome • Thrombotic microangiopathy • Shiga toxin
- Alternative pathway of complement • Eculizumab

KEY POINTS

- Hemolytic uremic syndrome (HUS) is the leading cause of acute kidney injury in children. Most cases are caused by Shiga-toxin-producing bacteria, especially Escherichia coli (STEC-HUS).
- Immediate outcome in STEC-HUS is often favorable but long-term renal sequelae are frequent and follow-up is necessary.
- Prevention of STEC-HUS relies on avoidance of undercooked bovine meat and unpasteurized dairy products, particularly before the age of 5 years.
- Atypical HUS (aHUS), which accounts for about 5% of cases, is mostly due to genetic and/or acquired abnormalities of the complement system.
- aHUS has a relapsing course with high risk of death, kidney failure and recurrence after renal transplantation.

The hemolytic uremic syndrome (HUS), defined by the simultaneous occurrence of microangiopathic hemolytic anemia, thrombocytopenia, and acute kidney injury, is a form of thrombotic microangiopathy affecting primarily the kidney.[1] The most common cause is HUS associated with Shiga toxin (Stx)-producing *Escherichia coli* infection (STEC-HUS). Other infections may cause HUS, and these include streptococcus pneumoniae and human immunodeficiency virus (HIV). Other causes of HUS, previously referred to as atypical HUS, include hereditary causes mainly due to complement gene variants, drug toxicity, and autoimmune diseases. A new classification of HUS based on the underlying mechanisms was recently proposed (**Fig. 1**).[2]

[a] Pediatric Nephrology, Necker Enfants Malades Hospital, Université Paris Cité, France;
[b] Néphrologie Pédiatrique, Hôpital Necker, 149 Rue de Sèvres, Paris 75015, France
* Corresponding author. Néphrologie Pédiatrique, Hôpital Necker, 149 Rue de Sèvres, Paris 75015, France.
E-mail address: pniaudet@gmail.com

Pediatr Clin N Am 69 (2022) 1181–1197
https://doi.org/10.1016/j.pcl.2022.07.006
0031-3955/22/© 2022 Elsevier Inc. All rights reserved.
pediatric.theclinics.com

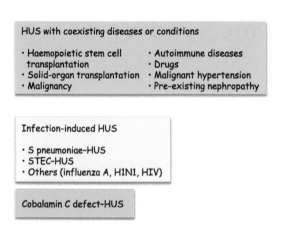

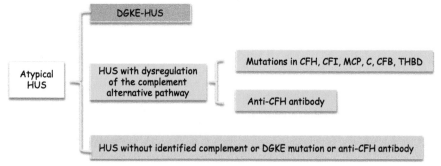

Fig. 1. Classification of various forms of hemolytic uremic syndrome. *Reprinted* with permission from Elsevier. The Lancet, Vol 390, Issue 10095, p,.681-696, Fadi Fakhouri et al., "Haemolytic uraemic syndrome", 2017. https://doi.org/10.1016/S0140-6736(17)30062-4.

INFECTION-INDUCED HEMOLYTIC UREMIC SYNDROME

HUS may occur following STEC or streptococcus pneumoniae infection and rarely with HIV, H1N1 influenza A, and SARS-CoV2 infections.

STEC-HUS

STEC-HUS is the most common form of HUS in children accounting for 90% of all cases. HUS develops in approximately 15% of children with STEC infection.

Epidemiology

Different *E coli* strains have been associated with both sporadic and epidemic STEC-HUS cases throughout the world. There are 2 clinically relevant categories of STEC: those that contain a gene encoding Stx 2 (with or without a gene encoding Stx1) and those that do not. Stx2 is associated with more severe forms of HUS.

The *E coli* serotype associated with HUS varies regionally and over time. In the United States and in Europe, *E coli* O157:H7 has been the most frequent strain associated with HUS in children. Almost all *E coli* O157:H7 contain a gene encoding Stx 2. However, other strains have become more common, including O26, O111, O121, O145, O91, O103, O104, and O80.[3] In Latin America, *E coli* O157:H7 remains the predominant strain (>70%). In Australia, approximately one-half of cases are due to *E coli* O111.

Although found in other animals, healthy cattle are the main vectors of STEC, with the bacteria being present in their intestine and feces.[4] Infection in humans occurs following ingestion of contaminated undercooked meat; unpasteurized milk or milk products; and contaminated water, fruits, or vegetables.[5] Secondary human to human contamination is also possible and may be a concern in day-care centers or in siblings.

Shigella dysenteriae type 1–associated HUS, also due to Shiga toxins, occurs in India, Bangladesh, and Southern Africa. Although the pathogenesis of disease is similar to that of HUS induced by *E coli* infection, the disease is usually more severe with an acute mortality rate of 15%, and greater than 40% of patients develop chronic kidney disease.

Pathophysiology

Stx-mediated injury to vascular endothelial cells in the kidney, brain, and other organs underlies the pathogenesis of HUS caused by STEC. These potent cytotoxins that are released in the gut by bacteria enter the blood stream and cause endothelial injury by binding to the globotriaosylceramide (Gb3) receptor on plasma membrane of the target cells.[6] In humans, Gb3 is a sphingolipid receptor expressed on endothelial cells, podocytes, and proximal tubular cells. Stx binding to Gb3 leads to Stx internalization by receptor-mediated endocytosis and its retrograde transport to the endoplasmic reticulum; this triggers a cascade of signaling events, involving NF-κB activation, which induces apoptosis and the binding of leukocytes to endothelial cells.[7] Activated endothelial cells become thrombogenic, initiating microvascular thrombus formation. In addition, Stxs activate complement and platelet thrombus formation on the endothelial cells.

Clinical manifestations

STEC-HUS principally affects children younger than 5 years. It usually occurs after a prodromal illness with abdominal pain, vomiting, and diarrhea that is frequently bloody. Five to ten days later, HUS develops with the onset of microangiopathic hemolytic anemia with fragmented erythrocytes called schistocytes (**Fig. 2**) and negative Coombs tests, thrombocytopenia, and acute kidney injury. Despite thrombocytopenia, there is usually no purpura or active bleeding. Although the degree of anemia or thrombocytopenia is unrelated to the severity of kidney dysfunction, an increased white blood cell count is associated with a worse prognosis. The hematologic manifestations of STEC-HUS usually resolve completely within 1 to 2 weeks. The kidney involvement ranges from hematuria, usually microscopic, and proteinuria, to severe kidney failure and oligoanuria that occurs in one-half of the cases. Hypertension is

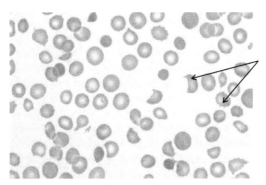

Fig. 2. Red blood cell fragmentation (schistocytes).

common. Dialysis is required in as many as 50% of children during the acute phase, for a mean period of 10 days. The short-term renal prognosis is generally favorable. However, the risk of kidney failure 20 years after the recovery of STEC-HUS is not negligible, and kidney histology showing glomerular microangiopathy affecting greater than 50% of glomeruli (**Fig. 3**), arterial microangiopathy, and/or cortical necrosis (**Fig. 4**) at disease onset indicates a poorer long-term prognosis.

STEC-HUS often affects other organ systems (**Fig. 5**).[8] Central nervous system involvement, which occurs in 20% to -50% of children, is the most serious complication associated with increased morbidity and mortality.[9] Patients may present with seizures, coma, stroke, hemiparesis, facial palsy, pyramidal or extrapyramidal syndromes, dysphasia, diplopia, and cortical blindness. Brain MRI typically reveals bilateral hyperintensity on T2-weighted and hypointensity on T1-weighted images of basal ganglia, thalami, and brainstem, sometimes extending to the surrounding white matter. In addition, MRI may display images of high blood pressure complications such as reversible posterior leukoencephalopathy syndrome and cerebral hemorrhage.

Gastrointestinal manifestations include severe hemorrhagic colitis, bowel necrosis and perforation, rectal prolapse, peritonitis, and intussusception. Cardiac ischemia and dysfunction may occur. Transient and rarely permanent diabetes mellitus may occur. Hepatomegaly and/or increased serum transaminases are frequently observed. Over the years, the mortality rate has dropped to about 5% and is mostly due to neurologic or cardiac involvement.[10] Persistent oligoanuria (>5 days of anuria and >10 days of oliguria), dehydration, elevated white blood cell count greater than 20,000 per mm^3, and hematocrit greater than 23% are other risk factors for mortality and long-term complications from HUS.

The evaluation for STEC infection includes testing for Stxs (polymerase chain reaction for the presence of ST-1 and/or ST-2 genes) in the stool and stool cultures. Results from stool cultures may be unreliable because the bacteria are present in stool for a few days only and, even if present, may not be detected by culture from stool samples. Serum antibodies to lipopolysaccharide of STEC persist for several weeks and may be of added value in the diagnosis of STEC infection.

Treatment

Patients with HUS can become profoundly anemic very quickly. Packed red blood cells should be transfused when the hemoglobin level is less than 6 g/dL or hematocrit less

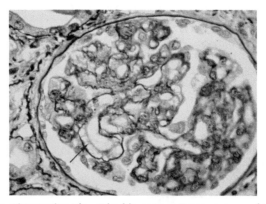

Fig. 3. Thrombotic microangiopathy: "double contour" appearance of the capillary walls with a widening of the subendothelial space. These lesions affect a variable proportion of glomeruli.

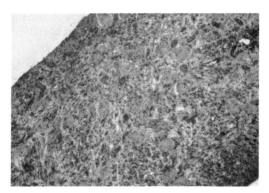

Fig. 4. Cortical necrosis.

than 18% to avoid cardiovascular and pulmonary complications. The goal is not to restore the hemoglobin level to normal because the increased volume may cause heart failure, pulmonary edema, and hypertension. Blood products should be volume reduced and preferably depleted of leukocytes and platelets to avoid alloimmunization.

Platelet transfusion is reserved for patients with clinically significant bleeding or if an invasive procedure is required. Significant bleeding is infrequent because the platelet count rarely falls less than 10,000/mm³, and platelet production and function are normal. Platelet transfusion may induce antihuman leukocyte antigen antibodies, which may be deleterious later if the patient progresses to end-stage kidney failure and requires kidney transplantation.

Fluid management is based on the intravascular volume status of the patient and kidney function. Patients with decreased intravascular volume are repleted to a euvolemic state, whereas those with increased intravascular volume and diminished urine

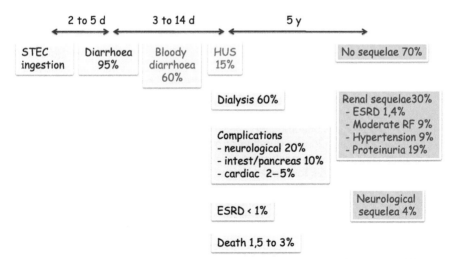

Fig. 5. Complement pathway. The black loop represents the complement amplification loop. Black stars represent known genes which mutations cause aHUS. Black squares indicate drugs targeting the complement system, used in aHUS. CFB, complement factor B; CFD, complement factor D; CFH, complement factor H; CFI, complement factor I; MAC, membrane attack complex; MCP, membrane cofactor protein; THBD, thrombomodulin.

output are fluid restricted. Observational studies have reported that an early volume expansion may reduce the risk of CNS involvement, need of kidney replacement therapy, and long-term renal sequelae.

There is no evidence that early dialysis affects the clinical outcome. As a result, the indications for dialysis in children with HUS are similar to those in children with other forms of acute kidney injury. In most young children, peritoneal dialysis is preferred. However, there is no evidence of increased benefit of peritoneal dialysis as compared with hemodialysis.

Management of hypertension is directed toward correcting the fluid status and using antihypertensive agents such as the calcium channel blockers. Randomized trials have not shown any benefits from antithrombotic or antifibrinolytic agents, plasma infusions, tissue-type plasminogen activator, and oral Stx-binding agents.[1] Patients with severe neurological manifestations may be treated with eculizumab[11,12] and immunoadsorption if they do not respond to eculizumab.[13]

Prevention

Prevention of STEC-HUS rests in part on measures aimed at reducing the risk of STEC infection. These measures include meticulous hygiene when cooking and changing diapers and avoidance of undercooked meat and unpasteurized milk products in young children. STEC infection may also occur through water contamination, direct contact with infected animals, or person–person spread.

Several studies have provided evidence supporting the possibility of preventing or reducing the severity of HUS by early intravascular volume expansion with intravenous isotonic solutions in patients with STEC who are volume depleted.[14] Once a patient is infected with STEC, attempts to prevent progression from the bloody diarrheal phase to the HUS have been unsuccessful. Administration of antimotility drugs (such as anticholinergic agents or narcotics) do not reduce the progression to HUS caused by STEC infection, but on the contrary seem to increase the risk for HUS.[15] The impact of antibiotic administration during the bloody diarrheal phase remains uncertain. There are clinical observational data that suggest administration of beta-lactams, and trimethoprim/sulfamethoxazole is associated with increased risk of developing HUS,[16] whereas fosfomycin may reduce the risk for HUS.[17]

Pneumococcal-Associated Hemolytic Uremic Syndrome

Pneumococcal-associated HUS accounts for about 5% of all childhood cases of HUS. Patients present with pneumonia (70%) or meningitis (20%–30%). In comparison to STEC HUS, children with pneumococcal-associated HUS are younger, have more severe disease onset with longer duration of oliguria and thrombocytopenia, and are likely to require more blood transfusions.[18]

The pathogenesis of this form of HUS remains unclear. It has been proposed that desialylation by neuraminidase results in exposing the Thomsen-Friedenreich antigen (T antigen) on red blood cells, platelets, and glomeruli, resulting in polyagglutination of patient's red cells and hemolysis.[19] In addition, an activation of the alternative pathway probably plays a role.[20]

The management of pneumococcal-associated HUS is supportive. In addition, empiric antibiotic therapy for invasive pneumococcal disease should be initiated with both vancomycin and a broad-spectrum cephalosporin. It is recommended to avoid plasma infusion or plasmapheresis because of concerns that plasma, which contains natural immunoglobulin M (IgM) class antibodies to the Thomsen-Friedenreich antigen, may aggravate hemolysis.[21] The mortality related to the underlying infection and the long-term risk of chronic kidney disease is higher as compared with patients with STEC HUS.

ATYPICAL HEMOLYTIC UREMIC SYNDROME

Atypical hemolytic uremic syndrome (aHUS) is a heterogeneous group of disorders that includes all forms of HUS that are not caused by infections or coexisting medical conditions.[2] It is a rare condition with an estimated incidence of 0.25 to 2 per million per year and accounts for 10% of all cases of HUS diagnosed in childhood.[22] The proposed mechanism for complement-mediated aHUS is the unregulated activation of the complement system triggered by infections, immunizations, or pregnancy, in a susceptible individual with inherited (genetic) or acquired (autoimmune) disruption of the alternate complement pathway (**Fig. 6**). An uninhibited continuous activation of the alternative pathway with subsequent formation of the membrane attack complex on endothelial cells, red blood cells, and platelets causes renal and extrarenal endothelial damage, activation of the coagulation cascade, and thrombotic microangiopathy.[23]

Nowadays, a hereditary abnormality in the alternative complement pathway is identified in approximately 60% of the patients with aHUS.[24] Other hereditary causes of complement-independent aHUS have been described. These include intracellular defects of vitamin B12 or lipid metabolisms. Untreated, aHUS has a poor prognosis with high risk of relapses, progression to kidney failure, and a significant mortality, risks that

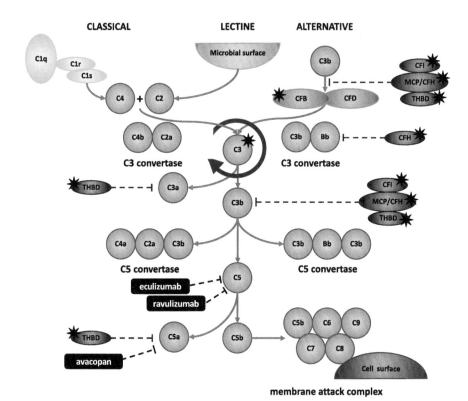

Fig. 6. Clinical presentation and evolution of STEC-HUS.

vary depending on the underlying cause.[25] Extrarenal manifestations of aHUS are frequent in children.[26] These include neurological involvement in up to 27% of cases, cardiovascular complications in 7%, and gastrointestinal symptoms in 10% to 80% of cases, which seem to be particularly frequent in case of anticomplement factor H (CFH) antibodies.[27]

Given the frequency of prodromal diarrhea in children with aHUS, it may be difficult to differentiate typical and atypical HUS at the disease onset.[25] The diagnostic workup should include a detailed assessment of complement function, including a CH50 assay (a functional hemolytic test that explores the classic and common final pathways) combined with a quantitative measurement of C3 and C4 fractions, factor H, factor B, and factor I proteins, and study of CD46 expression on the cell surface.[2] In addition, anti-factor H autoantibody detection should be performed urgently, as identification of high levels would require specific therapy. Genetic testing in patients with aHUS is essential for prognostic assessment and necessary for the long-term treatment of patients, as it may guide treatment duration.[2] Differential diagnoses such as ADAMTS13 deficiency or autoantibodies should also be promptly ruled out.

Complement Gene Variants

Complement acts as a major defense system against microorganisms in humans through spontaneous hydrolysis of C3 and deposition of C3b on multiple cells that are in contact with the plasma. Because of its permanent activation and amplification ability, complement system needs to be finely regulated so that its activation occurs only at the microbial surfaces but is inhibited at intact host cell surfaces. The variants causing aHUS ultimately lead to a permanent and uncontrolled activation of the alternative pathway of complement and thereby damage to host cells.

Genetically predisposed aHUS may occur due to loss-of-function variants of inhibitory genes (eg, *CFH*, *CFI*, *MCP*, or *THBD*) or gain-of-function variants in activating genes (eg, *CFB* and *C3*).[28] Even in these inherited conditions, aHUS can manifest at any age on triggering events. The predominant mode of inheritance is autosomal dominance, although a subset of patients has homozygous *CFH* or *CD46* variants and typically have earlier disease onset and more severe phenotypes. The penetrance of the disease is low, as less than 20% of family members, carrying the same variant as the patient, present with aHUS manifestations.[29]

CFH gene variants (encoding complement factor H, reported mutation frequency 20%–30%)

CFH encodes complement factor H, a complement alternative pathway inhibitor in the fluid phase and on cell surfaces. It binds to C3b, accelerates the decay of the C3bBb convertase, and also serves as a cofactor for complement factor I, another C3b inhibitor. *CFH* is the most frequently mutated gene in patients with aHUS, accounting for approximately 20% to 30% of all incident patients.[22,30] *CFH* pathogenic variants have been identified in approximately 25% of sporadic cases and 40% of familial aHUS cases.[31] They are distributed throughout the gene, but most are found in the carboxy-terminus, encoding short consensus repeats 19 and 20 that bind C3b[32] and endothelia.[33] Some variants cause a quantitative deficiency of protein in the plasma, whereas others induce a functional defect of the protein even when the level is normal.

The aHUS manifestations typically occur either before the age of 4 years or in the second to fourth decades.[30] Homozygous *CFH* variants are almost exclusively seen in infants, and heterozygous variants are found in all age groups, usually with incomplete penetrance.[34] Severe hypertension is commonly observed. Hemolytic anemia is marked at disease onset and during relapses, with haptoglobin and CH50 levels remaining low throughout the course of the disease. Among all aHUS patients, those with *CFH* variants have the worst outcome with the highest risk of developing kidney failure or death within one year of diagnosis.[35] Moreover, they have a high risk of post-kidney transplant recurrence and poor allograft survival in the absence of specific treatment.[30]

CD46 gene variants (previously known as membrane cofactor protein, 5%–15%)
CD46 (or membrane cofactor protein [MCP]) is a cofactor of complement factor I in the degradation of C3b. The mutations causing aHUS most commonly result in decreased cell surface levels of CD46 or a reduced ability to control activation of the alternative complement pathway on host cells without quantitative deficiency.[36] CD46-associated aHUS is characterized by an early onset in childhood, frequent relapses, a favorable renal course in most patients, and a low recurrence rate in the kidney allograft.[37]

CFI gene variants (complement factor I, 5%–10%)
Complement factor I inactivates C3b fragments by proteolytic cleavage in the presence of its serum cofactor (factor H) or membrane cofactor (CD46). The products of C3b degradation are unable to reconstitute a C3 convertase. Most patients bear heterozygous *CFI* variants, yielding a quantitative or qualitative factor I defect.[38,39] Of note, an additional genetic risk factor for HUS is sometimes identified in patients with *CFI* variants.[40] aHUS associated with *CFI* variants are less severe than aHUS related to *CFH* variants but more severe than aHUS due to *CD46* variants. The reported progression to kidney failure is 50% to 60% within 2 years of presentation,[40,41] with one-third of patients recovering from the initial thrombotic microangiopathy presentation without disease recurrence.[40] Recurrence occurs after kidney transplantation in 45% to 80% of patients and ultimately leads to graft loss.

C3 gene variants (complement factor 3, 4%–7%)
Although these variants are spread throughout the protein, there is a reported cluster in the thioester-containing domain that is essential for C3 activation.[40] Similar to patients with *CFH*-related aHUS, the renal prognosis of aHUS caused by *C3* variants is guarded in the absence of specific treatment.[42]

CFB gene variants (complement factor B, 1%–2%)
Gain-of-function *CFB* variants have been more rarely reported, either enhancing formation or delaying inactivation of the C3bBb convertase. They are associated with progression to kidney failure in 70% of patients, a very high risk of posttransplant aHUS recurrence and subsequent graft loss.[43,44]

THBD gene variants (thrombomodulin, 0%–5%)
Thrombomodulin serves as a cofactor for thrombin-catalyzed activation of protein C and is a natural anticoagulant. In addition, it enhances complement factor I–mediated degradation of C3b. One study reported 6 heterozygous *THBD* gene variants in 7 patients in a cohort of 152 patients with aHUS (5%). In vitro functional studies demonstrated that thrombomodulin mutants were less effective in inactivating C3b than the normal protein and resulted in deregulation of the complement system. Nevertheless, pathogenic variants in this gene have rarely been found by other groups, and their pathogenicity is still a matter of debate. Whether eculizumab is efficient in such cases deserves clarification.

Treatment

Symptomatic treatment is similar to STEC-HUS as detailed earlier.

Plasma therapy was once the cornerstone for the treatment of aHUS, despite the lack of a high level of evidence for its efficacy. The advantages of plasma exchanges compared with plasma infusion included removal of defective mutant proteins and autoantibodies, administration of functioning complement proteins, and a lower risk of volume overload and hypertension in patients with acute kidney injury. However, this treatment was suboptimal, given the low remission rate in less than 50% of patients and the high morbidity and mortality rates depending on the affected complement gene.[35,45,46] Indeed, the incidence of kidney failure or death was approximately 40% at onset and 65% within 1 year.[47] The remission rate was higher in cases of *CFH* variants than with *CFI* or *MCP* variants. The procedure was sometimes tolerated poorly with frequent allergic reactions, and its long-term hospital-based administration had a negative impact on the quality of life, schooling, and social activities of children.

The prognosis of aHUS has improved considerably with the advent of complement inhibitors. The first to be approved for this indication was eculizumab in 2011.[47] Eculizumab is a recombinant humanized monoclonal anti-C5 antibody that inhibits the terminal part of the complement pathway, from the formation of C5a to the membrane-attack-complex assemblage. In the majority of children treated with eculizumab, the reported outcome is favorable in both acute and chronic settings with a rapid and sustained improvement of hematological and renal parameters during the first and subsequent episodes of aHUS, including those occurring after renal transplantation.[48,49] Consequently, in 2014 an international consensus recommended its use as first-line treatment in children with a clinical diagnosis of aHUS.[2] It should be started promptly within 24 to 48 hours of diagnosis, as early initiation is associated with better recovery of kidney function. It is not necessary to wait for the results of genetic testing to initiate treatment, as this can take a long time, and eculizumab is effective in a number of children without any identified genetic variants. Currently, there are 2 drugs that act by targeting and inhibiting the C5/C5a axis and are suitable for the treatment of aHUS and these include eculizumab, and ravulizumab.[50] Other drugs are being investigated.

The most frequent and potentially fatal side effects of complement inhibitors are infections and in particular meningococcal meningitis. Children treated with complement blockers should therefore be vaccinated against all strains of meningococcus and pneumococcus, at best before the initiation of treatment, and receive antibiotic prophylaxis. With these precautions, drug-related infections are rare, and patients recover without any sequelae. Hepatotoxicity has also been reported but it is difficult to determine whether it is treatment related or related to preexisting hepatic thrombotic microangiopathy; this suggests an overall favorable risk profile for eculizumab.[2,47,48]

Considering the prohibitive cost, twice-monthly intravenous administration, and high infectious risks, several studies have investigated the safety of dose spacing or discontinuation of eculizumab in selected patients.[51] Fakhouri and colleagues[52] demonstrated in a prospective trial that eculizumab can be stopped safely in the absence of any causal variant or in the case of a *MCP* variant, provided that the relapses are closely monitored, and eculizumab restarted promptly in case of confirmed relapse. This study also revealed that restarting eculizumab promptly at the onset of a relapse was associated with a recovery of normal kidney function. These data are consistent with other retrospective series.[53–57] Until more robust data are available on the optimal administration and discontinuation of complement inhibitor therapy, the decision to withdraw therapy should be made carefully.

Monitoring of complement activity is warranted during eculizumab therapy to ensure its effectiveness. Of note, CH50 cannot be used for patients with complete CFH deficiency because it is permanently low. The interval between doses can be extended if adequate complement blockade is maintained. CH50 should be less than 10% for complete blockade, but an activity less than 30% seems to be associated with sustained disease remission despite reduced frequency of eculizumab administration.[58]

When eculizumab is not available, plasma exchange remains the preferred intervention, and it should also be started promptly within 24 to 48 hours of diagnosis to enhance efficacy.[59] Liver transplant is an alternative curative intervention when disease is driven by a protein synthetized by the liver (FH, FB, C3, and FI).

Variants in Complement-Independent Genes

The variants of these genes, which are transmitted as autosomal recessive traits, do not lead to overt complement dysfunction and therefore do not theoretically respond to complement inhibitors.

cblC gene variants (cobalamin-C)

Renal thrombotic microangiopathy has been described as a complication of cobalamin-C (cblC) deficiency due to cblC gene variants since the 1990s.[60] These variants underlie the combined methylmalonic aciduria (MMA) and homocystinuria, a genetically heterogeneous disorder of cobalamin (cbl; vitamin B12) metabolism. The majority of patients have an early onset in infancy, mostly within their first 4 months and many in their first days of life.[61] In addition to acute metabolic decompensations, patients may display intrauterine growth retardation, congenital heart disease, visual impairment, and nystagmus due to optic atrophy and retinopathy. They develop a progressive complex neurological phenotype with developmental delay, behavior perturbances, and peripheral neuropathy. Fulminant, often lethal manifestations with early onset aHUS and pulmonary hypertension have been reported, some with missed diagnosis or delayed treatment.[62] The diagnosis should be suspected in the presence of megaloblastosis. The specific treatment consisting of hydroxocobalamin and betaine may prevent metabolic crises and improve kidney function including in dialysis-dependent infants and should therefore be promptly initiated in all infants with unclear aHUS while waiting for the results of blood/plasma homocysteine levels and/or genetic testing of the MMACHC gene.[61]

DGKE gene variants (diacylglycerol kinase ε, 1%–17%)

Diacylglycerol kinase ε is an intracellular lipid kinase that phosphorylates diacylglycerol to phosphatidic acid, resulting in protein kinase C activation. The exact mechanism by which DGKE deficiency drives aHUS has not yet been unraveled. Such variants were reported in infants (median age 9 months) affected with aHUS and a particular phenotype characterized by persistent proteinuria, hematuria, and severe hypertension with progressive chronic kidney disease.[63,64] The kidney histology is also characteristic with respect to glomerular cellularity, split glomerular basement membranes, swelling of endothelial cells, and widening of the glomerular basement membrane internal lamina rara in the absence of electron-dense deposition.[63] Treatment with eculizumab does not seem to result in long-term clinical improvement in children with DGKE variants, and relapses have been described despite complement blockade[65]; this suggests that complement inhibitors should be withheld in such cases to avoid unwarranted side effects. Remarkably, no relapses have been published in transplanted patients.

Atypical Hemolytic Uremic Syndrome with Anticomplement Autoantibodies

Autoantibodies directed against complement regulators (factor H, factor I) account for approximately 6% to 25% of cases of aHUS with a pediatric onset.[66,67]

Anticomplement factor H autoantibodies

Anti-CFH IgGs are by far the most common autoantibodies identified in patients with aHUS. These antibodies cause aHUS in 5% to 25% of patients in Europe but greater than 50% of patients in South Asia.[68] They bind to multiple factor H domains, thereby perturbing its interaction with C3b and cell surfaces, ultimately reducing the ability of factor H to prevent damage.[69] More than 90% patients bear a homozygous deletion of *CFHR1* and *CFHR3* genes.[70] Of note, this deletion is also found in 2% to 5% of healthy individuals in the general population. At the disease onset, the majority of patients exhibit hallmarks of alternative complement pathway activation (decreased C3 and/ or factor B levels), and a subgroup of patients also have a decrease in factor H levels.[27] Other autoantibodies such as antinuclear antibodies may be present in some patients.

CFH antibody–mediated aHUS typically manifest in school-aged children (7– 10 years). Most cases present with a full triad of HUS manifestations, and a prodromal diarrhea has been reported in up to 80% cases, along with other infectious triggers in some patients.[27] Extrarenal complications are frequent and more than half of the patients require initial dialysis. Relapses are common and typically occur within the first 2 years after initial presentation, and the risk of kidney failure or death is higher in the absence of adequate treatment. The risk of post-kidney transplant recurrence is high.

Besides symptomatic treatments, the specific management of CFH antibody–mediated aHUS is challenging and evolving with the availability of complement inhibitors. The goals of treatment are to induce a rapid and sustained remission without disease recurrence. There is currently no consensus on the optimal regimen. The classical approach consisted of plasma exchanges aiming to rapidly remove circulating anti-CFH antibodies,[71] followed by immunosuppressive therapy to reduce the production of anti-CFH antibodies.[2] Dragon-Durey and colleagues[69] reviewed the treatment efficacy in published series and showed a 17% to 29% risk of relapse and 35% to 46% risk of chronic kidney disease stage 4 or 5 or death in case of supportive care or plasmapheresis-based protocols as opposed to 10% and 14% if plasma exchanges were combined to immunosuppressants.

Various combinations of immunosuppressants have been reported to be effective and these include corticosteroids, intravenous cyclophosphamide, rituximab, and oral mycophenolate mofetil.[72] For instance, a combination of 2 to 4 plasma exchanges and 2 mini-pulses of cyclophosphamide with a short trial of oral steroids has been shown to allow sustained treatment-free remission for up to 15 years.[42] At present, following the aforementioned international recommendation, eculizumab is often started before the identification of anti-CFH antibodies.[2] Thus, when the diagnosis is confirmed, 2 approaches are possible: (1) switch eculizumab to start plasma exchanges and immunosuppressants, especially if the child has a central line in place for dialysis, to reduce the burden of long-term eculizumab therapy; (2) continue eculizumab in combination with other immunosuppressants to avoid the possible complications of a central venous line access.[73] When antibody levels remain persistently low on immunosuppressants, experts suggest to stop eculizumab with close monitoring before discontinuation of other immunosuppressive drugs. Conversely, eculizumab alone without immunosuppression, although effective in controlling the disease and improving organ function, does not decrease the anti-CFH antibody titer and must therefore be continued indefinitely; otherwise there is a high risk of relapse.[74] Future research should seek to clearly define the optimal treatment of CFH antibody–mediated aHUS.

Anticomplement factor I autoantibodies
Recently, anti-CFI autoantibodies have been described in a few children who notably had 2 copies of the *CFHR1* and *CFHR3* genes and low levels of factor H. They seem to be more common in India and in children younger than 2 years, whereas children older than 2 years have predominantly anti-CFH antibodies.[75] Plasmapheresis carried out in 2 children resulted in a rapid improvement.

SUMMARY

HUS is due to a thrombotic microangiopathy affecting mainly the kidney. In children, HUS is most often secondary to an infection from STEC. Risk factors for poor outcomes include increased leukocyte count, the need for dialysis and its duration, and the extent of glomerular involvement. Early volume expansion improves the short- and long-term outcomes. During the past 10 years, complement dysregulation has been identified as the main cause of atypical HUS, enabling breakthroughs in the diagnosis and the therapy with monoclonal anti-C5 antibodies.

CLINICS CARE POINTS

- In STEC-HUS, early volume expansion can reduce the risk of complications.
- To avoid cardiovascular and pulmonary complications, the packed red blood cells (RBC) should be avoided unless hemoglobin level is <6 g/dL or hematocrit <18 percent."
- Platelet transfusion is reserved for patients with clinically significant bleeding or if an invasive procedure is required.
- There is no benefit in using antithrombotic or antifibrinolytic agents, plasma infusions, tissue-type plasminogen activator, and oral Shiga toxin-binding agents
- Plasma infusion and plasmapheresis should be avoided in pneumococcal- associated HUS because it may aggravate hemolysis due to the presence of antibodies to the Thomsen-Friedenreich antigen
- Monoclonal complement inhibitor is the first-line treatment in patients with atypical-HUS.
- A prompt plasma exchange is recommended if monoclonal complement inhibitor is not available

REFERENCES

1. Fakhouri F, Zuber J, Fremeaux-Bacchi V, et al. Haemolytic uraemic syndrome. Lancet 2017;390(10095):681–96.
2. Loirat C, Fakhouri F, Ariceta G, et al. An international consensus approach to the management of atypical hemolytic uremic syndrome in children. Pediatr Nephrol (Berlin, Germany) 2016;31(1):15–39.
3. Gould LH, Mody RK, Ong KL, et al. Increased recognition of non-O157 Shiga toxin-producing Escherichia coli infections in the United States during 2000-2010: epidemiologic features and comparison with E. coli O157 infections. Foodborne Pathog Dis 2013;10(5):453–60.
4. Kim JS, Lee MS, Kim JH. Recent Updates on Outbreaks of Shiga Toxin-Producing Escherichia coli and Its Potential Reservoirs. Front Cell Infect Microbiol 2020; 10:273.
5. Vaillant V, Espie E, de Valk H, et al. Undercooked ground beef and person-to-person transmission as major risk factors for sporadic hemolytic uremic

syndrome related to Shiga-toxin producing Escherchia coli infections in children in France. Pediatr Infect Dis J 2009;28(7):650–3.

6. Psotka MA, Obata F, Kolling GL, et al. Shiga toxin 2 targets the murine renal collecting duct epithelium. Infect Immun 2009;77(3):959–69.

7. Zoja C, Buelli S, Morigi M. Shiga toxin-associated hemolytic uremic syndrome: pathophysiology of endothelial dysfunction. Pediatr Nephrol (Berlin, Germany) 2010;25(11):2231–40.

8. Khalid M, Andreoli S. Extrarenal manifestations of the hemolytic uremic syndrome associated with Shiga toxin-producing Escherichia coli (STEC HUS). Pediatr Nephrol (Berlin, Germany) 2019;34(12):2495–507.

9. Nathanson S, Kwon T, Elmaleh M, et al. Acute neurological involvement in diarrhea-associated hemolytic uremic syndrome. Clin J Am Soc Nephrol 2010; 5(7):1218–28.

10. Brown CC, Garcia X, Bhakta RT, et al. Severe acute neurologic involvement in children with hemolytic-uremic syndrome. Pediatrics 2021;147(3). e2020013631.

11. Percheron L, Gramada R, Tellier S, et al. Eculizumab treatment in severe pediatric STEC-HUS: a multicenter retrospective study. Pediatr Nephrol (Berlin, Germany) 2018;33(8):650–3.

12. Lapeyraque AL, Malina M, Fremeaux-Bacchi V, et al. Complement blockade in severe shiga-toxin-associated HUS. N Engl J Med 2011;364(26):2561–3.

13. Greinacher A, Friesecke S, Abel P, et al. Treatment of severe neurological deficits with IgG depletion through immunoadsorption in patients with Escherichia coli O104:H4-associated haemolytic uraemic syndrome: a prospective trial. Lancet 2011;378(9797):1166–73.

14. Grisaru S, Xie J, Samuel S, et al. Associations between hydration status, intravenous fluid administration, and outcomes of patients infected with shiga toxin-producing escherichia coli: a systematic review and meta-analysis. JAMA Pediatr 2017;171(1):68–76.

15. Bell BP, Griffin PM, Lozano P, et al. Predictors of hemolytic uremic syndrome in children during a large outbreak of Escherichia coli O157:H7 infections. Pediatrics 1997;100(1):E12.

16. Wong CS, Jelacic S, Habeeb RL, et al. The risk of the hemolytic-uremic syndrome after antibiotic treatment of Escherichia coli O157:H7 infections. N Engl J Med 2000;342(26):1930–6.

17. Ikeda K, Ida O, Kimoto K, et al. Effect of early fosfomycin treatment on prevention of hemolytic uremic syndrome accompanying Escherichia coli O157:H7 infection. Clin Nephrol 1999;52(6):357–62.

18. Copelovitch L, Kaplan BS. Streptococcus pneumoniae-associated hemolytic uremic syndrome. Pediatr Nephrol (Berlin, Germany) 2008;23(11):1951–6.

19. Geary DF. Hemolytic uremic syndrome and streptococcus pneumoniae: improving our understanding. J Pediatr 2007;151(2):113–4.

20. Scobell RR, Kaplan BS, Copelovitch L. New insights into the pathogenesis of Streptococcus pneumoniae-associated hemolytic uremic syndrome. Pediatr Nephrol (Berlin, Germany) 2020;35(9):1585–91.

21. Spinale JM, Ruebner RL, Kaplan BS, et al. Update on Streptococcus pneumoniae associated hemolytic uremic syndrome. Curr Opin Pediatr 2013;25(2):203–8.

22. Noris M, Remuzzi G. Genetics and genetic testing in hemolytic uremic syndrome/ thrombotic thrombocytopenic purpura. Semin Nephrol 2010;30(4):395–408.

23. Goodship TH, Cook HT, Fakhouri F, et al. Atypical hemolytic uremic syndrome and C3 glomerulopathy: conclusions from a "Kidney Disease: improving Global Outcomes" (KDIGO) Controversies Conference. Kidney Int 2017;91(3):539–51.

24. Lemaire M, Noone D, Lapeyraque AL, et al. Inherited kidney complement diseases. Clin J Am Soc Nephrol 2021;16(6):942–56.
25. Loirat C, Fremeaux-Bacchi V. Atypical hemolytic uremic syndrome. Orphanet J Rare Dis 2011;6:60.
26. Fidan K, Goknar N, Gulhan B, et al. Extra-Renal manifestations of atypical hemolytic uremic syndrome in children. Pediatr Nephrol (Berlin, Germany) 2018;33(8): 1395–403.
27. Dragon-Durey MA, Sethi SK, Bagga A, et al. Clinical features of anti-factor H autoantibody-associated hemolytic uremic syndrome. J Am Soc Nephrol 2010; 21(12):2180–7.
28. Noris M, Brioschi S, Caprioli J, et al. Familial haemolytic uraemic syndrome and an MCP mutation. Lancet 2003;362(9395):1542–7.
29. Ardissino G, Longhi S, Porcaro L, et al. Risk of Atypical HUS Among Family Members of Patients Carrying Complement Regulatory Gene Abnormality. Kidney Int Rep 2021;6(6):1614–21.
30. Kavanagh D, Goodship TH, Richards A. Atypical hemolytic uremic syndrome. Semin Nephrol 2013;33(6):508–30.
31. Maga TK, Nishimura CJ, Weaver AE, et al. Mutations in alternative pathway complement proteins in American patients with atypical hemolytic uremic syndrome. Hum Mutat 2010;31(6):E1445–60.
32. Jokiranta TS, Jaakola VP, Lehtinen MJ, et al. Structure of complement factor H carboxyl-terminus reveals molecular basis of atypical haemolytic uremic syndrome. EMBO J 2006;25(8):1784–94.
33. Lehtinen MJ, Rops AL, Isenman DE, et al. Mutations of factor H impair regulation of surface-bound C3b by three mechanisms in atypical hemolytic uremic syndrome. J Biol Chem 2009;284(23):15650–8.
34. Pickering MC, Cook HT. Translational mini-review series on complement factor H: renal diseases associated with complement factor H: novel insights from humans and animals. Clin Exp Immunol 2008;151(2):210–30.
35. Fremeaux-Bacchi V, Fakhouri F, Garnier A, et al. Genetics and outcome of atypical hemolytic uremic syndrome: a nationwide French series comparing children and adults. Clin J Am Soc Nephrol 2013;8(4):554–62.
36. Fang CJ, Fremeaux-Bacchi V, Liszewski MK, et al. Membrane cofactor protein mutations in atypical hemolytic uremic syndrome (aHUS), fatal Stx-HUS, C3 glomerulonephritis, and the HELLP syndrome. Blood 2008;111(2):624–32.
37. Klambt V, Gimpel C, Bald M, et al. Different approaches to long-term treatment of aHUS due to MCP mutations: a multicenter analysis. Pediatr Nephrol (Berlin, Germany) 2021;36(2):463–71.
38. Kavanagh D, Kemp EJ, Mayland E, et al. Mutations in complement factor I predispose to development of atypical hemolytic uremic syndrome. J Am Soc Nephrol 2005;16(7):2150–5.
39. Fremeaux-Bacchi V, Dragon-Durey MA, Blouin J, et al. Complement factor I: a susceptibility gene for atypical haemolytic uraemic syndrome. J Med Genet 2004;41(6):e84.
40. Bienaime F, Dragon-Durey MA, Regnier CH, et al. Mutations in components of complement influence the outcome of Factor I-associated atypical hemolytic uremic syndrome. Kidney Int 2010;77(4):339–49.
41. Sellier-Leclerc AL, Fremeaux-Bacchi V, Dragon-Durey MA, et al. Differential impact of complement mutations on clinical characteristics in atypical hemolytic uremic syndrome. J Am Soc Nephrol 2007;18(8):2392–400.

42. Zuber J, Fakhouri F, Roumenina LT, et al. Use of eculizumab for atypical haemolytic uraemic syndrome and C3 glomerulopathies. Nat Rev Nephrol 2012;8(11): 643–57.

43. Goicoechea de Jorge E, Harris CL, Esparza-Gordillo J, et al. Gain-of-function mutations in complement factor B are associated with atypical hemolytic uremic syndrome. Proc Natl Acad Sci United States America 2007;104(1):240–5.

44. Roumenina LT, Jablonski M, Hue C, et al. Hyperfunctional C3 convertase leads to complement deposition on endothelial cells and contributes to atypical hemolytic uremic syndrome. Blood 2009;114(13):2837–45.

45. Noris M, Caprioli J, Bresin E, et al. Relative role of genetic complement abnormalities in sporadic and familial aHUS and their impact on clinical phenotype. Clin J Am Soc Nephrol 2010;5(10):1844–59.

46. Loirat C, Macher MA, Elmaleh-Berges M, et al. Non-atheromatous arterial stenoses in atypical haemolytic uraemic syndrome associated with complement dysregulation. Nephrol Dial Transpl 2010;25(10):3421–5.

47. Legendre CM, Licht C, Muus P, et al. Terminal complement inhibitor eculizumab in atypical hemolytic-uremic syndrome. N Engl J Med 2013;368(23):2169–81.

48. Licht C, Greenbaum LA, Muus P, et al. Efficacy and safety of eculizumab in atypical hemolytic uremic syndrome from 2-year extensions of phase 2 studies. Kidney Int 2015;87(5):1061–73.

49. Greenbaum LA, Fila M, Ardissino G, et al. Eculizumab is a safe and effective treatment in pediatric patients with atypical hemolytic uremic syndrome. Kidney Int 2016;89(3):701–11.

50. Rondeau E, Scully M, Ariceta G, et al. The long-acting C5 inhibitor, Ravulizumab, is effective and safe in adult patients with atypical hemolytic uremic syndrome naive to complement inhibitor treatment. Kidney Int 2020;97(6):1287–96.

51. Macia M, de Alvaro Moreno F, Dutt T, et al. Current evidence on the discontinuation of eculizumab in patients with atypical haemolytic uraemic syndrome. Clin Kidney J 2017;10(3):310–9.

52. Fakhouri F, Fila M, Hummel A, et al. Eculizumab discontinuation in children and adults with atypical hemolytic-uremic syndrome: a prospective multicenter study. Blood 2021;137(18):2438–49.

53. Ardissino G, Testa S, Possenti I, et al. Discontinuation of eculizumab maintenance treatment for atypical hemolytic uremic syndrome: a report of 10 cases. Am J Kidney Dis 2014;64(4):633–7.

54. Fakhouri F, Fila M, Provot F, et al. Pathogenic Variants in Complement Genes and Risk of Atypical Hemolytic Uremic Syndrome Relapse after Eculizumab Discontinuation. Clin J Am Soc Nephrol 2017;12(1):50–9.

55. Merrill SA, Brittingham ZD, Yuan X, et al. Eculizumab cessation in atypical hemolytic uremic syndrome. Blood 2017;130(3):368–72.

56. Wijnsma KL, Duineveld C, Wetzels JFM, et al. Eculizumab in atypical hemolytic uremic syndrome: strategies toward restrictive use. Pediatr Nephrol (Berlin, Germany) 2019;34(11):2261–77.

57. Ariceta G. Optimal duration of treatment with eculizumab in atypical hemolytic uremic syndrome (aHUS)-a question to be addressed in a scientific way. Pediatr Nephrol (Berlin, Germany) 2019;34(5):943–9.

58. Ardissino G, Tel F, Sgarbanti M, et al. Complement functional tests for monitoring eculizumab treatment in patients with atypical hemolytic uremic syndrome: an update. Pediatr Nephrol (Berlin, Germany) 2018;33(3):457–61.

59. Bagga A, Khandelwal P, Mishra K, et al. Hemolytic uremic syndrome in a developing country: Consensus guidelines. Pediatr Nephrol (Berlin, Germany) 2019; 34(8):1465–82.
60. Geraghty MT, Perlman EJ, Martin LS, et al. Cobalamin C defect associated with hemolytic-uremic syndrome. J Pediatr 1992;120(6):934–7.
61. Huemer M, Baumgartner MR. The clinical presentation of cobalamin-related disorders: From acquired deficiencies to inborn errors of absorption and intracellular pathways. J Inherit Metab Dis 2019;42(4):686–705.
62. Beck BB, van Spronsen F, Diepstra A, et al. Renal thrombotic microangiopathy in patients with cblC defect: review of an under-recognized entity. Pediatr Nephrol (Berlin, Germany) 2017;32(5):733–41.
63. Lemaire M, Fremeaux-Bacchi V, Schaefer F, et al. Recessive mutations in DGKE cause atypical hemolytic-uremic syndrome. Nat Genet 2013;45(5):531–6.
64. Ozaltin F, Li B, Rauhauser A, et al. DGKE variants cause a glomerular microangiopathy that mimics membranoproliferative GN. J Am Soc Nephrol 2013;24(3): 377–84.
65. Brocklebank V, Kumar G, Howie AJ, et al. Long-term outcomes and response to treatment in diacylglycerol kinase epsilon nephropathy. Kidney Int 2020;97(6): 1260–74.
66. Dragon-Durey MA, Loirat C, Cloarec S, et al. Anti-Factor H autoantibodies associated with atypical hemolytic uremic syndrome. J Am Soc Nephrol 2005;16(2): 555–63.
67. Hofer J, Janecke AR, Zimmerhackl LB, et al. Complement factor H-related protein 1 deficiency and factor H antibodies in pediatric patients with atypical hemolytic uremic syndrome. Clin J Am Soc Nephrol 2013;8(3):407–15.
68. Puraswani M, Khandelwal P, Saini H, et al. Clinical and immunological profile of anti-factor H antibody associated atypical hemolytic uremic syndrome: a nationwide database. Front Immunol 2019;10:1282.
69. Durey MA, Sinha A, Togarsimalemath SK, et al. Anti-complement-factor H-associated glomerulopathies. Nat Rev Nephrol 2016;12(9):563–78.
70. Dragon-Durey MA, Blanc C, Garnier A, et al. Anti-factor H autoantibody-associated hemolytic uremic syndrome: review of literature of the autoimmune form of HUS. Semin Thromb Hemost 2010;36(6):633–40.
71. Schwartz J, Winters JL, Padmanabhan A, et al. Guidelines on the use of therapeutic apheresis in clinical practice-evidence-based approach from the Writing Committee of the American Society for Apheresis: the sixth special issue. J Clin Apher 2013;28(3):145–284.
72. Sinha A, Gulati A, Saini S, et al. Prompt plasma exchanges and immunosuppressive treatment improves the outcomes of anti-factor H autoantibody-associated hemolytic uremic syndrome in children. Kidney Int 2014;85(5):1151–60.
73. Hackl A, Ehren R, Kirschfink M, et al. Successful discontinuation of eculizumab under immunosuppressive therapy in DEAP-HUS. Pediatr Nephrol (Berlin, Germany) 2017;32(6):1081–7.
74. Brocklebank V, Johnson S, Sheerin TP, et al. Factor H autoantibody is associated with atypical hemolytic uremic syndrome in children in the United Kingdom and Ireland. Kidney Int 2017;97(6):1260–74.
75. Govindarajan S, Rawat A, Ramachandran R, et al. Anti-complement factor I antibody associated atypical hemolytic uremic syndrome - A new insight for future perspective! Immunobiology 2020;225(5):152000.

Vasculitis and Kidney Disease

Manpreet K. Grewal, MD[a,b], Matthew D. Adams, MD[c],
Rudolph P. Valentini, MD[a,b],*

KEYWORDS

- Pediatric vasculitis • Kidney disease • Necrotizing glomerulonephritis

KEY POINTS

- Vasculitis is typically classified according to the size of blood vessel involvement into small, medium, or large vessel vasculitis.
- Vasculitis may occur secondary to infections, medications, underlying connective tissue disease, systemic diseases, or malignancy.
- Kidney manifestations include acute glomerulonephritis in the setting of small vessel vasculitis or hypertension in the medium and large vessel forms of vasculitis.
- A kidney biopsy is often needed in the setting of acute glomerulonephritis for diagnosis and management decisions.
- Pulmonary renal syndrome can be seen in ANCA-associated vasculitis, anti-GBM disease, and sometimes in patients with SLE.

INTRODUCTION

Vasculitis is characterized by an inflammation of the blood vessels of various sizes; it may be primary or secondary, and the latter is caused by a variety of conditions such as infections, adverse drug reaction, underlying connective tissue disease, systemic diseases (eg, systemic lupus erythematosus, sarcoidosis, rheumatoid arthritis), or malignancy. Renal vasculitis may be restricted to kidneys only or it can occur as part of a broader multiorgan vasculitis. The inflammatory process causes damage to the renal vasculature and parenchyma and presents clinically as acute glomerulonephritis (AGN). Patients may also present with acute kidney injury, particularly those with a rapidly progressive clinical course, also called *rapidly progressive glomerulonephritis* (RPGN).

[a] Division of Nephrology and Hypertension, Department of Pediatrics, Children's Hospital of Michigan, 3901 Beaubien Boulevard, MI, 48201, USA; [b] Department of Pediatrics, Central Michigan University College of Medicine, 1280 East Campus Drive, Mount Pleasant, MI 48858, USA; [c] Department of Pediatrics, Wayne State University School of Medicine, 540 East Canfield Street, Detroit, MI 48201, USA
* Corresponding author.
E-mail address: rvalenti@dmc.org

Pediatr Clin N Am 69 (2022) 1199–1217
https://doi.org/10.1016/j.pcl.2022.07.009
0031-3955/22/© 2022 Elsevier Inc. All rights reserved.
pediatric.theclinics.com

The 2 most commonly used classifications for pediatric vasculitis are the updated Chapel Hill consensus conference criteria for systemic vasculitis (2012) (**Box 1**)[1] and the EULAR (European League against Rheumatism)/PRES (Pediatric Rheumatology European Society)/PRINTO (Pediatric Rheumatology International Trials Organization) (2006) classification for childhood vasculitis (**Box 2**).[2] Both sets of criteria are similar in terms of broad categorization of vasculitis into small, medium, or large vessel depending on the caliber of the affected vessels but differ in that the 2012 Chapel Hill criteria further subdivides the small vessel vasculitis (SVV) into pauci-immune antineutrophil cytoplasmic autoantibody (ANCA) and immune complexes types.

Of the various types of vasculitis, the SVV is the commonest one in children. The SVV with kidney involvement include conditions such as Henoch-Schönlein purpura (HSP), granulomatosis with polyangiitis (GPA), microscopic polyangiitis (MPA), eosinophilic granulomatosis with polyangiitis (EGPA), and anti-glomerular basement membrane (anti-GBM) disease.[1,2] These conditions typically affect the glomerular capillaries and manifest clinically as glomerulonephritis. The forms of vasculitis involving the medium to larger vessels include classic polyarteritis nodosa (PAN) and Takayasu arteritis (TA), which predominantly result in renal ischemia and hypertension. Kawasaki disease (KD) is a medium vessel vasculitis with limited kidney involvement.

Diagnosis of Vasculitis

Classification criteria have been developed to aid in the diagnosis of renal vasculitis, but failure to meet classification criteria does not necessarily preclude a specific diagnosis.[3] A combination of clinical symptoms, physical findings, laboratory testing for serologic markers, and, depending on the severity of kidney involvement, a kidney biopsy is needed to establish a diagnosis. Tests are also needed to assess and monitor the kidney function and the potential complications, which include

- Kidney function and serum electrolytes
- Complete blood cell count
- Inflammatory markers: erythrocyte sedimentation rate (ESR)/C-reactive protein
- Urinalysis (UA), urine protein/creatinine ratio
- Serologic markers include C3 and C4, anti-GBM, Smith, ribonuclear protein, angiotensin-converting enzyme (ACE), lysozyme, ANCA titers including anti-proteinase 3 (PR-3) antibodies, and anti-myeloperoxidase (MPO) antibodies. In addition, ANA (antinuclear antibody) and anti-double-stranded DNA should be measured to rule out other diseases such as systemic lupus erythematosus.
- Kidney biopsy: Histopathologic diagnosis using a kidney biopsy is the most valuable diagnostic test for renal vasculitis. Light microscopic findings of necrotizing GN can be seen in SVV, whereas the histology of a granuloma can differentiate GPA and EGPA from MPA.[1] Immunofluorescence (IF) staining for the presence or absence of immune complexes can assist in the diagnosis of the underlying cause for the renal vasculitis.
- Renal ultrasonography: In a patient with hypertension with or without azotemia, and minimal urinary findings, a renal ultrasonography with Doppler can be helpful to look at kidney size and renal blood flow. More sophisticated cross-sectional imaging such as computed tomography angiography (CTA) and magnetic resonance angiography (MRA) are far superior to ultrasonography if suspicion for PAN is high. Consultation with radiology locally to determine recommendations for CTA versus MRA versus traditional renal angiography can be considered because angiography is typically the diagnostic study of choice to diagnose PAN.[4]

SMALL VESSEL VASCULITIS

Small vessel vasculitis affects small arteries, arterioles, capillaries, and postcapillary venules. Based on the underlying immunopathology, SVV can be immune complex mediated or ANCA-associated pauci-immune types.[1]

Immune Complex-Mediated Disease

These diseases result from the presence of antigen-antibody complement complexes in blood vessels, leading to activation of the complement cascade and subsequent damage. These immune complexes can either form in circulation (eg, HSP) and then deposit in the vasculature or may result from in situ formation (eg, anti-GBM disease). Histopathologic specimens show granular deposits visible on IF and electron-dense deposits on electron microscopy (EM). The most common immune complex-mediated systemic vasculitis with kidney involvement include:

- HSP
- Anti-GBM disease

Henoch-Schönlein purpura

HSP classically involves skin, gastrointestinal (GI) tract, musculoskeletal system, and the kidneys. HSP is the most common pediatric vasculitis with an incidence of 10 to 20 children per 100,000 per year.[5] HSP is commonly seen in children younger than 10 years but has also been reported in older children and adults.[6] HSP occurs mostly during winter and spring, and upper respiratory tract infection or group A streptococcal infections are commonly reported triggers.[6] Malignancies, vaccinations, medications, and infections with other organisms like coxsackievirus, hepatitis A, hepatitis B, mycoplasma, parvovirus B19, Campylobacter, varicella, and adenovirus have also been reported as triggers for HSP.[6-8]

The clinical presentation of HSP can include palpable purpura, joint pain, colicky abdominal pain, and GI bleeding. Kidney involvement is seen in nearly 30% to 50% of the patients,[9,10] and risk factors for kidney involvement include older age at onset, severe GI symptoms, elevated white blood cell count, elevated platelet count, high anti-streptolysin O (ASO) titer, and low serum C3 levels.[11,12] Of note, the overwhelming majority of patients with HSP have a normal C3. Spectrum of kidney involvement in HSP nephritis includes microscopic hematuria with or without proteinuria, overt AGN with renal insufficiency and hypertension, or nephrotic syndrome (NS).[13] The common clinical pattern in patients with HSP nephritis is an acute presentation followed by complete remission. A few patients, though, achieve only a partial remission or develop a relapsing course following an initial remission with progression to IgA nephropathy.[13]

Owing to asymptomatic nature of kidney disease in most cases, an initial urinalysis should be obtained in all patients with HSP. If it is normal or reveals only microscopic hematuria, regular monitoring with urinalysis and blood pressure checks is warranted:

- Weekly for the first month after disease onset
- Every 2 weeks between 1 and 3 months
- Monthly up to 6 to 12 months, although newer studies have suggested that a shorter duration of follow-up to 6 months is sufficient[14,15]

Patients with proteinuria, combined hematuria/proteinuria, NS, azotemia, or hypertension may require a kidney biopsy. Light microscopy findings on kidney biopsy may include focal, necrotizing, and crescentic glomerulonephritis. IF typically shows immune complexes in mesangium and capillary walls with prominent IgA deposition,

---

Box 1
Chapel Hill consensus conference criteria for systemic vasculitis (2012)

Large vessel vasculitis
- Takayasu arteritis
- Giant cell arteritis

Medium vessel vasculitis
- Polyarteritis nodosa
- Kawasaki disease

Small vessel vasculitis
- Antineutrophil cytoplasmic antibody–associated vasculitis
  - Microscopic polyangiitis
  - Granulomatosis with polyangiitis (Wegener)
  - Eosinophilic granulomatosis with polyangiitis (Churg-Strauss)
- Immune complex vasculitis
  - Henoch-Schönlein purpura (IgA vasculitis)
  - Cryoglobulinemic vasculitis
  - Hypocomplementemic urticarial vasculitis (anti-C1q vasculitis)
  - Anti-glomerular basement membrane disease

Variable vessel vasculitis
- Behcet's disease
- Cogan's syndrome

Single-organ vasculitis
- Cutaneous leukocytoclastic angiitis
- Cutaneous arteritis
- Primary central nervous system vasculitis
- Isolated aortitis
- Others

Vasculitis associated with systemic disease
- Lupus vasculitis
- Rheumatoid vasculitis
- Sarcoid vasculitis
- Others

Vasculitis associated with probable etiology
- Hepatitis C virus–associated cryoglobulinemic vasculitis
- Hepatitis B virus–associated vasculitis
- Syphilis-associated aortitis
- Drug-associated immune complex vasculitis
- Drug-associated ANCA-associated vasculitis
- Cancer-associated vasculitis
- Others

Adapted from Jennette JC, Falk RJ, Bacon PA, et al. 2012 revised International Chapel Hill Consensus Conference Nomenclature of Vasculitides. *Arthritis Rheum.* 2013;65(1):1-11.

---

and less intense staining for C3 and IgG.[16] The International Study of Kidney Disease in Children classification of HSP nephritis is the most commonly used classification system for grading of kidney biopsies in patients with HSP nephritis.[17,18] The severity of disease (often based on degree of crescentic involvement) helps guide treatment decisions and therapy selections.

For most patients HSP is self-limited allowing patients to be cared for in an ambulatory setting with rest and adequate hydration and in those without kidney involvement, nonsteroidal anti-inflammatory drugs for the management of mild to moderate pain. Glucocorticoids are recommended in the management of severe

---

Box 2
European League against Rheumatism/Pediatric Rheumatology European Society/Pediatric Rheumatology International Trials Organization (2006) classification for childhood vasculitis

- Predominantly large vessel vasculitis
  - Takayasu arteritis

- Predominantly medium vessel vasculitis
  - Childhood polyarteritis nodosa
  - Cutaneous polyarteritis
  - Kawasaki disease

- Predominantly small vessel vasculitis
  - Granulomatous
    - Wegener granulomatosis
    - Churg-Strauss syndrome
  - Nongranulomatous
    - Microscopic polyangiitis
    - Henoch-Schönlein purpura
    - Isolated cutaneous leucocytoclastic vasculitis
    - Hypocomplementemic urticarial vasculitis

- Other vasculitides
  - Behçet disease
  - Vasculitis secondary to infection (including hepatitis B–associated polyarteritis nodosa), malignancies, and drugs including hypersensitivity vasculitis
  - Vasculitis associated with connective tissues diseases
  - Isolated vasculitis of the central nervous system
  - Cogan syndrome
  - Unclassified

Adapted from Ozen S, Ruperto N, Dillon MJ, et al. EULAR/PReS endorsed consensus criteria for the classification of childhood vasculitides. Ann Rheum Dis. 2006;65(7):936-941.

---

pain or GI symptoms and in those with severe life-threatening disease.[19] In patients with HSP nephritis without RPGN, the 2021 Kidney Disease: Improving Global Outcomes (KDIGO) guidelines recommend managing patients with proteinuria greater than 0.5 g/d with ACE inhibitors for a minimum of 3 months.[20] However, this approach may result in a delay in management of acute glomerular inflammation and thus might not prevent the development of sclerotic changes. As a result, in patients with NS, acute kidney injury, and certainly in those with evidence of crescentic RPGN on kidney biopsy, commencement of immunosuppressive therapy with glucocorticoids is needed; of note, patients with NS may warrant oral prednisone (2 mg/kg/d in divided doses, maximum dose 60 mg daily), but patients with RPGN would be treated with intravenous pulse methylprednisolone (10–30 mg/kg/d; maximum of 250–1000 mg dose/d × 3 days).[21–23] Additional treatment with cyclophosphamide (CYP) or azathioprine (AZA) may be necessary in patients with RPGN depending on the degree of crescentic involvement.[23]

Anti-glomerular basement membrane disease

Anti-GBM disease also called Goodpasture disease is rare in children. This disease is caused by antibodies directed against GBM antigen. The incidence of anti-GBM disease is 0.5 to 1 per million per year in adults and even lower in children.[24,25] The circulating autoantibodies react with a component of GBM in the kidneys and alveolar basement membrane (ABM) in the lung. These antibodies cross the fenestrated glomerular endothelium and interact with the sequestered epitope contained within non-collagenous domain (NC1) of α3 chain of type IV collagen.[26] Endothelial injury from cigarette smoking, hydrocarbon exposure, or viral infections has been implicated in the exposure of the sequestered epitope of endothelial basement membrane.[27] Human leukocyte antigen (HLA) has also been found to have a role in the pathogenesis of this condition with a positive association with HLA DRB1*1501 and HLA DR4 and a negative association with HLA DR1 and DR7.[28,29]

The disease spectrum varies widely, and clinical presentation may vary from overt kidney failure with limited or no pulmonary involvement to pulmonary hemorrhage with minimal or no kidney involvement.[30] The renal manifestations can range from asymptomatic hematuria with proteinuria to RPGN, which is the clinical presentation in nearly 80% of the cases. Pulmonary symptoms commonly include chest pain, shortness of breath, wheezing, and hemoptysis due to pulmonary hemorrhage, which is seen in about 40% to 60% of the patients.[31] When presenting concurrently, the terminology of pulmonary-renal syndrome is commonly used. Other conditions that cause pulmonary renal syndromes include ANCA-associated vasculitis (AAV), SLE, cryoglobulinemic vasculitis, and HSP.[32]

Laboratory studies reveal anemia (out of proportion to hemoptysis or kidney failure), whereas serologic studies including ANA, rheumatoid factor, and ASO titers usually give negative results. ESR is usually only mildly elevated. Most pertinent to the diagnosis is the presence of anti-GBM antibodies, either in serum or on kidney biopsy specimens. Serologic testing for anti-GBM antibodies using indirect IF or radioimmunoassay should be obtained immediately, although in nearly 10% of patients circulating antibodies may be negative.[26,33] ANCA is elevated in 20% to 30% patients with anti-GBM disease: usually pANCA/MPO-ANCA.[34] On kidney biopsy, light microscopy most commonly reveals a focal necrotizing and crescentic glomerulonephritis. IF demonstrates linear IgG deposition along glomerular capillary basement membrane. Absence of electron-dense deposits on EM is characteristic of this disease.[26] In patients with pulmonary involvement, chest radiographs show patchy/diffuse infiltrates with sparing of upper lung fields, not limited by fissures.

Management of anti-GBM disease requires a 2-pronged approach involving removal of the pathogenic antibody using plasma exchange (PE) and inhibiting new antibody production using immunosuppression. Daily PE for 14 days or until circulating antibodies can no longer be detected is recommended. Each PE session typically consists of an exchange volume of 40 to 50 mL/kg of ideal body weight and replacement with albumin or fresh frozen plasma. Immunosuppressive therapy with corticosteroids and CYP are used to suppress the ongoing antibody synthesis. Prednisone is given at a dose of 1 mg/kg/dose (80 mg maximum), tapered to 20 mg by 6 weeks, and then tapered slowly thereafter. CYP is given at 2 to 3 mg/kg/d and continued for 3 to 4 months. Anti-GBM titer, kidney function, and chest radiograph should be monitored intermittently to decide on the duration of various therapies.[20,26,30]

Although anti-GBM disease is uncommon in pediatrics, renal outcome has been poor in most instances and has usually been associated with progressive kidney disease.[35,36] Early diagnosis and prompt treatment offers the best opportunity to reduce morbidity and mortality of this disease in children.

Pauci-immune Disease (Antineutrophil Cytoplasmic Autoantibody-Associated Disease)

SVV with minimal or no immune deposits on IF on kidney biopsy is classified as pauci-immune. Most such cases are ANCA associated, but a small number are ANCA negative. ANCA are antibodies directed against antigens found in the cytoplasmic granules of polymorphonuclear cells. There are 2 types of ANCA, which are classified by immune staining of ethanol-fixed human neutrophils—*perinuclear* or pANCA is typically directed against MPO antigen and *cytoplasmic* or cANCA is typically directed against PR3 antigen. AAV is composed of 3 systemic diseases, that is, GPA, EGPA, and MPA and 1 renal limited disease, that is, necrotizing and crescentic glomerulonephritis (NCGN). These diseases are further characterized by the presence or absence of granulomas on histology.

- Granulomatous disease
  - GPA
  - EGPA
- Nongranulomatous disease
  - MPA
  - NCGN

Granulomatosis with polyangiitis

GPA (previously known as Wegener granulomatosis) is granulomatous inflammation of small vessels that is uncommon in children with a reported incidence of less than 1 per 100,000 children.[37,38] According to the 2014 United States Renal Data System Annual Data Report, GPA was the underlying cause of end-stage kidney disease (ESKD) in 56 pediatric patients (median age: 16 years) between 2008 and 2012.[39] The disease is more commonly seen in Caucasians and has a female preponderance.[40,41]

The disease is characterized by necrotizing granulomatous lesions of the respiratory tract, necrotizing vasculitis involving both small- and medium-sized vessels, and focal necrotizing glomerulonephritis. Clinically, upper and lower respiratory tract involvement in the form of recurrent sinusitis (most common), recurrent epistaxis, chronic otitis media, conductive hearing loss, or subglottic stenosis are the most common presenting symptoms.[42] Asymptomatic to fulminant pulmonary involvement in the form of stridor, hoarseness of voice, cough, dyspnea, pleuritic chest pain, and hemoptysis are commonly reported.[43] Chest radiographic findings of bilateral pulmonary infiltrates suggestive of pulmonary hemorrhage (**Fig. 1**) can be seen in severe cases. Constitutional symptoms of fever, malaise, arthralgias, and weight loss can also be present for months before presentation. Ocular manifestations include conjunctivitis, blepharitis, episcleritis, scleritis, and keratitis.[44] Mucocutaneous lesions, neurologic, and cardiovascular involvement can also be present.[41]

Kidney involvement in GPA can range from asymptomatic microscopic hematuria to a necrotizing and crescentic GN, which can be rapidly progressive (ie, RPGN) (**Fig. 2**). Older studies reported AGN in only a small number of children with GPA at disease presentation, which increased to nearly 60% during the course of the disease.[42] However, in a recent meta-analysis, kidney involvement was reported in 65% of patients at the time of presentation.[45] Long-term outcomes in GPA in children are difficult to assess due to the rarity of the disease, but Rottem and colleagues[42] in their pediatric series of 23 patients with GPA reported development of chronic kidney disease in 57% of the patients.

Besides the basic workup for autoimmune diseases, diagnosis of GPA involves serologic testing for ANCA with characteristic positivity of cANCA. cANCA testing in GPA is not specific for PR3, but in patients with vasculitis approximately 90% of cANCA are PR3-ANCA.[46] Results of ANCA testing vary depending on the severity and activity of disease with 90% positivity in patients with active generalized (sinopulmonary and renal) GPA, whereas nearly 30% to 40% in remission will still be cANCA positive.[47] Kidney biopsy is required in patients with azotemia or hematuria with proteinuria and typically shows a pauci-immune necrotizing and crescentic glomerulonephritis. Kidney biopsies in patients with GPA rarely show granulomas[47] unlike a lung or sinus biopsy, which may be needed for diagnosis in patients with minimal renal disease.

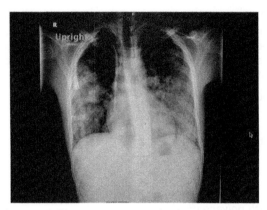

Fig. 1. Bilateral pulmonary infiltrates suggestive of pulmonary hemorrhage in patient with ANCA-associated glomerulonephritis.

Eosinophilic granulomatosis with polyangiitis

EGPA (previously called Churg-Strauss disease) is a pauci-immune AAV, which is rare in children. EGPA is characterized by systemic necrotizing vasculitis with hypereosinophilia, eosinophilic tissue infiltrates, and extravascular granulomas and occurs almost exclusively in patients with asthma.[48]

The disease commonly affects the lungs, skin, peripheral nerves, heart, and GI tract, whereas kidney involvement is less commonly reported in children. Kidney involvement when present ranges from asymptomatic hematuria with proteinuria to RPGN, which is the most common presentation. In a recent pediatric series of 13 patients with EGPA, only 1 had kidney involvement in the form of proteinuria and hypertension.[49] In adults, the most common presentation of kidney disease is RPGN, which accounts for nearly 50% to 75% of the cases with kidney involvement.[50,51]

ANCA positivity has been reported in about 40% of adult patients with EGPA, usually pANCA[52,53]; one pediatric study revealed a 30% ANCA (+) rate in 14 children with

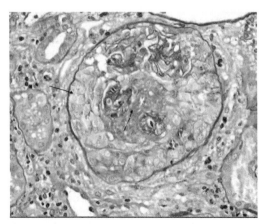

Fig. 2. Kidney biopsy demonstrating glomerulus with cellular crescent (*solid arrow*) and necrosis (*dotted arrow*). Light microscopy with hematoxylin & eosin stain (original magnification × 400). (Used with permission, Courtesy of Arkana Laboratories, Little Rock, Arkansas.)

EGPA.[54] Clinical phenotype of the patients also correlates to their ANCA status because kidney involvement has been seen predominantly in ANCA-positive patients, whereas extrarenal manifestations are more common in ANCA-negative patients.[51,52] Kidney biopsy findings can range from pauci-immune necrotizing GN with intense eosinophilic inflammatory infiltrate to acute interstitial nephritis with predominant eosinophilic infiltration. A few cases of membranous and membranoproliferative GN have also been reported.[51,52]

Microscopic polyangiitis
MPA is a multisystem, necrotizing pauci-immune ANCA vasculitis, which differs from EGPA and GPA by the absence of granulomas on histopathology. The disease is rare in children, and its incidence has not been determined.[55] Among children, it has a higher female preponderance,[55–57] as opposed to adults where the disease is more common in males. MPA is most often a primary vasculitis; however, MPA can also occur secondary to antithyroid drugs like propylthiouracil and methimazole.[57–59]

MPA has significant overlap with GPA in terms of organ involvement and most commonly affects the renal and pulmonary vascular beds, but unlike GPA, it does not affect the upper airway.[56] Kidney involvement results in hematuria with proteinuria, acute kidney injury clinically presenting as RPGN. Macroscopic hematuria has been reported in up to 30% patients.[56] ANCA testing typically reveals pANCA in greater than 80% of the patients.[57,58] Histologically, cellular, fibrocellular, or fibrous crescents are seen on kidney biopsy specimens in 80% to 90% of patients at presentation.[57,58,60] Besides the classical crescentic necrotizing GN, segmental or global glomerular sclerosis, fibrinoid necrosis, and interstitial fibrosis are other histopathologic lesions that are commonly seen on kidney biopsies.[57,58,60]

Long-term outcomes in pediatric patients have been reported in few recent case series. Although nearly 90% patients seem to achieve remission with initial therapy, about 20% to 50% of these patients have been reported to develop advanced chronic kidney disease over long-term follow-up.[57,58,60]

Necrotizing and crescentic glomerulonephritis
The renal limited NCGN is a rare entity that is characterized by isolated kidney involvement in patients with circulating ANCAs.[61,62] The serologic studies in these patients reveal either MPO or PR-3 ANCA with nearly 80% patients positive for MPO ANCA.[63] Clinically, these patients may present later in the course of their illness because kidney disease is often asymptomatic and lack of any other organ involvement results in delay in seeking medical attention. As a result, on histopathology specimens, a greater component of glomerulosclerosis may be noted when compared with GPA and MPA, which are more symptomatic and hence likely to be diagnosed sooner.[64]

TREATMENT STRATEGIES IN PAUCI-IMMUNE ANTINEUTROPHIL CYTOPLASMIC AUTOANTIBODY GLOMERULONEPHRITIS

In patients with suspected AAV and severe renal involvement, prompt treatment is recommended to prevent disease progression; this can occur without a renal biopsy if patient is too unstable to undergo this procedure; similarly, empirical treatment pulse methylprednisolone can be initiated in such a patient while awaiting the kidney biopsy result to be finalized.[21] The management includes induction and maintenance phases. The induction phase involves use of glucocorticoids with either CYP or rituximab to induce remission. Most centers often use pulse methylprednisolone at a dose of 10 to 30 mg/kg (maximum 1 g/d) in 3 successive daily doses followed by daily prednisone at 1 to 2 mg/kg/d. Two landmark trials reported that CYP and rituximab have similar efficacy for induction. The Rituximab in ANCA-Associated Vasculitis (RAVE) trial demonstrated that rituximab was not inferior to oral CYP in inducing remission when given as 4 doses of 375 mg/m^2/dose weekly.[65] The second study was the RTUXIVAS trial, which compared rituximab with 2 doses of intravenous (IV) CYP versus IV CYP alone and concluded that no difference in rate of sustained remission was observed between the 2 groups at 12 and 24 months of follow-up.[66] However, there is paucity of data on the use of rituximab in patients with severe kidney disease (serum creatinine level > 4 mg/dL) making CYP the preferred agent. The current KDIGO guidelines recommend reducing prednisone to 5 mg/d by 6 months following induction with CYP, whereas in cases in which rituximab is used for induction, prednisolone can be completely stopped by 6 months.

The maintenance phase of treatment involves transitioning the patient to a relatively less toxic regimen at 6 months to 1 year, using rituximab or AZA and low-dose glucocorticoids. AZA dose is 2 mg/kg/d, whereas rituximab can be dosed on a fixed schedule or upon reappearance of CD19 B cells and/or ANCA.[21] Rituximab is recommended as a preferred agent for maintenance therapy in patients in whom rituximab was used as the induction agent.[20,67,68]

Plasmapheresis is recommended for patients with severe kidney dysfunction (creatinine level > 5.7 mg/dL in adults), pulmonary hemorrhage, and concomitant anti-GBM disease.[20,69] More recently, a novel therapeutic agent mepolizumab, which is a monoclonal antibody targeting interleukin (IL)-5, has been approved for use in relapsing or refractory EGPA.[70]

SMALL VESSEL VASCULITIS AND CORONAVIRUS DISEASE 2019

Viral infections are well known triggers of autoimmunity leading to the development of autoimmune diseases.[71] Cytokine storm leading to activation of innate and adaptive immune systems has been well described with coronavirus doseas3 2019 (COVID-19).[72] An unchecked activation of the immune system has been hypothesized as the underlying cause of development of various autoimmune diseases reported in adult patients with COVID-19. In pediatric age group, several case reports of ANCA-associated SVV secondary to COVID-19 infection have been reported.[73–75] Scattered case reports of ANCA-associated SVV in adults following vaccination for COVID-19 have also been described, although no such pediatric data has been reported so far.[76,77]

MEDIUM VESSEL VASCULITIS

Medium vessel vasculitis mainly affects the visceral arteries (eg, coronary, hepatic, mesenteric, and renal) and veins and their main branches. The common medium vessel vasculitis in children include

- PAN
- KD

Polyarteritis Nodosa

PAN causes focal necrotizing injury to the vessel wall leading to aneurysm formation. Aneurysms can further lead to infarction, hemorrhage, and organ dysfunction. The disease is commonly seen in association with hepatitis B infection in adults, but this association is less commonly seen in children. The typical age of presentation in children is around 9 years.[78,79]

Clinical features include constitutional symptoms of fever, malaise, weight loss, and arthralgias along with signs and symptoms of multisystem involvement. Cutaneous involvement in the form of livedo reticularis, tender subcutaneous nodules, and skin ulcerations can be seen,[80] and is often considered a separate entity. Mononeuritis multiplex may lead to sensory and motor deficits. Hypertension from renal artery involvement is a well-known presentation; patients can also present with proteinuria, flank pain, hematuria, and rarely retroperitoneal hemorrhage from aneurysmal rupture.[81]

Interlobar and arcuate arteries are most commonly involved when compared with the main renal artery. Diagnostic angiography of vessels involving the kidney or intestinal vessels will often show segmental narrowing and variations in the caliber of arteries, together with pruning of the peripheral vascular tree.[82] Selective renal angiography is often required to detect very small peripheral aneurysms. Kidney biopsy may reveal necrotizing vasculitis without a crescentic or necrotizing glomerulonephritis. ANCA is typically negative in PAN; as such, the presence of cANCA or pANCA should raise the possibility of GPA or MPA as an alternative diagnosis.[83]

Corticosteroids and usually an alkylating agent such as CYP or AZA are the mainstay of treatment with improving prognosis with the use of immunosuppressive therapy.[83]

Kawasaki Disease

KD is a febrile vasculitis that predominantly affects young children aged less than 5 years with predominant involvement of the coronary vasculature.[84] Urinary tract and renal involvement in KD is uncommon and ranges from sterile pyuria secondary to urethritis (most common) to acute kidney injury, tubular abnormalities, nephritic/NS, or vascular abnormalities including stenosis or aneurysms.[85] The underlying mechanisms of renal involvement in KD are not well understood, but CD 8 T cell activation, inflammation of renal vessels, and immune-complex-mediated kidney injury are hypothesized to contribute to the development of kidney and urinary tract manifestations.[85]

LARGE VESSEL VASCULITIS

Large vessel vasculitis affect the aorta and its major branches. The only large vessel vasculitis seen in the pediatric age group is TK.

Takayasu Arteritis

TK is a granulomatous inflammatory condition that progressively involves the aorta, carotids, and sometime the renal arteries leading to a panarteritis causing stenosis and aneurysm formation. TK is also known as the pulseless disease, due to the involvement of aortic arch and subclavian vessels resulting in arterial narrowing and decreased brachial pulses. TK occurs more commonly in females with most cases being diagnosed between age 10 and 20 years.[86–88]

The diagnosis of TK can be made based on the EULAR/PRINTO/PRES criteria for TA in children,[3] which requires the presence of angiographic abnormalities of the aorta or its main branches in the form of aneurysm/dilatation, narrowing, occlusion, or arterial wall thickening not due to fibromuscular dysplasia and at least 1 of the following 5 features:

- Pulse deficit (lost/decreased/unequal peripheral artery pulse[s]) and/or claudication induced by activity
- Systolic blood pressure difference greater than 10 mm Hg between any limbs
- Bruits or thrills over the aorta and/or its major branches

- Hypertension
- Elevated acute-phase reactants

Hypertension is the most common presenting complaint in pediatric age group. Kidney involvement is most commonly in the form of renin-mediated renovascular hypertension secondary to renal artery stenosis/narrowing.[89,90]

Corticosteroids and CYP are the mainstay of treatment during the induction phase, whereas cytotoxic agents like methotrexate, AZA, and mycophenolate mofetil are used during the maintenance phase. Treatment of hypertension mainly includes vasodilators, beta-blockers, and diuretics. ACE inhibitors can be used but require extreme caution due to the risk of precipitating acute kidney injury.[91] The long-term prognosis of TKA is generally quite good with 5-year survival rates of approximately 95%.

MONOGENETIC VASCULOPATHIES

The monogenetic vasculopathies are a heterogeneous group of disorders including type 1 interferonopathies,[92] which may have renal involvement,[93,94] adenosine deaminase 2 (ADA2) deficiency,[95] and complement deficiency in lupus.[96] These are a heterogeneous group of disorders that tend to be characterized by multiorgan inflammation and systemic vasculitis. Their causes are diverse, and the treatments and outcomes depend on the specific mutations. Genetic studies such as genome-wide association studies and whole exome sequencing are making significant contributions to our understanding of systemic vasculitis and helping define newer entities.

Deficiency of adenosine deaminase 2 (DADA2): DADA2 is a monogenetic, autosomal recessive disease of ADA2 deficiency. ADA2 is secreted into the extracellular space by macrophage and myeloid cells and catalyzes the conversion of adenosine and 2′-deoxyadenosine to inosine and 2′-deoxyinosine. The pathophysiology of DADA2 is complex and not completely understood, but adenosine has both proinflammatory and anti-inflammatory effects, and ADA2 is important in removing extracellular adenosine. As such, adenosine level increases in the setting of DADA2 and proinflammatory effects come to dominate, which results in systemic vasculitis mimicking PAN, and presenting symptoms may include skin rashes, abdominal pain, fever, hypertension, and stroke. Like ADA1 deficiency, DADA2 can lead to immune deficiencies such as hypogammaglobulinemia and lymphopenia.[97,98]

STING-associated vasculopathy with onset in infancy (SAVI): SAVI is caused by dominant gain-of-function mutation in TMEM1723 and a subsequent overproduction of type I interferons (IFN). The type I IFN family is a multigene cytokine family that encodes 13 partially homologous IFNα subtypes in humans, a single IFNβ, and several poorly defined single gene products IFNε, IFNτ, IFNκ, IFNω, IFNδ, and IFNζ. This family usually presents in infancy with systemic inflammation, interstitial lung disease, cold-induced vasculitis, and glomerulonephritis.[99,100]

IL-1 diseases: These disease are caused by a heterogeneous group of mutations located on different genes with a common pathway of inflammasome activation and IL-1 beta and IL-18 overproduction. The most common presentations are as periodic fever syndromes, characterized by recurrent fevers, rash, and serositis. All have been reported in the literature to have occasional small and medium vessel vasculitis as a complication. However, it is chronic infantile neurologic cutaneous and articular disease that almost always presents as neonatal vasculitis with chronic inflammation and multisystem organ involvement. For all the IL-1 beta disease states, the vasculitis is commonly treated with anakinra, an IL-1 receptor antagonist, or canakinumab, a human monoclonal antibody directed against IL-1 beta.[97]

SUMMARY

Vasculitis should be included in the differential diagnosis of the pediatric patient presenting with systemic symptoms including fevers, rashes, joint pains, hemoptysis, abdominal pain, edema, or cola-colored urine. Although not all symptoms will be present at disease onset, serial examinations and a high index of suspicion should be present in the pediatric patient who is not showing signs of improvement. Proper investigation of these patients includes a history and physical examination followed by laboratory and potential imaging investigations to look for markers of inflammation, including underlying causes such as ANCA titers. Furthermore, one must be cognizant of the risks for hypertension and acute kidney injury with timely referral to a pediatric nephrologist and pediatric rheumatologist for consultation, possible renal biopsy, and institution of time-sensitive immunosuppressive therapies. With timely diagnosis and referral, the pediatric patient with vasculitis has the best likelihood of recovery, but a small minority will progress to ESKD and/or have chronic pulmonary or otolaryngology disease states.

CLINICS CARE POINTS

- Patients with suspected vasculitis require a UA and urine protein/creatinine ratio to screen for occult renal disease.

- Initial UA can be done at point of care to provide preliminary information

- Patients with an active urinary sediment (hematuria and/or proteinuria) should be referred to nephrology to be considered for a renal biopsy to substantiate the histologic diagnosis and drive therapeutic decision making.

- Blood work for the patient with systemic symptoms and suspicion for vasculitis should include complete blood count, serum urea nitrogen, creatinine, albumin, and serologies for underlying causes including ANCA (anti-MPO and anti-PR 3), complement components 3 and 4, antinuclear antibody, and anti-double-stranded DNA.

- Patients with suspected vasculitis and respiratory symptoms (cough, shortness of breath, or hemoptysis) require a chest radiograph to screen for pulmonary hemorrhage.

- Patients with suspected RPGN or pulmonary-renal syndrome require urgent referral to a specialty pediatric center for consultation and possible hospitalization.

DISCLOSURE

All the authors report no conflicts of interest in this work.

REFERENCES

1. Jennette JC, Falk RJ, Bacon PA, et al. 2012 revised International Chapel Hill Consensus Conference Nomenclature of Vasculitides. Arthritis Rheum 2013; 65(1):1–11. https://doi.org/10.1002/art.37715.
2. Ozen S, Ruperto N, Dillon MJ, et al. EULAR/PReS endorsed consensus criteria for the classification of childhood vasculitides. Ann Rheum Dis 2006;65(7): 936–41. https://doi.org/10.1136/ard.2005.046300.
3. Ozen S, Pistorio A, Iusan SM, et al. EULAR/PRINTO/PRES criteria for Henoch-Schönlein purpura, childhood polyarteritis nodosa, childhood Wegener granulomatosis and childhood Takayasu arteritis: Ankara 2008. Part II: Final classification criteria. Ann Rheum Dis 2010;69(5):798–806. https://doi.org/10.1136/ard. 2009.116657.

4. Chung SA, Gorelik M, Langford CA, et al. 2021 American College of Rheumatology/Vasculitis Foundation Guideline for the Management of Polyarteritis Nodosa. Arthritis Rheumatol 2021;73(8):1384–93. https://doi.org/10.1002/art.41776.

5. Hetland LE, Susrud KS, Lindahl KH, et al. Henoch-Schönlein Purpura: A Literature Review. Acta Derm Venereol 2017;97(10):1160–6. https://doi.org/10.2340/00015555-2733.

6. Chan H, Tang YL, Lv XH, et al. Risk Factors Associated with Renal Involvement in Childhood Henoch-Schönlein Purpura: A Meta-Analysis. PLoS One 2016;11(11):e0167346. https://doi.org/10.1371/journal.pone.0167346.

7. Ghrahani R, Ledika MA, Sapartini G, et al. Age of onset as a risk factor of renal involvement in Henoch-Schönlein purpura. Asia Pac Allergy 2014;4(1):42–7. https://doi.org/10.5415/apallergy.2014.4.1.42.

8. Reamy BV, Williams PM, Lindsay TJ. Henoch-Schönlein purpura. Am Fam Physician 2009;80(7):697–704.

9. Sohagia AB, Gunturu SG, Tong TR, et al. Henoch-schonlein purpura-a case report and review of the literature. Gastroenterol Res Pract 2010;2010:597648. https://doi.org/10.1155/2010/597648.

10. Greer JM, Longley S, Edwards NL, et al. Vasculitis associated with malignancy. Experience with 13 patients and literature review. Medicine (Baltimore) 1988;67(4):220–30. https://doi.org/10.1097/00005792-198807000-00003.

11. Trapani S, Micheli A, Grisolia F, et al. Henoch Schonlein purpura in childhood: epidemiological and clinical analysis of 150 cases over a 5-year period and review of literature. Semin Arthritis Rheum 2005;35(3):143–53. https://doi.org/10.1016/j.semarthrit.2005.08.007.

12. Chang WL, Yang YH, Wang LC, et al. Renal manifestations in Henoch-Schönlein purpura: a 10-year clinical study. Pediatr Nephrol 2005;20(9):1269–72. https://doi.org/10.1007/s00467-005-1903-z.

13. Davin JC. Henoch-Schonlein purpura nephritis: pathophysiology, treatment, and future strategy. Clin J Am Soc Nephrol 2011;6(3):679–89. https://doi.org/10.2215/CJN.06710810.

14. Narchi H. Risk of long term renal impairment and duration of follow up recommended for Henoch-Schonlein purpura with normal or minimal urinary findings: a systematic review. Arch Dis Child 2005;90(9):916–20. https://doi.org/10.1136/adc.2005.074641.

15. Wang H, Das L, Hoh SF, et al. Urinalysis monitoring in children with Henoch-Schönlein purpura: Is it time to revise? Int J Rheum Dis 2019;22(7):1271–7. https://doi.org/10.1111/1756-185X.13552.

16. Jelusic M, Sestan M, Cimaz R, et al. Different histological classifications for Henoch-Schönlein purpura nephritis: which one should be used? Pediatr Rheumatol Online J 2019;17(1):10. https://doi.org/10.1186/s12969-019-0311-z.

17. Counahan R, Winterborn MH, White RH, et al. Prognosis of Henoch-Schönlein nephritis in children. Br Med J 1977;2(6078):11–4. https://doi.org/10.1136/bmj.2.6078.11.

18. Haas M. IgA nephropathy and Henoch-Schönlein Purpura nephritis. In: Jennette JC, Olson JC, Schwartz MM, et al, editors. Heptinstall's pathology of the kidney. Philadelphia: Lippincott, Williams & Wilkins; 2007. p. 423–86.

19. Weiss PF, Klink AJ, Localio R, et al. Corticosteroids may improve clinical outcomes during hospitalization for Henoch-Schönlein purpura. Pediatrics 2010;126(4):674–81. https://doi.org/10.1542/peds.2009-3348.

20. Kidney Disease: Improving Global Outcomes (KDIGO) Glomerular Diseases Work Group. KDIGO 2021 Clinical Practice Guideline for the Management of Glomerular Diseases. Kidney Int 2021;100(4S):S1–276. https://doi.org/10. 1016/j.kint.2021.05.021.
21. Niaudet P, Habib R. Methylprednisolone pulse therapy in the treatment of severe forms of Schönlein-Henoch purpura nephritis. Pediatr Nephrol 1998;12(3): 238–43. https://doi.org/10.1007/s004670050446.
22. Davin JC, Coppo R. Henoch-Schönlein purpura nephritis in children. Nat Rev Nephrol 2014;10(10):563–73. https://doi.org/10.1038/nrneph.2014.126.
23. Ozen S, Marks SD, Brogan P, et al. European consensus-based recommendations for diagnosis and treatment of immunoglobulin A vasculitis-the SHARE initiative. Rheumatology (Oxford) 2019;58(9):1607–16. https://doi.org/10.1093/rheumatology/kez041.
24. Fischer EG, Lager DJ. Anti-glomerular basement membrane glomerulonephritis: a morphologic study of 80 cases. Am J Clin Pathol 2006;125(3):445–50. https://doi.org/10.1309/nptp-4ukv-7ju3-elmq.
25. USRDS U.S. Renal Data System 2015 Annual Data Report: pediatric ESRD. National Institutes of Health, National Institute of Diabetes and Digestive and Kidney Disease, Bethesda. Available at: https://www.usrds.org/media/2293/vol2_usrds_esrd_15.pdf. Accessed January 20, 2022.
26. McAdoo SP, Pusey CD. Anti-Glomerular Basement Membrane Disease. Clin J Am Soc Nephrol 2017;12(7):1162–72. https://doi.org/10.2215/CJN.01380217.
27. Bombassei GJ, Kaplan AA. The association between hydrocarbon exposure and anti-glomerular basement membrane antibody-mediated disease (Goodpasture's syndrome). Am J Ind Med 1992;21(2):141–53. https://doi.org/10. 1002/ajim.4700210204.
28. Ooi JD, Chang J, O'Sullivan KM, et al. The HLA-DRB1*15:01-restricted Goodpasture's T cell epitope induces GN. J Am Soc Nephrol 2013;24(3):419–31. https://doi.org/10.1681/ASN.2012070705.
29. Pedchenko V, Kitching AR, Hudson BG. Goodpasture's autoimmune disease - A collagen IV disorder. Matrix Biol 2018;71-72:240–9. https://doi.org/10.1016/j.matbio.2018.05.004.
30. Dowsett T, Oni L. Anti-glomerular basement membrane disease in children: a brief overview. Pediatric Nephrology (Berlin, Germany) 2021. https://doi.org/10.1007/s00467-021-05333-z. PMID: 34767075; PMCID: PMC8586640.
31. West SC, Arulkumaran N, Ind PW, et al. Pulmonary-renal syndrome: A life threatening but treatable condition. Postgrad Med J 2013;89(1051):274.
32. Savage CO, Pusey CD, Bowman C, et al. Antiglomerular basement membrane antibody mediated disease in the British Isles 1980-4. Br Med J (Clin Res Ed) 1986;292(6516):301–4. https://doi.org/10.1136/bmj.292.6516.301.
33. Salama AD, Dougan T, Levy JB, et al. Goodpasture's disease in the absence of circulating anti-glomerular basement membrane antibodies as detected by standard techniques. Am J Kidney Dis 2002;39(6):1162–7. https://doi.org/10. 1053/ajkd.2002.33385.
34. Li JN, Cui Z, Wang J, et al. Autoantibodies against Linear Epitopes of Myeloperoxidase in Anti-Glomerular Basement Membrane Disease. Clin J Am Soc Nephrol 2016;11(4):568–75. https://doi.org/10.2215/CJN.05270515.
35. Menzi CP, Bucher BS, Bianchetti MG, et al. Management and outcomes of childhood Goodpasture's disease. Pediatr Res 2018;83(4):813–7. https://doi.org/10. 1038/pr.2017.315.

36. Williamson SR, Phillips CL, Andreoli SP, et al. A 25-year experience with pediatric anti-glomerular basement membrane disease. Pediatr Nephrol 2011;26(1): 85–91. https://doi.org/10.1007/s00467-010-1663-2.

37. Cotch MF, Hoffman GS, Yerg DE, et al. The epidemiology of Wegener's granulomatosis. Estimates of the five-year period prevalence, annual mortality, and geographic disease distribution from population-based data sources. Arthritis Rheum 1996;39(1):87–92. https://doi.org/10.1002/art.1780390112.

38. Koldingsnes W, Nossent H. Epidemiology of Wegener's granulomatosis in northern Norway. Arthritis Rheum 2000;43(11):2481–7. https://doi.org/10.1002/1529-0131(200011)43:11<2481::AID-ANR15>3.0.CO;2-6.

39. Saran R, Li Y, Robinson B, et al. US Renal Data System 2014 Annual Data Report: Epidemiology of Kidney Disease in the United States. Am J Kidney Dis 2015;66(1 Suppl 1):Svii-S305. https://doi.org/10.1053/j.ajkd.2015.05.001 [published correction appears in Am J Kidney Dis. 2015 Sep;66(3):545].

40. Cabral DA, Uribe AG, Benseler S, et al. Classification, presentation, and initial treatment of Wegener's granulomatosis in childhood. Arthritis Rheum 2009; 60(11):3413–24. https://doi.org/10.1002/art.24876.

41. Bohm M, Gonzalez Fernandez MI, Ozen S, et al. Clinical features of childhood granulomatosis with polyangiitis (wegener's granulomatosis). Pediatr Rheumatol Online J 2014;12(18). https://doi.org/10.1186/1546-0096-12-18.

42. Rottem M, Fauci AS, Hallahan CW, et al. Wegener granulomatosis in children and adolescents: clinical presentation and outcome. J Pediatr 1993;122(1): 26–31. https://doi.org/10.1016/s0022-3476(05)83482-1.

43. Gómez-Puerta JA, Hernández-Rodríguez J, López-Soto A, et al. Antineutrophil cytoplasmic antibody-associated vasculitides and respiratory disease. Chest 2009;136(4):1101–11. https://doi.org/10.1378/chest.08-3043.

44. Kubaisi B, Abu Samra K, Foster CS. Granulomatosis with polyangiitis (Wegener's disease): An updated review of ocular disease manifestations. Intractable Rare Dis Res 2016;5(2):61–9. https://doi.org/10.5582/irdr.2016.01014.

45. Iudici M, Quartier P, Terrier B, et al. Childhood-onset granulomatosis with polyangiitis and microscopic polyangiitis: systematic review and meta-analysis. Orphanet J Rare Dis 2016;11(1):141. https://doi.org/10.1186/s13023-016-0523-y.

46. Jennette JC, Falk RJ. Small-vessel vasculitis. N Engl J Med 1997;337(21): 1512–23. https://doi.org/10.1056/NEJM199711203372106.

47. Lynch JP 3rd, Hoffman GS. Wegener's granulomatosis: controversies and current concepts. Compr Ther 1998;24(9):421–40.

48. Vaglio A, Buzio C, Zwerina J. Eosinophilic granulomatosis with polyangiitis (Churg-Strauss): state of the art. Allergy 2013;68(3):261–73. https://doi.org/10.1111/all.12088.

49. Eleftheriou D, Gale H, Pilkington C, et al. Eosinophilic granulomatosis with polyangiitis in childhood: retrospective experience from a tertiary referral centre in the UK. Rheumatology (Oxford) 2016;55(7):1263–72. https://doi.org/10.1093/rheumatology/kew029.

50. Sinico RA, Di Toma L, Maggiore U, et al. Renal involvement in Churg-Strauss syndrome. Am J Kidney Dis 2006;47(5):770–9. https://doi.org/10.1053/j.ajkd.2006.01.026.

51. Durel CA, Sinico RA, Teixeira V, et al. Renal involvement in eosinophilic granulomatosis with polyangiitis (EGPA): a multicentric retrospective study of 63 biopsy-proven cases. Rheumatology (Oxford) 2021;60(1):359–65. https://doi.org/10.1093/rheumatology/keaa416.

52. Sinico RA, Di Toma L, Maggiore U, et al. Prevalence and clinical significance of antineutrophil cytoplasmic antibodies in Churg-Strauss syndrome. Arthritis Rheum 2005;52(9):2926–35. https://doi.org/10.1002/art.21250.

53. Dunogué B, Pagnoux C, Guillevin L. Churg-strauss syndrome: clinical symptoms, complementary investigations, prognosis and outcome, and treatment. Semin Respir Crit Care Med 2011;32(3):298–309. https://doi.org/10.1055/s-0031-1279826.

54. Fina A, Dubus JC, Tran A, et al. Eosinophilic granulomatosis with polyangiitis in children: Data from the French RespiRare® cohort. Pediatr Pulmonol 2018; 53(12):1640–50. https://doi.org/10.1002/ppul.24089.

55. Arulkumaran N, Jawad S, Smith SW, et al. Long- term outcome of paediatric patients with ANCA vasculitis. Pediatr Rheumatol Online J 2011;9(12). https://doi.org/10.1186/1546-0096-9-12.

56. Cabral DA, Canter DL, Muscal E, et al. Comparing Presenting Clinical Features in 48 Children With Microscopic Polyangiitis to 183 Children Who Have Granulomatosis With Polyangiitis (Wegener's): An ARChiVe Cohort Study. Arthritis Rheumatol 2016;68(10):2514–26. https://doi.org/10.1002/art.39729.

57. Sun L, Wang H, Jiang X, et al. Clinical and pathological features of microscopic polyangiitis in 20 children. J Rheumatol 2014;41(8):1712–9. https://doi.org/10.3899/jrheum.131300.

58. Li Q, Yu LC, Li FX, et al. The Clinical and Pathological Features of Children With Microscopic Polyangiitis. Front Pediatr 2021;9:645785. https://doi.org/10.3389/fped.2021.645785.

59. Dedeoglu F. Drug-induced autoimmunity. Curr Opin Rheumatol 2009;21(5): 547–51. https://doi.org/10.1097/BOR.0b013e32832f13db.

60. Basu B, Mahapatra TK, Mondal N. Favourable renal survival in paediatric microscopic polyangiitis: efficacy of a novel treatment algorithm. Nephrol Dial Transpl 2015;30(Suppl 1):i113–8. https://doi.org/10.1093/ndt/gfv016.

61. Khan AJJ, Khan NAJ. Renal limited ANCA-positive vasculitis: a rare manifestation of a rare disease. J Investig Med High Impact Case Rep 2020;8. https://doi.org/10.1177/2324709620974874. 2324709620974874.

62. Sato N, Yokoi H, Imamaki H, et al. Renal-limited vasculitis with elevated levels of multiple antibodies. CEN Case Rep 2017;6(1):79–84. https://doi.org/10.1007/s13730-017-0248-3.

63. Seo P, Stone JH. The antineutrophil cytoplasmic antibody-associated vasculitides. Am J Med 2004;117(1):39–50. https://doi.org/10.1016/j.amjmed.2004.02.030.

64. Novick TK, Chen M, Scott J, et al. Patient Outcomes in Renal-Limited Antineutrophil Cytoplasmic Antibody Vasculitis With Inactive Histology. Kidney Int Rep 2018;3(3):671–6. https://doi.org/10.1016/j.ekir.2018.01.012. Published 2018 Feb 21.

65. Stone JH, Merkel PA, Spiera R, et al. Rituximab versus cyclophosphamide for ANCA-associated vasculitis. N Engl J Med 2010;363(3):221–32. https://doi.org/10.1056/NEJMoa0909905.

66. Jones RB, Tervaert JW, Hauser T, et al. Rituximab versus cyclophosphamide in ANCA-associated renal vasculitis. N Engl J Med 2010;363(3):211–20. https://doi.org/10.1056/NEJMoa0909169.

67. Guillevin L, Pagnoux C, Karras A, et al. Rituximab versus azathioprine for maintenance in ANCA-associated vasculitis. N Engl J Med 2014;371(19):1771–80. https://doi.org/10.1056/NEJMoa1404231.

68. Smith RM, Jones RB, Specks U, et al. Rituximab as therapy to induce remission after relapse in ANCA-associated vasculitis. Ann Rheum Dis 2020;79(9):1243–9. https://doi.org/10.1136/annrheumdis-2019-216863.

69. Walsh M, Merkel PA, Peh CA, et al. Plasma Exchange and Glucocorticoids in Severe ANCA-Associated Vasculitis. N Engl J Med 2020;382(7):622–31. https://doi.org/10.1056/NEJMoa1803537.

70. Bettiol A, Urban ML, Dagna L, et al. Mepolizumab for Eosinophilic Granulomatosis With Polyangiitis: A European Multicenter Observational Study. Arthritis Rheumatol 2022;74(2):295–306. https://doi.org/10.1002/art.41943.

71. Sfriso P, Ghirardello A, Botsios C, et al. Infections and autoimmunity: the multifaceted relationship. J Leukoc Biol 2010;87(3):385–95. https://doi.org/10.1189/jlb.0709517.

72. Ragab D, Salah Eldin H, Taeimah M, et al. The COVID-19 Cytokine Storm; What We Know So Far. Front Immunol 2020;11:1446. https://doi.org/10.3389/fimmu.2020.01446.

73. Reiff DD, Meyer CG, Marlin B, et al. New onset ANCA-associated vasculitis in an adolescent during an acute COVID-19 infection: a case report. BMC Pediatr 2021;21(1):333. https://doi.org/10.1186/s12887-021-02812-y.

74. Wintler T, Zherebtsov M, Carmack S, et al. Acute PR3-ANCA vasculitis in an asymptomatic COVID-19 teenager. J Pediatr Surg Case Rep 2021;75:102103. https://doi.org/10.1016/j.epsc.2021.102103.

75. Powell WT, Campbell JA, Ross F, et al. Acute ANCA Vasculitis and Asymptomatic COVID-19. Pediatrics 2021;147(4). https://doi.org/10.1542/peds.2020-033092. e2020033092.

76. Hakroush S, Tampe B. Case Report: ANCA-Associated Vasculitis Presenting With Rhabdomyolysis and Pauci-Immune Crescentic Glomerulonephritis After Pfizer-BioNTech COVID-19 mRNA Vaccination. Front Immunol 2021;12:762006. https://doi.org/10.3389/fimmu.2021.762006.

77. Feghali EJ, Zafar M, Abid S, et al. De-novo Antineutrophil Cytoplasmic Antibody-Associated Vasculitis Following the mRNA-1273 (Moderna) Vaccine for COVID-19. Cureus 2021;13(11):e19616. https://doi.org/10.7759/cureus.19616.

78. Ozen S, Anton J, Arisoy N, et al. Juvenile polyarteritis: results of a multicenter survey of 110 children. J Pediatr 2004;145(4):517–22. https://doi.org/10.1016/j.jpeds.2004.06.046.

79. Besbas N, Ozen S, Saatci U, et al. Renal involvement in polyarteritis nodosa: evaluation of 26 Turkish children. Pediatr Nephrol 2000;14(4):325–7. https://doi.org/10.1007/s004670050769.

80. Sheth AP, Olson JC, Esterly NB. Cutaneous polyarteritis nodosa of childhood. J Am Acad Dermatol 1994;31(4):561–6. https://doi.org/10.1016/s0190-9622(94)70216-0.

81. Pagnoux C, Seror R, Henegar C, et al. Clinical features and outcomes in 348 patients with polyarteritis nodosa: a systematic retrospective study of patients diagnosed between 1963 and 2005 and entered into the French Vasculitis Study Group Database. Arthritis Rheum 2010;62(2):616–26. https://doi.org/10.1002/art.27240.

82. Brogan PA, Davies R, Gordon I, et al. Renal angiography in children with polyarteritis nodosa. Pediatr Nephrol 2002;17(4):277–83. https://doi.org/10.1007/s00467-002-0823-4.

83. Dillon MJ, Eleftheriou D, Brogan PA. Medium-size-vessel vasculitis. Pediatr Nephrol 2010;25(9):1641–52. https://doi.org/10.1007/s00467-009-1336-1.

84. Burns JC, Glodé MP. Kawasaki syndrome. Lancet 2004;364(9433):533–44. https://doi.org/10.1016/S0140-6736(04)16814-1.
85. Watanabe T. Kidney and urinary tract involvement in kawasaki disease. Int J Pediatr 2013;2013:831834. https://doi.org/10.1155/2013/831834.
86. Kerr GS, Hallahan CW, Giordano J, et al. Takayasu arteritis. Ann Intern Med 1994;120(11):919–29. https://doi.org/10.7326/0003-4819-120-11-199406010-00004.
87. Hong CY, Yun YS, Choi JY, et al. Takayasu arteritis in Korean children: clinical report of seventy cases. Heart Vessels Suppl 1992;7:91–6. https://doi.org/10.1007/BF01744551.
88. Szugye HS, Zeft AS, Spalding SJ. Takayasu Arteritis in the pediatric population: a contemporary United States-based single center cohort. Pediatr Rheumatol Online J 2014;12:21. https://doi.org/10.1186/1546-0096-12-21.
89. Cakar N, Yalcinkaya F, Duzova A, et al. Takayasu arteritis in children. J Rheumatol 2008;35(5):913–9.
90. Russo RAG, Katsicas MM. Takayasu Arteritis. Front Pediatr 2018;6:265. https://doi.org/10.3389/fped.2018.00265.
91. de Graeff N, Groot N, Brogan P, et al. European consensus-based recommendations for the diagnosis and treatment of rare paediatric vasculitides - the SHARE initiative. Rheumatology (Oxford) 2019;58(4):656–71. https://doi.org/10.1093/rheumatology/key322 [published correction appears in Rheumatology (Oxford). 2020 Apr 1;59(4):919].
92. Volpi S, Picco P, Caorsi R, et al. Type I interferonopathies in pediatric rheumatology. Pediatr Rheumatol Online J 2016;14(1):35. https://doi.org/10.1186/s12969-016-0094-4.
93. Fenaroli P, Rossi GM, Angelotti ML, et al. Collapsing Glomerulopathy as a Complication of Type I Interferon-Mediated Glomerulopathy in a Patient With RNASEH2B-Related Aicardi-Goutières Syndrome. Am J Kidney Dis 2021;78(5):750–4. https://doi.org/10.1053/j.ajkd.2021.02.330.
94. Abid Q, Best Rocha A, Larsen CP, et al. APOL1-Associated Collapsing Focal Segmental Glomerulosclerosis in a Patient With Stimulator of Interferon Genes (STING)-Associated Vasculopathy With Onset in Infancy (SAVI). Am J Kidney Dis 2020;75(2):287–90. https://doi.org/10.1053/j.ajkd.2019.07.010.
95. Meyts I, Aksentijevich I. Deficiency of Adenosine Deaminase 2 (DADA2): Updates on the Phenotype, Genetics, Pathogenesis, and Treatment. J Clin Immunol 2018;38(5):569–78. https://doi.org/10.1007/s10875-018-0525-8.
96. Sharma M, Vignesh P, Tiewsoh K, et al. Revisiting the complement system in systemic lupus erythematosus. Expert Rev Clin Immunol 2020;16(4):397–408. https://doi.org/10.1080/1744666X.2020.1745063.
97. Jain A, Misra DP, Sharma A, et al. Vasculitis and vasculitis-like manifestations in monogenic autoinflammatory syndromes. Rheumatol Int 2018;38(1):13–24. https://doi.org/10.1007/s00296-017-3839-6.
98. Pinto B, Deo P, Sharma S, et al. Expanding spectrum of DADA2: a review of phenotypes, genetics, pathogenesis and treatment. Clin Rheumatol 2021;40(10):3883–96. https://doi.org/10.1007/s10067-021-05711-w.
99. McNab F, Mayer-Barber K, Sher A, et al. Type I interferons in infectious disease. Nat Rev Immunol 2015;15(2):87–103. https://doi.org/10.1038/nri3787.
100. Kim H, Sanchez GA, Goldbach-Mansky R. Insights from Mendelian Interferonopathies: Comparison of CANDLE, SAVI with AGS, Monogenic Lupus. J Mol Med (Berl) 2016;94(10):1111–27.

Update on Pediatric Acute Kidney Injury

Priyanka Khandelwal, MD, DM[a], Nadia McLean, MBBS, DM[b], Shina Menon, MD[c],*

KEYWORDS

- Acute kidney injury • Biomarkers • Electronic alert • CKD

KEY POINTS

- Serum creatinine, a marker of kidney function, has significant limitations in the diagnosis of acute kidney injury (AKI).
- It is recommended to use the definition and staging proposed by Kidney Disease: Improving Global Outcome (KDIGO) for AKI in children.
- More than 10% to 20% fluid overload may represent a critical threshold for intervention.
- Children with severe AKI or repeated episodes of AKI may be at higher risk of developing chronic kidney disease.
- Long-term follow-up is advisable in those at risk of developing chronic kidney disease.

INTRODUCTION

Acute kidney injury (AKI) is common in children and is associated with significant morbidity and mortality. Since the publication of a review titled "Acute Kidney Injury in Children: An Update on Diagnosis and Treatment" in this journal in 2013,[1] there have been new developments in our understanding of the epidemiology and impact of AKI in children. In this review, the authors aim to provide an update on pediatric AKI (prevalence, outcomes, and complications) and review the recent research in diagnostics and the management.

EVOLVING DEFINITIONS OF ACUTE KIDNEY INJURY

Over the last 2 decades, various attempts have been made to standardize the diagnosis of AKI to help improve the clinical outcomes across different patient populations. The very first step for a standardized definition of AKI was taken by the Acute Dialysis

[a] Division of Nephrology, Department of Pediatrics, All India Institute of Medical Sciences, Academic Block, Ansari Nagar, New Delhi 110029, India; [b] Cornwall Regional Hospital, c/o Cornwall Regional Hospital, PO Box 900, Mount Salem, Montego Bay #2 PO, St. James, Jamaica, West Indies; [c] Department of Pediatrics, Division of Nephrology, University of Washington, Seattle Children's Hospital, 4800 Sand Point Way NE, Mailstop OC9.820, Seattle, WA 98103, USA
* Corresponding author.
E-mail address: shina.menon@seattlechildrens.org

Pediatr Clin N Am 69 (2022) 1219–1238
https://doi.org/10.1016/j.pcl.2022.08.003
0031-3955/22/© 2022 Elsevier Inc. All rights reserved.
pediatric.theclinics.com

Quality Initiative (ADQI) in 2004 with the proposal of the RIFLE criteria that used 3 AKI staging strata (Risk, Injury, Failure) and 2 outcome strata (Loss and End-Stage Kidney Disease)[2]; this was later modified for use in pediatrics, pRIFLE (**Table 1**).[3] Arikan and colleagues showed that worse pRIFLE class significantly predicted increased risk of mortality, even after adjustment for severity of illness.[3] Because even a small increase in serum creatinine (SCr) by 0.3 mg/dL was shown to be independently associated with adverse outcomes in adults,[4] the RIFLE criteria were accordingly expanded by the Acute Kidney Injury Network (AKIN) in 2007.[5] In an attempt to unify these definitions, the Kidney Disease: Improving Global Outcome (KDIGO) consensus classification was proposed in 2012.[6] It defined AKI by an increase in serum creatinine by greater than 0.3 mg/dL within 48 hours or more than or equal to 1.5-fold increase in the prior 7 days or decrease in urine output by less than 0.5 mL/kg/h for 6 to 12 hours.[6] The degree of increase in serum creatinine from baseline or the severity and duration of oliguria is used for staging (see **Table 1**).

Recognizing that the duration of AKI also predicts adverse outcomes, the ADQI in 2017 proposed that the definition of AKI be limited to 7 days and acute kidney disease (AKD) be used for persistence of deranged kidney function beyond this period till the chronic kidney disease (CKD) criterion of 90 days.[7] The KDIGO has recently harmonized the definition of AKD to include abnormalities of kidney function and/or structure with a duration of 3 months or less that may or may not include prior AKI.[8]

LIMITATIONS OF SERUM CREATININE

Unfortunately, SCr has several notable limitations for defining AKI. Creatinine needs to be checked in steady state to accurately reflect renal function, and it increases only after the loss of at least 50% of renal function, which may take 24 to 48 hours after the injury has occurred.[9] Thus, SCr often does not reflect the acute changes seen with AKI in both critical and noncritical hospitalized patients. Serum creatinine level depends on muscle mass, which may decrease during prolonged critical illness.[10] Furthermore, fluid overload, a common phenomenon during critical illness, may dilute SCr, as it is distributed over total body water.[11] A baseline creatinine value is required for the diagnosis of AKI, which may not always be available for pediatric patients. In such cases, various methods have been recommended to estimate baseline creatinine and these include back-calculating from a "normal" estimated glomerular filtration rate (eGFR)[12] or using an age and sex appropriate normative value.[13] Accordingly, the reported incidence of AKI ranges from 4.6% to 43.1% in noncritical hospitalized children and 12.2% to 87.8% in critically ill children, depending on the baseline used.[12]

Attempts have been made in recent times to improve on these challenges associated with SCr. Xu and colleagues developed the pediatric reference change value optimized criterion for AKI in children (pROCK) by undertaking a statistical process to define age-based 95% confidence threshold of serum creatinine.[14] Using the pROCK criteria, AKI was defined as follows:

- Stage 1: serum creatinine increase of 0.23 mg/dL and a 30% increase over baseline
- Stage 2: serum creatinine increase of 0.45 mg/dL and $\geq$60% increase over baseline
- Stage 3: serum creatinine increase of 0.91 mg/dL and a $\geq$120% increase over baseline

The pROCK criteria were noted to be more specific for patients with low and very variable serum creatinine who might be misclassified as AKI stage I by KDIGO or

Table 1
Commonly used definitions for acute kidney injury (all ages)

Class/stage[a]	pRIFLE[3]		AKIN[5]		KDIGO[6]		Neonatal Modifications[20]	
	Estimated CCl	Urine output	Serum creatinine	Urine output	Serum creatinine	Urine output	Serum creatinine	Urine output
Risk/I	eCCl decreased by ≥25%	<0.5 mL/kg/h for ≥8 h	SCr increase ≥0.3 mg/dL or 150%–200% in ≤48 h	<0.5 mL/kg/h for 8 h	SCr increase ≥0.3 mg/dL in 48 h or 1.5–1.9 times in 7 d	<0.5 mL/kg/h for 6–12 h	SCr increase ≥0.3 mg/dL in 48 h or 1.5–1.9 times over baseline (previous lowest value) in 7 d	<1 mL/kg/h for 24 h
Injury/II	eCCl decreased by ≥50%	<0.5 mL/kg/h for ≥16 h	SCr increase >200%–300%	<0.5 mL/kg/h for 16 h	SCr increase 2.0–2.9 times	<0.5 mL/kg/h for >12 h	SCr increase 2.0–2.9 times	<0.5 mL/kg/h for ≥24 h
Failure/III	eCCl decreased by ≥75% or eCCl <35 mL/min/1.73 m²	<0.3 mL/kg/h for 24 h or anuria for 12 h	SCr increase >300% or SCr ≥4 mg/dL	<0.5 mL/kg/h for 24 h or <0.3 mL/kg/h for 12 h	SCr increase ≥3.0 times or SCr ≥4.0 mg/dL or eCCl <35 mL/min/1.73 m² or need for renal replacement therapy	<0.3 mL/kg/h for 24 h or anuria for 12 h	SCr increase ≥3.0 times or SCr ≥2.5 mg/dL or need for renal replacement therapy	<0.3 mL/kg/h for 24 h

Abbreviations: AKIN, acute kidney injury network; eCCl, estimated creatinine clearance; KDIGO, kidney disease improving global outcomes; pRIFLE, pediatric version of the RIFLE criteria (Risk, Injury, Failure, and 2 outcome criteria, Loss and End-Stage Kidney Disease); SCr, serum creatinine.

[a] Class risk, injury, and failure (pRIFLE) correspond to stage 1, 2, and 3 (AKIN and KDIGO), respectively.

pRIFLE (5.3% vs 10.2% or 15.2%, respectively).[14] pROCK seeks to improve the specificity of AKI diagnosis. However, given that SCr may not increase until 50% kidney function is lost, a more sensitive definition such as the one by KDIGO may allow early identification and monitoring of affected patients.

Another novel concept is that of kinetic eGFR (KeGFR), which has been proposed to estimate the kidney function when the creatinine is not yet at steady state.[15] The KeGFR method relies on a combination of various factors including initial creatinine content, rate of creatinine production, volume of distribution, and the change in SCr over time. It allows one to estimate kidney function when the creatinine is changing rapidly. Since the initial description,[15] KeGFR has been used in adults as well as in children for the diagnosis of AKI.[16,17]

URINE OUTPUT AS A CRITERION FOR ACUTE KIDNEY INJURY

Although urine output (UOP) has been a key component of all AKI definitions, it may get overlooked in some studies due to the challenges associated with either extracting UOP data from the electronic health record or collecting urine in younger pediatric patients, who may not have a urinary catheter, particularly outside the critical care setting. However, recent studies emphasize the impact of oliguria on diagnosis of AKI. The multinational prospective, Assessment of Worldwide AKI, Renal Angina and Epidemiology (AWARE) study showed that 18% of patients had severe AKI (KDIGO stage 2 or 3) as diagnosed by UOP criterion, which would have been missed by using the SCr criterion only.[18] Kaddourah and colleagues also showed that 28-day mortality was similar for patients who met either SCr or UOP criterion (6.7% vs 7.8%) but was significantly higher in those who met both criteria (38.1%; $P < .001$).[19]

CHALLENGES IN NEONATES

In addition to the issues discussed earlier that can make the diagnosis of AKI difficult, there are additional challenges unique to the neonatal population. The diagnosis of AKI requires a change in SCr from a steady state baseline, which is not seen in neonates, as their SCr is physiologically decreasing postnatally. The neonatal modification of the KDIGO definition is commonly used in clinical practice. It defines AKI based on an increase in SCr level from the previous lowest or trough value and/or a decrease in UOP (see **Table 1**).[6] The UOP criteria were modified over time keeping in mind neonatal physiology. The neonatal AKI workgroup sponsored by the National Institute of Diabetes and Digestive and Kidney Diseases recommended additional research in this area and continued work on developing a standard definition based on rational understanding of neonatal physiology.[20] Since then, attempts have been made to optimize the AKI definition in neonates. Askenazi and colleagues did a secondary analysis of the multicenter Assessment of Worldwide Acute Kidney Injury Epidemiology in Neonates study (AWAKEN) study and suggested using SCr thresholds based on gestational age (GA). The optimal SCr thresholds for the prediction of mortality were greater than or equal to 0.6 mg/dL for infants with less than or equal to 29 weeks GA and greater than or equal to 0.3 mg/dL for those with greater than 29 weeks GA.[21]

INCIDENCE OF ACUTE KIDNEY INJURY

The multicenter, prospective AWARE study was a landmark study that looked at the epidemiology of AKI in critically ill hospitalized patients.[18] Kaddourah and colleagues reported 4683 patients, aged 3 months to 25 years, admitted to pediatric intensive care units (ICUs) and expected to require a stay of 48 hours or longer. AKI occurred in 26.9% (n = 1261) and severe AKI (KDIGO stage 2 or 3) in 11.6% (n = 543) of the cases. The adjusted odds ratio for death by day 28 for patients with severe AKI was 1.77 (95% confidence interval, 1.17–2.68).[18] Other studies using a standardized definition of AKI criteria report incidence rates ranging from 10% to 40% in critically ill children.[3,18,22]

A recent retrospective cross-sectional study that looked at the incidence of AKI using an SCr-based electronic-alert (e-alert) algorithm across 6 hospitals in England reported an incidence of 10.8%, in patients younger than 6 years and with AKI stage 1.[23] A prospective national cohort study using the Welsh electronic AKI reporting system reported an incidence of 77.3 cases of AKI per 1,00,000 person-years; 84% with stage 1 AKI.[24] Thirty-day mortality was 1.7% but was significantly higher in hospital (2.1%) as compared with community-acquired AKI (0.8%, $P < .001$) and correlated with the severity of AKI at presentation.

There are limited data on the global burden of AKI, particularly from lower- and middle-income countries (LMIC). A systematic review and meta-analyses of large cohort studies from 2004 to 2012 by Susantitaphong and colleagues showed pooled incidence rates of 33.7% in children (95% confidence interval [CI], 26.9–41.3) and a pooled AKI-associated mortality rate of 13.8% (95% CI, 8.8–21.0).[25] However, greater than 80% of the studies included in this systematic review came from the high-income countries (HIC), and nations that spend greater than or equal to 5% of the gross domestic product on total health expenditure.[25]

Neonatal AKI is also common and an independent risk factor for mortality and longer hospital stay. The Assessment of Worldwide Acute Kidney injury Epidemiology in Neonates (AWAKEN) study, which was a 3-month retrospective cohort analysis of critically ill neonates from 24 centers looked at more than 2000 neonates and reported an AKI incidence of 29·9%.[26] Rates varied by gestational age groups (in ≥22 to <29 weeks GA = 47·9%; ≥29 to <36 weeks GA = 18·3%; and ≥36 weeks GA = 36·7%), and neonates with AKI had higher mortality compared with those without AKI with an adjusted odds ratio (OR) of 4·6 (95% CI, 2.5–8.3).[26]

CAUSE

The cause of AKI may vary based on multiple factors such as community versus hospital-acquired, HIC versus LMIC, or ICU versus non-ICU hospitalized patients. Acute tubular injury due to renal ischemia caused by hypoperfusion, cardiac surgery, sepsis, nephrotoxic drugs, or toxins is a major cause of AKI in HIC.[27] In LMIC, AKI is often due to systemic sepsis; diarrhea; infections such as malaria, leptospirosis, and dengue; use of nephrotoxic agents; and primary kidney disease.[28–30] In the International Society of Nephrology (ISN) 0by25 Global Snapshot study, Macedo and colleagues demonstrated that 80% of AKI cases in LMIC occurred before hospitalization.[28] The cause of AKI also varies based on where the AKI develops: within the community versus in hospitals. In the ISN Global Snapshot study, primary glomerulopathy and hypotension/shock were the most common causes of community-based AKI, and a significant proportion of hospital-acquired AKI was caused by postsurgical complications.[28] Further details on common causes of AKI in children are shown in **Table 2**.

PATHOPHYSIOLOGY

Several excellent reviews have been published describing the pathophysiology of AKI, including molecular and cellular mechanisms.[31–35] Traditionally AKI has been classified as prerenal, renal (intrinsic), and postrenal. Prerenal AKI is characterized by renal

Table 2
Common causes of acute kidney injury in children

Classification	Mechanism	Cause
Prerenal (functional)	Volume depletion Decreased cardiac output Peripheral vasodilation Renal vasoconstriction	Gastroenteritis, vomiting, hemorrhage, diuretics, septic shock, burns, nephrotic syndrome Congestive heart failure (congenital heart disease, myocarditis), arrythmia, postcardiac surgery Sepsis, hepatorenal syndrome Sepsis, nonsteroidal antiinflammatory drugs, angiotensin-converting enzyme inhibitors, calcineurin inhibitors, postcardiac surgery, hepatorenal syndrome
Intrinsic renal	Acute tubular necrosis	Prolonged ischemia, prerenal cause; medications (aminoglycosides, amphotericin, acyclovir, cisplatin, radiocontrast); toxins (ethylene glycol, methanol, heavy metals, myoglobin, hemoglobin, tumor lysis syndrome)
	Vascular Glomerulonephritis Interstitial nephritis Infection	Renal vein or renal artery thrombosis; renal artery stenosis; hemolytic uremic syndrome Immune mediated, vasculitis Drug induced, idiopathic Pyelonephritis, malaria, leptospirosis
Postrenal	Obstructive	Posterior urethral valves, urethral stricture; ureteral obstruction: stenosis, stone, ureterocele

hypoperfusion, often without damage to the renal parenchyma, and as an adaptive response to extrarenal insults. Several pathophysiological pathways exist for acute tubular injury (inflammatory, immunologic, and autoregulatory). Briefly, an ischemic trigger activates neurohormonal mechanisms to release vasoactive molecules causing renal vasoconstriction and subsequent decline in GFR. Persistence of the ischemic insult leads to a final common pathophysiological pathway of proximal tubular injury by apoptosis or necrosis (acute tubular necrosis) and consequent inflammatory response. Ischemia-reperfusion injury and microvascular/endothelial cell injury occurs chiefly within the corticomedullary junction of the kidney. Kidneys have an excellent capacity for recovery from ATN, which is marked by tubular cell dedifferentiation and proliferation and normalization of blood flow and cellular homeostasis. Incomplete recovery is characterized by persistent tubulointerstitial inflammation, proliferation of fibroblasts, and excessive deposition of extracellular matrix, leading to chronic damage.

- *Cardiorenal syndrome* is an important cause of AKI in children. It occurs due to complex bidirectional acute (types 1, 3) or chronic (types 2, 4) injury to heart and kidney, usually following myocarditis, congenital heart disease, and cardiopulmonary bypass.[36] AKI in cardiorenal syndrome occurs due to several pathogenetic mechanisms including ischemia-reperfusion injury (hypotension, low cardiac output, aggressive postoperative diuresis), inflammation, oxidative stress, hemolysis, and nephrotoxins.[37]

- Pathophysiology of *sepsis*-associated AKI is complex and poorly understood; in addition to hypoperfusion, interplay of microvascular dysfunction, dysregulated inflammation, and metabolic reprograming are the chief mechanisms.[38]
- Mechanisms of *drug-induced nephrotoxicity* include the following: (1) dose-dependent proximal tubular injury due to intratubular accumulation of drugs and their metabolites; (2) tubular obstruction by crystals or casts containing drugs and their metabolites (dose dependent); and (3) dose-independent interstitial nephritis.[39]
- Transplants, both solid organ and hematopoietic stem cell transplantation (HSCT), may be complicated by AKI due to one or several causes unique to such patients. These causes include use of nephrotoxic drugs (calcineurin inhibitors, conditioning regimens, antibiotics/antifungals), infections (sepsis, cytomegalovirus infection), and thrombotic microangiopathy. In addition, sinusoidal obstruction syndrome and acute graft-versus-host disease may cause AKI after HSCT.[40]

ADVANCES IN DIAGNOSIS

Although creatinine is the most used diagnostic marker for AKI, it has significant drawbacks as discussed earlier. One of the biggest issues with creatinine is that it is a marker of kidney function, not kidney injury. In the past few years, multiple biomarkers of structural injury have been identified. These include neutrophil gelatinase–associated lipocalin, tissue inhibitor of metalloproteinases-2, insulin-like growth factor–binding protein 7, and C-C motif chemokine ligand 14. These biomarkers have been studied for AKI prediction, early detection, and diagnosis of subclinical cases. Here the authors focus on 2 biomarkers that are currently available for clinical use.

Functional and damage biomarkers can be combined to identify different AKI phenotypes; this was initially proposed by the 10th Acute Disease Quality Initiative (ADQI) consensus conference and more recently updated by the 23rd ADQI conference.[41,42] Using these biomarkers, 4 different phenotypes can be identified (**Fig. 1**).

Those with normal functional markers and negative damage markers are considered as having no AKI. Elevation in kidney injury biomarkers in the absence of changes in functional markers (SCr and UOP) is called "subclinical AKI." Patients with a change in functional markers without an elevation in kidney injury biomarkers are considered as having "functional AKI"; these often include patients who were traditionally considered as having "prerenal" or fluid responsive AKI. Finally, the last quadrant includes patients who have a change in functional markers as well as elevation of injury markers. This combination of functional and damage biomarkers allows earlier diagnosis and better delineation of the AKI syndrome.

It is important to understand that this process is dynamic, and patients may move from one subtype to another.

Neutrophil gelatinase–associated lipocalin (NGAL): NGAL is one of the most widely studied AKI biomarkers in children.[43] It is a protein produced by neutrophils that works to inhibit bacterial growth, chelate iron, and induce epithelial cell growth. In the event of tubular injury, NGAL is upregulated and released into urine. By chelating iron, it protects the tubules from further injury. High NGAL levels in AKI may be from both increased renal and extrarenal expression and decreased tubular reabsorption.[44] NGAL was first studied as an AKI biomarker in the pediatric cardiac surgery population by Mishra and colleagues who showed that its level 2 hours after cardiopulmonary bypass initiation was a powerful and independent predictor of AKI on multivariable

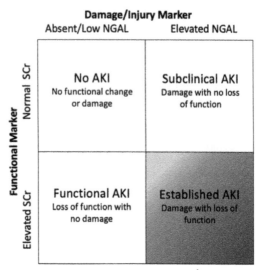

Fig. 1. Using functional and damage biomarkers to identify different AKI phenotypes. Adapted from 10th and 23rd Acute Disease Quality Initiative (ADQI) consensus conference.[41,42] Using these biomarkers, 4 different phenotypes can be identified as shown.

analysis with an area under the receiver operating characteristic curves (AUC-ROCs) of 0.998.[45] A subsequent multicenter cohort study of 311 children undergoing surgery for congenital cardiac lesions showed moderate accuracy of urine NGAL for diagnosis of severe AKI, with AUC of 0.71.[46]

The performance of NGAL has been less accurate in more heterogeneous populations. Elevated levels of NGAL have been reported in multiple non-AKI–like conditions including urinary tract infections, sepsis, and malignancy. Although not yet approved for use in the United States by the Food and Drug Administration, it is being used by some centers to predict AKI, diagnose subclinical AKI, and determine recovery, particularly in combination with a risk stratification construct as renal angina index (RAI).[47]

Tissue inhibitor of metalloproteinases-2 (TIMP-2) and insulin like growth factor–binding protein 7 (IGFBP7): TIMP-2 and IGFBP7, together known as Nephrocheck, are proteins expressed and secreted by renal tubular cells during cell stress or injury.[48] TIMP-2, expressed in many normal tissues, and expressed and secreted by distal tubular cells, is an inhibitor of matrix metalloproteinase. IGFBP7, expressed across the entire tubule and secreted by proximal tubular cells, regulates insulin-like growth factors in tissues and stimulates cell adhesion. During early AKI, they block cyclin-dependent protein kinase complexes and lead to G1 cell-cycle arrest.

After their initial identification out of more than 300 candidate biomarkers, TIMP-2 and IGFBP7 underwent validation in multicenter studies.[49,50] These studies showed that the product of the 2 markers ([TIMP-2] × [IGFBP7]) was superior to others in predicting KDIGO stage 2 or 3 AKI within 12 hours.[50] These data also led to the establishment of 2 cutoffs for [TIMP-2] × [IGFBP7], based on sensitivity and specificity for assessment of risk for AKI.[50] A cutoff of 0.3 $(ng/mL)^2/1000$ had high sensitivity and high negative predictive values of 89% and 97%, respectively, whereas a cutoff of 2 $(ng/mL)^2/1000$ had high specificity and moderate positive predictive values of 95% and 49%, respectively.[49] In adult patients at high risk for AKI after cardiopulmonary bypass, Meersch and colleagues used [TIMP-2] × [IGFBP7] for randomizing them to receive standard of care management (control) or rigorous implementation of KDIGO clinical practice guidelines (intervention).[51] The rate of severe AKI was less in the intervention group when compared with the control, with an absolute risk reduction of 16.6% (95% CI, 5.5%–27.9%; $P = .004$).[51]

RENAL ANGINA

RAI is a risk stratification construct that combines patient risk factors and early signs of kidney injury (fluid overload and changes in creatinine) for prediction of severe (stage 2 or 3) ICU day 3 AKI.[52] Typically calculated 12 hours after admission to an ICU, patients are given a risk score and an injury score, which are then multiplied to get an RAI. A score of 8 or more indicates the presence of renal Angina (**Fig. 2**). An RAI less than 8 has high negative predictive value for day 3 AKI. In a single-center study, Menon and colleagues showed that incorporation of a urine NGAL with RAI improved the AUC-ROC for severe ICU day 3 AKI from 0.8 to 0.97.[53] In the AWARE study, the RAI demonstrated better prediction for severe AKI than an elevation of SCr from baseline, with an adjusted OR of 3.21 (95% CI, 2.20–4.67).[54] More recently, RAI has been modified for other clinical settings. One such modification, "acute RAI" (aRAI), successfully identified on arrival to the emergency department, pediatric patients with sepsis who were at greatest risk of inpatient AKI.[55] For prediction of inpatient AKI, aRAI had an AUC of 0.92 (95% CI, 0.86–0.98), sensitivity of 94%, and a negative predictive value of 99% as compared with a sensitivity of 59% and negative predictive value of 93% for doubling of creatinine from baseline.[55]

FUROSEMIDE STRESS TEST

A furosemide challenge is commonly used in a patient with AKI in the clinical setting. Chawla and colleagues described a standardized furosemide stress test (FST) in adult

Risk Strata	
Risk Criteria	**Score**
ICU Admission	1
Stem Cell or Solid Organ Transplant	3
Mechanical Ventilation and Vasoactive Medication Use	5

Risk X Injury
Score Range: 1–40

Injury Strata		
Change in Serum Creatinine from Baseline	**% Fluid Overload**	**Score**
Decreased or no change	<5%	1
> 1X- 1.49X	> 5-10%	2
> 1.5X – 1.99X	10-15%	4
> 2X	≥ 15%	8

Fig. 2. Renal angina index, a risk stratification construct that combines patient risk factors and early signs of kidney injury (fluid overload and changes in creatinine) for prediction of severe (stage 2 or 3) ICU day 3 AKI.[52] Patients are assigned a risk score and an injury score, which are then multiplied to get an RAI, with a score of 8 or more indicating the presence of renal angina.

patients, wherein a dose of furosemide (1 mg/kg in loop diuretic naïve and 1.5 mg/kg in those who have previously received a loop diuretic) was administered and a UOP less than 200 mL in 2 h after furosemide administration predicted progression to AKI stage 3 with a specificity of 84.1% and a sensitivity of 87.1%.[56] It has since been used to improve risk stratification and combined with NGAL and [TIMP-2]X [IGFBP7] for more accurate assessment of the risk of severe AKI.[57]

In recent years, FST has also been used in pediatric patients. In a retrospective study of 568 infants who underwent CPB and received routine postoperative furosemide (0.8–1.2 mg/kg per dose between 8 and 24 hours after surgery), lack of furosemide responsiveness (defined as UOP <1 mL/kg/h) predicted AKI development (AUC-ROC of 0.74 at 2 hours and 0.77 at 6 hours).[58] Patients with UOP greater than 1 mL/kg/h were unlikely to have AKI (negative predictive value, 97%). In a multicenter, retrospective chart review of consecutive children undergoing cardiac surgery requiring CPB across 4 hospitals, Penk and colleagues found that low urine flow rates at 2 and 6 hours after furosemide administration (mean dose of 0.9 ± 0.3 mg/kg) were independently associated with development of AKI (2-hour odds ratio, 1.2, $P = .002$; 6-hour odds ratio, 1.40, $P < .001$).[59] However, there is no standard definition of the dose of furosemide and the response in pediatrics, and more prospective studies are needed to standardize this.

CLINICAL DECISION SUPPORT SYSTEMS

With the widespread use of electronic medical records (EMR), clinical decision support systems that include electronic alerts (e-alerts) have been used to improve recognition of patients with AKI. Despite extensive studies on the implementation of electronic alerts, their overall impact on clinical outcomes has been variable. These systems may be used to either identify patients at risk for AKI or to detect patients already with AKI. The 15th ADQI consensus conference recognized AKI alerts as an opportunity to prompt earlier evaluation and intervention and recommended linking alerts to actionable interventions.[60] One such successful intervention was the Nephrotoxic Injury Negated by Just in Time Action (NINJA) program, a prospective quality improvement project that works to reduce nephrotoxic medication–associated AKI among noncritically ill hospitalized children.[61] Since initiation, it was successful in reducing the number of AKI days per 100 days by 42% in its first year and has been successfully replicated across 9 pediatric institutions.[61,62]

Others have looked at the use of e-alerts in those who develop AKI. The Welsh AKI group studied AKI alerts in pediatric patients in hospital and community setting over a period of 30 months.[13] They reported better identification of AKI with an e-alert and an incidence rate of 1.37 cases per 1000 person-years. Another prospective study aimed to determine whether an AKI alert paired with a standardized care pathway would improve AKI detection and renal outcomes.[63] In this study with 239 unique AKI alerts, the intervention/alert phase was associated with a significant increase in AKI documentation, intake and output charting, as well as adjustments to fluid and medications. Sandokji and colleagues worked on an AKI prediction model using variables from the EMR and a machine learning–based algorithm.[64] Using this model, they reported an AUC of 0.79 (95% CI, 0.74–0.83) for predicting stage 2 or 3 AKI in children.

MANAGEMENT

Management of AKI includes its prevention and providing supportive care once AKI develops. The KDIGO AKI guidelines recommend using AKI staging to guide management.[6] It is hoped that as biomarkers become more widely available, identification of different AKI phenotypes will improve, allowing for use of more targeted therapies.

Patients with any stage of AKI should have careful monitoring of their fluid balance, thoughtful assessment of medications, and discontinuation or avoidance of nephrotoxic agents. Regarding nephrotoxic medications, it is critical to assess the risks versus benefits. Patients should receive potentially nephrotoxic medications only if they absolutely need them and only for the needed duration.[61] Education of clinicians and careful monitoring of kidney function in patients who are receiving nephrotoxic agents has been shown to reduce the risk and progression of AKI.[61]

Fluid Balance

There is a delicate balance that needs to be maintained regarding the volume status of a patient with AKI. Fluid management should be personalized based on patient's clinical status and disease trajectory. Various models of fluid management have been proposed for critically ill patients. One such model comprises 3 phases: fluid resuscitation/repletion, fluid balance maintenance, and fluid removal/recovery.[65] Although optimization of intravascular circulating volume and correction of intravascular hypovolemia is crucial for the prevention and management of AKI, unrestrained fluid administration may result in progression of AKI and worse outcomes. Thus, after initial resuscitation and adequate repletion, it is important to maintain a net even fluid balance, prevent further fluid overload (FO), and work on de-escalation and mobilization of accumulated fluid.

Stewart and colleagues, through the acute respiratory distress syndrome (ARDS) Clinical Trials Network Fluid and Catheter Treatment Trial (FACTT), showed that surgical patients receiving a conservative fluid management strategy had more ventilator-free days, and ICU-free days, but there was no effect on dialysis-free days.[66] In one systematic review and meta-analysis that looked at conservative or deresuscitative fluid strategies in adults and children with ARDS and sepsis, no significant difference in mortality was noted with conservative or deresuscitative strategies (pooled risk ratio 0.92, 95% CI, 0.82–1.02).[67] However, the conservative or deresuscitative strategy resulted in increased ventilator-free days and reduced length of ICU stay compared with a liberal strategy or standard care.[67]

FO occurs in 10% to 80% patients in the ICU due to systemic inflammation, capillary leak, disordered fluid homeostasis, and AKI. It is an independent but modifiable predictor of mortality. A metanalysis of 11 studies, including more than 3000 critically ill pediatric patients, showed 6% increase in odds of in-hospital mortality for every 1% increase in percentage FO.[68] Fluid overload can be calculated using the cumulative fluid balance[69] or based on daily weights[70]:

- Percent Fluid Overload (%FO) = [Daily input (Liters) - Daily output (Liters) x 100]/ ICU admission weight (kilograms)
- Percent Fluid Overload (%FO) = [Daily Weight – ICU admission weight x 100]/ ICU admission weight (kilograms)

There is also a concern that FO might put patients at risk of being underdiagnosed with AKI or lead to underestimation of its severity, as serum creatinine is influenced by the volume of distribution.[71] In a study of 92 patients undergoing arterial switch operation for transposition of the great vessels, correction of serum creatinine for the degree of fluid overload (by the following formula) refined the diagnosis of AKI and strengthened its association with morbidity.[72]

Corrected creatinine = serum creatinine (1 + net fluid balance/total body water)

where, total body water = 0.6 × weight (in kilograms)

Fluid accumulation *per se* renders an individual vulnerable to AKI and often predates it. It can also worsen AKI by increasing venous pressure and causing abdominal hypertension and interstitial edema.[73,74] Evidence in cardiac surgery patients shows an association between early postoperative FO and longer hospital stay, prolonged mechanical ventilation, and the development of AKI.[75] Although AKI and fluid overload are physiologically linked, a recent prospective study in 143 critically ill patients showed an association of fluid overload greater than 20% on day 3 of ICU stay with morbidity and mortality, which was independent of AKI status and severity of illness.[76] Overall, evidence suggests greater than 10% to 20% FO may represent a critical threshold at which outcomes are adversely affected and targeted interventions should be considered.[77]

Kidney replacement therapy (KRT): although the timing for initiation of KRT seems obvious in the presence of severe complications of AKI, including metabolic derangements and FO, there has been discussion whether early start of KRT, before the onset of these derangements, would improve the outcomes. A multicenter, Standard versus Accelerated Initiation of Renal-Replacement Therapy in Acute Kidney Injury (STARRT-AKI) randomized controlled trial compared an accelerated strategy (within 12 hours) versus standard (based on prespecified indication) strategy of KRT initiation.[78] It showed no difference in deaths at 90 days between the 2 groups. However, patients in the accelerated group had a higher dependence on KRT (10.4% vs 6%, RR, 1.74; 95% CI, 1.24–2.43) and more adverse events. Although there are no studies in children, looking at the timing of KRT initiation, Sutherland and colleagues showed that children with greater FO before initiation of continuous KRT (CKRT) had higher mortality than those with less fluid overload.[79] In this multicenter prospective observational study, those with 20% or greater FO fluid overload at CKRT initiation had an adjusted mortality OR of 8.5 (95% CI, 2.8–25.7) compared with those with less than 20% FO.

There is no evidence regarding the superiority of one dialysis modality over another in terms of outcomes in AKI. The decision on which modality is used is based on patient characteristics, institutional resources, and expertise. Each has advantages and disadvantages as discussed in **Table 3**.

CLINICAL OUTCOMES
Short-Term Outcomes

Despite advancements in diagnosis and management of AKI, the short- and medium-term outcomes following AKI remain unsatisfactory. Several studies have clearly demonstrated an independent association between pediatric and neonatal AKI and higher mortality,[3,18,26,80] longer hospital stay,[3,18,26,80] and need for mechanical ventilation.[18,80,81] The ISN 0 by 25 global snapshot study reported 7-day mortality of 17% to 25% in hospitalized children with AKI, 4.5% to 20.2% in community-acquired AKI, 25% in patients requiring KRT, and 40% in critically ill patients in resource-limited settings.[28]

Effect on Other Organs

AKI is now understood to be a systemic disorder with impact on other organs such as lungs, heart, liver, and brain. Pulmonary dysfunction is one of the most relevant organ effects of AKI in critically ill children. The AWARE study showed a stepwise increase in requirement of mechanical ventilation with worsening AKI severity (38.2%, 40.5%, and 50.2% in stage 1, 2, and 3, respectively vs 29.5% without AKI).[18] The association of

Table 3
Comparative features of dialysis modalities

	Peritoneal Dialysis (PD)	Intermittent Hemodialysis (IHD)	Continuous Kidney Replacement Therapy (CKRT)	Sustained Low-Efficiency Dialysis (SLED)
Principle	Diffusion and convection	Diffusion	Convection with or without diffusion	Diffusion
Efficiency	Slow clearance; ultrafiltration might not be accurate	Most rapid clearance; suitable for drug ingestion, hyperammonemia, tumor lysis syndrome; accurate ultrafiltration	Rapid clearance; suitable for removal of toxins/drugs requiring continuous convective clearance; accurate ultrafiltration	Rapid clearance; suitable for emergent situations; accurate ultrafiltration
Fluid and solute balance	Least hemodynamic compromise and fluctuations in solutes	Hypotension in small or critically ill children possible; causes large fluctuations in solutes	Suitable for hemodynamically unstable or intolerant to fluctuations in fluid balance and solutes	Risk of fluid and solute shifts lower than intermittent hemodialysis
Need for vascular access	Not required	Required	Required	Required
Need for systemic anticoagulation	Not required	Usually required	Required	Usually required
Need for intact peritoneal membrane	Required	Not required	Not required	Not required
Complexity; cost	Minimum equipment and training needs; feasible in small infants, neonates; inexpensive	Procedural simplicity compared with CKRT, requires facilities for dialysis water, less labor intensive than CKRT; expensive	Complex, no requirement for facilities for dialysis water, more labor intensive than IHD; expensive	Procedural simplicity compared with CKRT, requires IHD facilities, less labor intensive than CKRT; cheaper than CKRT
Disadvantages	Risk of peritonitis, increased intraabdominal pressure, peritoneal fluid leakage, catheter block; protein losses	Vascular access thrombosis, stenosis, infection; risk of hemodynamic instability	Vascular access thrombosis, stenosis, infection; hypothermia in small children; bradykinin release syndrome with AN-69 membranes	Vascular access thrombosis, stenosis, infection; lack of continuous dialyzing; loss of 15%–35% of amino acids; limited studies in children

prolonged ventilator dependence with AKI has been shown in other studies, including neonates.[80,82] A secondary analysis of the AWAKEN study showed an association of AKI with moderate to severe bronchopulmonary dysplasia in neonates born between 29 and 32 weeks.[83] AKI-induced generation of inflammatory cytokines and trafficking of T lymphocytes and neutrophils to the lungs propagates acute lung injury. Worsening of pulmonary edema occurs in the setting of AKI due to fluid overload, angiopoietin-2–induced vascular leak, and uremia-induced changes in expression of pulmonary epithelial sodium and aquaporin-5 channels.[84]

AKI may also play a role in propagating cardiac dysfunction. Although post-cardiac surgical AKI was found to be associated with an increased 5-year risk for myocardial infarction and heart failure in adults, long-term data in children are limited.[85] There are also emerging data that AKI may increase the risk of infection, and this may be mediated by neutrophil dysfunction.[86] Studies of neurocognitive outcomes following pediatric AKI are limited; medium- to long-term follow-up indicates development of new morbidity and worse functional outcome at discharge in CKRT survivors,[87] lower quality of life and poor physical performance at 3 month in survivors of sepsis-associated AKI,[88] and persistent neurocognitive problems at 2 years following AKI associated with severe malaria.[89] An analysis of premature neonates from the AWAKEN study showed that patients with AKI had 1.6 times higher odds to develop intraventricular hemorrhage.[90]

Acute Kidney Injury and Chronic Kidney Disease

The association between AKI and CKD has been clearly established in recent years. What remains less clear is whether AKI causes CKD or if it highlights preexisting CKD or lack of renal reserve. Most studies show that proteinuria, hypertension, and reduced eGFR are common following AKI.[91,92] Menon and colleagues compared 100 children who developed nephrotoxic AKI with matched non-AKI controls and reported significantly lower eGFR, more proteinuria, and a higher incidence of hypertension in those who experienced AKI.[93] Mammen and colleagues reviewed survivors of AKI stage 1 or higher, 1 to 3 years after ICU discharge. Although rates of hypertension (3.2%) and proteinuria (9.5%) were not very high, almost 40% of the children had an eGFR less than 90 mL/min/1.73 m^2.[94]

The KDIGO guidelines recommended a 3-month follow-up for all patients who developed AKI to assess for presence of CKD. However, most long-term follow-up studies show rates of follow-up of less than 50%.[93,94] Children who develop AKI need long-term observation and monitoring. AKI follow-up clinics have been established in some institutions.[95] The intensity and level of post-AKI and -AKD care may depend on the severity of AKI, recovery or lack of recovery of kidney function, and other comorbidities. In addition to such clinics, a systematic program to educate non-nephrologists and patients and a focus on patient-centered outcomes may help patients with AKI receive appropriate follow-up.

SUMMARY

Our understanding of AKI in children has advanced over the past decade. It has become obvious that AKI is not a single disease limited to the kidneys but a systemic syndrome that can affect multiple organs. The use of newer tools such as AKI risk stratification models, biomarkers, and electronic alerts allows us to consider a dynamic and multidimensional approach, which may further improve characterization and phenotyping of AKI. The management of AKI remains supportive, but these tools may also allow predictive enrichment and personalized pediatric AKI management in the future.

CLINICS CARE POINTS

- When evaluating a patient with AKI, recognize that serum creatinine has certain limitations in defining AKI and may not increase until 50% kidney function is lost.
- Patients at risk of AKI (those with critical illness, sepsis, receiving nephrotoxic medications) should have close monitoring of urine output and creatinine.
- Patients with any stage of AKI should have careful monitoring of their fluid balance, thoughtful assessment of medications, and discontinuation or avoidance of nephrotoxic agents.
- Patients with AKI should be followed-up for long-term consequences including proteinuria, hypertension, and CKD

REFERENCES

1. Fortenberry JD, Paden ML, Goldstein SL. Acute kidney injury in children: an update on diagnosis and treatment. Pediatr Clin North Am 2013;60(3):669–88.
2. Bellomo R, Ronco C, Kellum JA, et al. Acute Dialysis Quality Initiative w. Acute renal failure - definition, outcome measures, animal models, fluid therapy and information technology needs: the Second International Consensus Conference of the Acute Dialysis Quality Initiative (ADQI) Group. Crit Care 2004;8(4):R204–12.
3. Akcan-Arikan A, Zappitelli M, Loftis LL, et al. Modified RIFLE criteria in critically ill children with acute kidney injury. Kidney Int 2007;71(10):1028–35.
4. Chertow GM, Burdick E, Honour M, et al. Acute kidney injury, mortality, length of stay, and costs in hospitalized patients. J Am Soc Nephrol 2005;16(11):3365–70.
5. Mehta RL, Kellum JA, Shah SV, et al. Acute Kidney Injury Network: report of an initiative to improve outcomes in acute kidney injury. Crit Care 2007;11(2):R31.
6. Group KDIGOKAKIW. KDIGO Clinical Practice Guideline for Acute Kidney Injury. Kidney Int 2012;(2):1–138.
7. Chawla LS, Bellomo R, Bihorac A, et al. Acute kidney disease and renal recovery: consensus report of the Acute Disease Quality Initiative (ADQI) 16 Workgroup. Nat reviewsNephrology 2017;13(4):241–57.
8. Lameire NH, Levin A, Kellum JA, et al. Harmonizing acute and chronic kidney disease definition and classification: report of a Kidney Disease: Improving Global Outcomes (KDIGO) Consensus Conference. Kidney Int 2021;100(3):516–26.
9. Sutherland SM, Kwiatkowski DM. Acute Kidney Injury in Children. Adv chronic kidney Dis 2017;24(6):380–7.
10. Thongprayoon C, Cheungpasitporn W, Kashani K. Serum creatinine level, a surrogate of muscle mass, predicts mortality in critically ill patients. J Thorac Dis 2016;8(5):E305–11.
11. Liu KD, Thompson BT, Ancukiewicz M, et al. Acute kidney injury in patients with acute lung injury: impact of fluid accumulation on classification of acute kidney injury and associated outcomes. Crit Care Med 2011;39(12):2665–71.
12. Zappitelli M, Parikh CR, Akcan-Arikan A, et al. Ascertainment and epidemiology of acute kidney injury varies with definition interpretation. Clin J Am Soc Nephrol 2008;3(4):948–54.
13. Holmes J, Roberts G, May K, et al. The incidence of pediatric acute kidney injury is increased when identified by a change in a creatinine-based electronic alert. Kidney Int 2017;92(2):432–9.

14. Xu X, Nie S, Zhang A, et al. A New Criterion for Pediatric AKI Based on the Reference Change Value of Serum Creatinine. J Am Soc Nephrol 2018;29(9):2432–42.

15. Chen S. Retooling the creatinine clearance equation to estimate kinetic GFR when the plasma creatinine is changing acutely. J Am Soc Nephrol 2013;24(6): 877–88.

16. Pianta TJ, Endre ZH, Pickering JW, et al. Kinetic Estimation of GFR Improves Prediction of Dialysis and Recovery after Kidney Transplantation. PLoS One 2015; 10(5):e0125669.

17. Menon S, Basu RK, Barhight MF, et al. Utility of Kinetic GFR for Predicting Severe Persistent AKI in Critically Ill Children and Young Adults. Kidney360. 2021;2(5): 869–72.

18. Kaddourah A, Basu RK, Bagshaw SM, et al. Epidemiology of Acute Kidney Injury in Critically Ill Children and Young Adults. N Engl J Med 2017;376(1):11–20.

19. Kaddourah A, Basu RK, Goldstein SL, et al. Assessment of Worldwide Acute Kidney Injury RAaEI. Oliguria and Acute Kidney Injury in Critically Ill Children: Implications for Diagnosis and Outcomes. Pediatr Crit Care Med 2019;20(4):332–9.

20. Zappitelli M, Ambalavanan N, Askenazi DJ, et al. Developing a neonatal acute kidney injury research definition: a report from the NIDDK neonatal AKI workshop. Pediatr Res 2017;82(4):569–73.

21. Askenazi D, Abitbol C, Boohaker L, et al. Optimizing the AKI definition during first postnatal week using Assessment of Worldwide Acute Kidney Injury Epidemiology in Neonates (AWAKEN) cohort. Pediatr Res 2019;85(3):329–38.

22. Sutherland SM, Byrnes JJ, Kothari M, et al. AKI in hospitalized children: comparing the pRIFLE, AKIN, and KDIGO definitions. Clin J Am Soc Nephrol 2015;10(4):554–61.

23. Parikh RV, Tan TC, Salyer AS, et al. Community-Based Epidemiology of Hospitalized Acute Kidney Injury. Pediatrics 2020;146(3). https://doi.org/10.1542/peds. 2019-2821.

24. Gubb S, Holmes J, Smith G, et al. Acute Kidney Injury in Children Based on Electronic Alerts. J Pediatr 2020;220:14–20.e4.

25. Susantitaphong P, Cruz DN, Cerda J, et al. World incidence of AKI: a meta-analysis. Clin J Am Soc Nephrol 2013;8(9):1482–93.

26. Jetton JG, Boohaker LJ, Sethi SK, et al. Incidence and outcomes of neonatal acute kidney injury (AWAKEN): a multicentre, multinational, observational cohort study. LancetChild Adolesc Health 2017;1(3):184–94.

27. Hui-Stickle S, Brewer ED, Goldstein SL. Pediatric ARF epidemiology at a tertiary care center from 1999 to 2001. Am J Kidney Dis 2005;45(1):96–101.

28. Macedo E, Cerda J, Hingorani S, et al. Recognition and management of acute kidney injury in children: The ISN 0by25 Global Snapshot study. PLoS One 2018;13(5):e0196586.

29. Lameire NH, Bagga A, Cruz D, et al. Acute kidney injury: an increasing global concern. Lancet 2013;382(9887):170–9.

30. Abdelraheem MB. Acute kidney injury in low- and middle-income countries: investigations, management and prevention. Paediatr Int Child Health 2017; 37(4):269–72.

31. Ruas AFL, Lebeis GM, de Castro NB, et al. Acute kidney injury in pediatrics: an overview focusing on pathophysiology. Pediatr Nephrol 2021. https://doi.org/10. 1007/s00467-021-05346-8.

32. Basile DP, Anderson MD, Sutton TA. Pathophysiology of acute kidney injury. Compr Physiol 2012;2(2):1303–53.

33. Makris K, Spanou L. Acute Kidney Injury: Definition, Pathophysiology and Clinical Phenotypes. Clin Biochem Rev 2016;37(2):85–98.

34. Martensson J, Bellomo R. Pathophysiology of Septic Acute Kidney Injury. Contrib Nephrol 2016;187:36–46.

35. Pickkers P, Darmon M, Hoste E, et al. Acute kidney injury in the critically ill: an updated review on pathophysiology and management. Intensive Care Med 2021;47(8):835–50.

36. Ricci Z, Romagnoli S, Ronco C. Cardiorenal Syndrome. Crit Care Clin 2021;37(2): 335–47.

37. Wang Y, Bellomo R. Cardiac surgery-associated acute kidney injury: risk factors, pathophysiology and treatment. Nat Rev Nephrol 2017;13(11):697–711.

38. Manrique-Caballero CL, Del Rio-Pertuz G, Gomez H. Sepsis-Associated Acute Kidney Injury. Crit Care Clin 2021;37(2):279–301.

39. Kwiatkowska E, Domanski L, Dziedziejko V, et al. The Mechanism of Drug Nephrotoxicity and the Methods for Preventing Kidney Damage. Int J Mol Sci 2021;(11):22. https://doi.org/10.3390/ijms22116109.

40. Miyata MIK, Matsuki E, Watanabe M, et al. Recent Advances of Acute Kidney Injury in Hematopoietic Cell Transplantation. Front Immunol 2022. https://doi.org/10.3389/fimmu.2021.779881.

41. Ostermann M, Zarbock A, Goldstein S, et al. Recommendations on Acute Kidney Injury Biomarkers From the Acute Disease Quality Initiative Consensus Conference: A Consensus Statement. JAMA Netw Open 2020;3(10):e2019209.

42. Murray PT, Mehta RL, Shaw A, et al. Potential use of biomarkers in acute kidney injury: report and summary of recommendations from the 10th Acute Dialysis Quality Initiative consensus conference. Kidney Int 2014;85(3):513–21.

43. Greenberg JH, Parikh CR. Biomarkers for Diagnosis and Prognosis of AKI in Children: One Size Does Not Fit All. Clin J Am Soc Nephrol 2017;12(9):1551–7.

44. Skrypnyk NI, Gist KM, Okamura K, et al. IL-6-mediated hepatocyte production is the primary source of plasma and urine neutrophil gelatinase-associated lipocalin during acute kidney injury. Kidney Int 2020;97(5):966–79.

45. Mishra J, Dent C, Tarabishi R, et al. Neutrophil gelatinase-associated lipocalin (NGAL) as a biomarker for acute renal injury after cardiac surgery. Lancet 2005;365(9466):1231–8.

46. Parikh CR, Devarajan P, Zappitelli M, et al. Postoperative biomarkers predict acute kidney injury and poor outcomes after pediatric cardiac surgery. J Am Soc Nephrol 2011;22(9):1737–47.

47. Varnell CD, Goldstein SL, Devarajan P, et al. Impact of Near Real-Time Urine Neutrophil Gelatinase-Associated Lipocalin Assessment on Clinical Practice. Kidney Int Rep 2017;2(6):1243–9.

48. Sandokji I, Greenberg JH. Novel biomarkers of acute kidney injury in children: an update on recent findings. Curr Opin Pediatr 2020;32(3):354–9.

49. Hoste EA, McCullough PA, Kashani K, et al. Derivation and validation of cutoffs for clinical use of cell cycle arrest biomarkers. Nephrol Dial Transpl 2014; 29(11):2054–61.

50. Kashani K, Al-Khafaji A, Ardiles T, et al. Discovery and validation of cell cycle arrest biomarkers in human acute kidney injury. Crit Care 2013;17(1):R25.

51. Meersch M, Schmidt C, Hoffmeier A, et al. Prevention of cardiac surgery-associated AKI by implementing the KDIGO guidelines in high risk patients identified by biomarkers: the PrevAKI randomized controlled trial. Intensive Care Med 2017;43(11):1551–61.

52. Basu RK, Zappitelli M, Brunner L, et al. Derivation and validation of the renal angina index to improve the prediction of acute kidney injury in critically ill children. Kidney Int 2014;85(3):659–67.

53. Menon S, Goldstein SL, Mottes T, et al. Urinary biomarker incorporation into the renal angina index early in intensive care unit admission optimizes acute kidney injury prediction in critically ill children: a prospective cohort study. Nephrol Dial Transplant 2016;31(4):586–94.

54. Basu RK, Kaddourah A, Goldstein SL, et al. Assessment of a renal angina index for prediction of severe acute kidney injury in critically ill children: a multicentre, multinational, prospective observational study. Lancet Child Adolesc Health 2018;2(2):112–20.

55. Hanson HR, Carlisle MA, Bensman RS, et al. Early prediction of pediatric acute kidney injury from the emergency department: A pilot study. Am J Emerg Med 2021;40:138–44.

56. Chawla LS, Davison DL, Brasha-Mitchell E, et al. Development and standardization of a furosemide stress test to predict the severity of acute kidney injury. Crit Care 2013;17(5):R207.

57. Koyner JL, Davison DL, Brasha-Mitchell E, et al. Furosemide Stress Test and Biomarkers for the Prediction of AKI Severity. J Am Soc Nephrol 2015;26(8):2023–31.

58. Kakajiwala A, Kim JY, Hughes JZ, et al. Lack of Furosemide Responsiveness Predicts Acute Kidney Injury in Infants After Cardiac Surgery. Ann Thorac Surg 2017; 104(4):1388–94.

59. Penk J, Gist KM, Wald EL, et al. Furosemide response predicts acute kidney injury in children after cardiac surgery. J Thorac Cardiovasc Surg 2019;157(6): 2444–51.

60. Hoste EA, Kashani K, Gibney N, et al. Impact of electronic-alerting of acute kidney injury: workgroup statements from the 15(th) ADQI Consensus Conference. Can J kidney Health Dis 2016;3. https://doi.org/10.1186/s40697-016-0101-1. 10-016-0101-1. eCollection 2016.

61. Goldstein SL, Kirkendall E, Nguyen H, et al. Electronic Health Record Identification of Nephrotoxin Exposure and Associated Acute Kidney Injury. Pediatrics 2013. https://doi.org/10.1542/peds.2013-0794.

62. Goldstein SL, Dahale D, Kirkendall ES, et al. A prospective multi-center quality improvement initiative (NINJA) indicates a reduction in nephrotoxic acute kidney injury in hospitalized children. Kidney Int 2020;97(3):580–8.

63. Menon S, Tarrago R, Carlin K, et al. Impact of integrated clinical decision support systems in the management of pediatric acute kidney injury: a pilot study. Pediatr Res 2021;89(5):1164–70.

64. Sandokji I, Yamamoto Y, Biswas A, et al. A Time-Updated, Parsimonious Model to Predict AKI in Hospitalized Children. J Am Soc Nephrol 2020;31(6):1348–57.

65. Goldstein SL. Fluid management in acute kidney injury. J Intensive Care Med 2014;29(4):183–9.

66. Stewart RM, Park PK, Hunt JP, et al. Less is more: improved outcomes in surgical patients with conservative fluid administration and central venous catheter monitoring. J Am Coll Surg 2009;208(5):725–35 [discussion: 735–7].

67. Silversides JA, Major E, Ferguson AJ, et al. Conservative fluid management or deresuscitation for patients with sepsis or acute respiratory distress syndrome following the resuscitation phase of critical illness: a systematic review and meta-analysis. Intensive Care Med 2017;43(2):155–70.

68. Alobaidi R, Morgan C, Basu RK, et al. Association Between Fluid Balance and Outcomes in Critically Ill Children: A Systematic Review and Meta-analysis. JAMA Pediatr 2018;172(3):257–68.

69. Goldstein SL, Currier H, Graf C, et al. Outcome in children receiving continuous venovenous hemofiltration. Pediatrics 2001;107(6):1309–12.

70. Lombel RM, Kommareddi M, Mottes T, et al. Implications of different fluid overload definitions in pediatric stem cell transplant patients requiring continuous renal replacement therapy. Intensive Care Med 2012;38(4):663–9.

71. Goldstein SL. Urine Output Assessment in Acute Kidney Injury: The Cheapest and Most Impactful Biomarker. Front Pediatr 2019;7:565.

72. Basu RK, Andrews A, Krawczeski C, et al. Acute kidney injury based on corrected serum creatinine is associated with increased morbidity in children following the arterial switch operation. Pediatr Crit Care Med 2013;14(5):e218–24.

73. Godin M, Bouchard J, Mehta RL. Fluid balance in patients with acute kidney injury: emerging concepts. Nephron Clin Pract 2013;123(3–4):238–45.

74. Rajendram R, Prowle JR. Venous congestion: are we adding insult to kidney injury in sepsis? Crit Care 2014;18(1):104.

75. Hassinger AB, Wald EL, Goodman DM. Early postoperative fluid overload precedes acute kidney injury and is associated with higher morbidity in pediatric cardiac surgery patients. Pediatr Crit Care Med 2014;15(2):131–8.

76. Gist KM, Selewski DT, Brinton J, et al. Assessment of the Independent and Synergistic Effects of Fluid Overload and Acute Kidney Injury on Outcomes of Critically Ill Children. Pediatr Crit Care Med 2020;21(2):170–7.

77. Selewski DT, Goldstein SL. The role of fluid overload in the prediction of outcome in acute kidney injury. Pediatr Nephrol 2016. https://doi.org/10.1007/s00467-016-3539-6.

78. Bagshaw SM, Wald R, Adhikari NKJ, et al. Timing of Initiation of Renal-Replacement Therapy in Acute Kidney Injury. N Engl J Med 2020;383(3):240–51.

79. Sutherland SM, Zappitelli M, Alexander SR, et al. Fluid overload and mortality in children receiving continuous renal replacement therapy: the prospective pediatric continuous renal replacement therapy registry. Am J Kidney Dis 2010;55(2):316–25.

80. Alkandari O, Eddington KA, Hyder A, et al. Acute kidney injury is an independent risk factor for pediatric intensive care unit mortality, longer length of stay and prolonged mechanical ventilation in critically ill children: a two-center retrospective cohort study. Crit Care 2011;15(3):R146.

81. Fitzgerald JC, Basu RK, Akcan-Arikan A, et al. Acute Kidney Injury in Pediatric Severe Sepsis: An Independent Risk Factor for Death and New Disability. Crit Care Med 2016;44(12):2241–50.

82. Selewski DT, Jordan BK, Askenazi DJ, et al. Acute kidney injury in asphyxiated newborns treated with therapeutic hypothermia. J Pediatr 2013;162(4):725–9.e1.

83. Starr MC, Boohaker L, Eldredge LC, et al. Acute Kidney Injury and Bronchopulmonary Dysplasia in Premature Neonates Born Less than 32 Weeks' Gestation. Am J Perinatol 2020;37(3):341–8.

84. Alge J, Dolan K, Angelo J, et al. Two to Tango: Kidney-Lung Interaction in Acute Kidney Injury and Acute Respiratory Distress Syndrome. Front Pediatr 2021;9:744110.

85. Hansen MK, Gammelager H, Jacobsen CJ, et al. Acute Kidney Injury and Long-term Risk of Cardiovascular Events After Cardiac Surgery: A Population-Based Cohort Study. J Cardiothorac Vasc Anesth 2015;29(3):617–25.

86. Formeck CL, Joyce EL, Fuhrman DY, et al. Association of Acute Kidney Injury With Subsequent Sepsis in Critically Ill Children. Pediatr Crit Care Med 2021; 22(1):e58–66.

87. Smith M, Bell C, Vega MW, et al. Patient-centered outcomes in pediatric continuous kidney replacement therapy: new morbidity and worsened functional status in survivors. Pediatr Nephrol 2022;37(1):189–97.

88. Starr MC, Banks R, Reeder RW, et al. Severe Acute Kidney Injury Is Associated With Increased Risk of Death and New Morbidity After Pediatric Septic Shock. Pediatr Crit Care Med 2020;21(9):e686–95.

89. Conroy AL, Opoka RO, Bangirana P, et al. Acute kidney injury is associated with impaired cognition and chronic kidney disease in a prospective cohort of children with severe malaria. BMC Med 2019;17(1):98.

90. Stoops C, Boohaker L, Sims B, et al. The Association of Intraventricular Hemorrhage and Acute Kidney Injury in Premature Infants from the Assessment of the Worldwide Acute Kidney Injury Epidemiology in Neonates (AWAKEN) Study. Neonatology 2019;116(4):321–30.

91. Hessey E, Perreault S, Dorais M, et al. Acute Kidney Injury in Critically Ill Children and Subsequent Chronic Kidney Disease. Can J kidney Health Dis 2019;6. 2054358119880188.

92. Zappitelli M, Parikh CR, Kaufman JS, et al. Acute Kidney Injury and Risk of CKD and Hypertension after Pediatric Cardiac Surgery. Clin J Am Soc Nephrol 2020; 15(10):1403–12.

93. Menon S, Kirkendall ES, Nguyen H, et al. Acute kidney injury associated with high nephrotoxic medication exposure leads to chronic kidney disease after 6 months. J Pediatr 2014;165(3):522–7.e2.

94. Mammen C, Al Abbas A, Skippen P, et al. Long-term risk of CKD in children surviving episodes of acute kidney injury in the intensive care unit: a prospective cohort study. Am J Kidney Dis 2012;59(4):523–30.

95. Silver SA, Goldstein SL, Harel Z, et al. Ambulatory care after acute kidney injury: an opportunity to improve patient outcomes. Can J kidney Health Dis 2015;2. https://doi.org/10.1186/s40697-015-0071-8. 36-3015-0071-8. eCollection 2015.

Chronic Kidney Disease in Children

Judith Sebestyen VanSickle, MD*, Bradley A. Warady, MD

KEYWORDS

- Pediatrics • CKD • ESKD • Dialysis • Transplant

KEY POINTS

- Chronic kidney disease (CKD) in children occurs primarily due to congenital anomalies of the kidney and urinary tract.
- Complications of CKD include impaired growth and development, anemia, bone and mineral disorder, and cardiovascular disease.
- Adequate nutritional support, including salt supplementation in some cases, is essential for normal growth and development.
- Dialysis options include peritoneal and hemodialysis; peritoneal dialysis is the most frequent dialysis modality used for children worldwide.
- A multidisciplinary team approach by a pediatric nephrologist, trained nurse, social worker, dietitian, child life therapist, and a psychologist is essential.

INTRODUCTION AND OVERVIEW
Incidence and Prevalence of Chronic Kidney Disease

There are very few population-based studies of pediatric chronic kidney disease (CKD),[1,2] and most epidemiologic data are based on relatively small registries. One of the largest national studies, the Italian Pediatric Registry of Chronic Renal Failure (ItalKid) project, surveyed the incidence and prevalence of CKD in children, as defined by an estimated glomerular filtration rate (eGFR) less than 75 mL/min/1.73 m². They reported a CKD incidence of 12.1 per million of the age-related population (pmarp) and prevalence of 74.7 pmarp.[3] One of the reasons for lack of data is the asymptomatic nature of early CKD in children. However, a routine use of prenatal ultrasound evaluations has made the early diagnosis of CKD much more common. Also, an increasing number of premature and low-birth-weight infants, presumed to have a lower nephron endowment, as well as an increasing prevalence of obesity in children are likely to increase further the number of children with CKD.[4]

Children's Mercy Kansas City, University of Missouri - Kansas City School of Medicine, Division of Pediatric Nephrology, 2401 Gillham Road, Kansas City, MO 64108, USA
* Corresponding author.
E-mail address: jvansickle@cmh.edu

Pediatr Clin N Am 69 (2022) 1239–1254
https://doi.org/10.1016/j.pcl.2022.07.010
pediatric.theclinics.com
0031-3955/22/© 2022 Elsevier Inc. All rights reserved.

Cause of Chronic Kidney Disease

In adult and children, the normal eGFR is greater than90 mL/min/1.73 m^2. The National Kidney Foundation's Kidney Disease Outcomes Quality Initiative (NKF-K/DOQI) stages the severity of CKD for children older than 2 years and adults based on eGFR (**Table 1**).[1,2] Most recently, the U25 equations, based on serum creatinine and cystatin C, respectively, have been developed by the Chronic Kidney Disease in Children (CKiD) study for those children with mild to moderately impaired kidney function.[5] Formal staging of CKD in children younger than 2 years does not exist because of the normal physiologic maturation of kidney function during this time. Instead, the serum creatinine of such children should be compared with age-related mean values, and a level more than one standard deviation greater than the mean indicates CKD. Most pediatric CKD cases are a result of congenital anomalies of kidney and urinary tract (CAKUT) (49.1%) followed by focal segmental glomerulosclerosis (FSGS), particularly among older children (8.4%). Other causes of CKD in children are shown in (**Table 2**).[1]

Management of Chronic Kidney Disease

The rate of progression of pediatric CKD is variable and depends on several nonmodifiable and modifiable factors. Most importantly, glomerular diseases such as chronic glomerulonephritis and nephrotic syndrome are associated with more rapid progression of CKD as compared with a nonglomerular CAKUT disorders such as posterior urethral valves.[6] Studies have repeatedly shown a close correlation between the presence and severity of proteinuria and the rate of CKD progression. Early treatment of this modifiable risk factor with renin-angiotensin blockade using either an angiotensin converting enzyme inhibitor (ACEi) or an angiotensin receptor blocker (ARB) may be beneficial.[7] Intensified blood pressure control, ideally with ACEi or ARB, also slows the progression of CKD.[8] In the ESCAPE trial of children with CKD, a mean 24-hour ambulatory blood pressure (ABPM) between the 50th and 95th percentile was associated with a slower progression of CKD. The study also revealed that in the absence of 24-hour ABPM office blood pressure values should ideally be between the 50th and 70th percentile or at a minimum, less than the 90th percentile to help slow the progression of the CKD.[7] Furthermore, the severity of dyslipidemia also correlates with the degree of kidney function deterioration[9] and should be addressed, if present.

Table 1 Stages of chronic kidney disease[1,2]		
Stage	**Description**	**GFR (mL/ min/ 1.73 m^2)**
1	Kidney damage with normal GFR or increased GFR	>90
2	Kidney damage with mild decrease in GFR	60–89
3A	Moderate decrease in GFR	45–59
3B	Moderate decrease in GFR	30–44
4	Severe decrease in GFR	15–29
5	Kidney failure with need for kidney replacement therapy	< 15

GFR: glomerular filtration rate.

Table 2	
Causes of chronic kidney disease in children[1]	
Primary Diagnosis	**%**
CAKUT	49.1
FSGS	8.1
Other glomerular	11.6
Cystic kidney diseases	5.3
Renal infarct	2.2
Hemolytic uremic syndrome	2.0
Interstitial nephritis/pyelonephritis	1.5
Cystinosis	1.5
Wilms tumor	0.5
Sickle cell nephropathy	0.2
Diabetic nephropathy	0.2
Oxalosis	0.1
Other	15.1
Unknown	2.6

CAKUT: congenital anomalies of kidney and urinary tract.
FSGS: Focal segmental glomerulosclerosis.

Nutrition

Children with CKD require special considerations in terms of their dietary requirements. The child's age, gender, nutritional status, and growth parameters, along with the stage of CKD need to be considered when individualizing nutritional management.[10] Caloric and energy needs are similar to age-appropriate healthy children. However, many pediatric patients with CKD, especially those with advanced CKD or young infants, experience failure to thrive and require energy intake of at least 100% to 120% of daily recommended intake (DRI) to provide optimal growth.[11] In addition, the dietary protein intake in CKD and end-stage kidney disease (ESKD) is recommended to be 100% to 140% and 100% to 120% of DRI, respectively.[11] The greatest risk for malnutrition is during infancy. CAKUT may result in a high urine output, high renal sodium losses, and low total body water content. Gastric emptying can be delayed in uremia and may be associated with frequent emesis. These children may also have poor oral motor skills and be unable to feed from the breast or bottle to meet their nutritional needs. For these reasons, supplemental tube feeding, most often through a gastrotomy tube and under the guidance of a pediatric renal dietitian, is necessary. Prompt and careful management of the nutritional status of infants with CKD is necessary to optimize overall development.[12]

Chronic kidney disease—mineral bone disorder

The management of CKD-mineral bone disorder (MBD) in children is important because of the impact it can have on growth and cardiovascular disease (see later discussion). The calcium requirement is higher in children than in adults due to accelerated skeletal growth. However, the presence of hyperphosphatemia that often occurs with moderate to severe CKD in combination with a high dietary calcium intake may lead to vascular calcification. Phosphorus retention may occur as early as stage 2 CKD due to a decreased ability to excrete it in urine despite increased levels of fibroblast growth factor-23 and the parathyroid hormone (PTH), which are phosphaturic.[12]

Thus, dietary phosphorus should be restricted to 100% of DRI in children with mild CKD and to 80% of DRI for those with advanced CKD, often accompanied by the use of a phosphorus binder to achieve a normal age-based serum phosphorus level.[10–12] Education of families and patients about the phosphate content of common food (eg, dairy products) and snack items, as well as some medications, is essential. As shown in **Table 3**, an easy-to-use phosphorus-point system has been developed to help manage dietary phosphorus intake.[13]

Attention to the possibility of vitamin D 25 OH deficiency is also important because of its contribution to impaired enteral calcium absorption, the development of secondary hyperparathyroidism, and the subsequent increased risk for renal osteodystrophy and pathological fractures.[14] Treatment with cholecalciferol or ergocalciferol is indicated when the 25(OH)D level is less than 30 ng/mL.[15] In patients with persistent elevation of PTH despite good control of serum phosphorus and normal 25OH(D) levels, activated vitamin D therapy (eg, calcitriol) is recommended. Although hypocalcemia in patients with severe CKD is more prevalent, hypercalcemia may develop in a child who is immobilized or who is receiving a large quantity of calcium rich foods such as fish, green leafy vegetables, or high Ca-containing mineral water.[16]

Growth

Impaired growth, a CKD-related complication that is unique to children, can be observed in early stages of CKD but is more profound in young children with moderate to severe CKD.[10] In older children, a decrease in growth rate usually correlates with the decline in the GFR, although poor nutrition, uncontrolled CKD-MBD, and persistent metabolic acidosis can be contributing factors.[12] In infancy, nutritional adequacy is the most important factor influencing growth and it can be compromised by reduced intake, recurrent vomiting, and poor oral motor skills. Failure to address significant urinary loss of salt that can occur in polyuric kidney disorders can also result in poor growth.[11] The growth hormone/insulin-like growth factor (IGF) axis is also affected in CKD. An elevated level of circulating IGF binding proteins causes a decreased concentration of bioactive IGF-I and end-organ (bone) resistance to growth hormone.[12] The administration of recombinant growth hormone can result in improved height velocity.[12]

Neurocognitive development

Historically, infants with advanced CKD have higher rates of severe developmental delay with microcephaly and chronic seizures.[17] Etiologic factors included poor nutrition and exposure to poorly excreted aluminum present in some medications. As a result of advances in CKD care, such as early diagnosis, nutritional support, anemia management, and the avoidance of aluminum containing phosphate binders, significant neurocognitive impairment is significantly less common now.[17] The CKiD study demonstrated that significant developmental delay due to CKD is uncommon across the pediatric age range. Nevertheless, decreased kidney function, proteinuria, and hypertension remain risk factors that are associated with poor cognitive outcomes, and their presence should prompt a formal developmental evaluation.[18] Genomic variants associated with CKD have also been linked to impaired IQ, executive function, and behavioral problems in children.[19]

Cardiovascular complications

Left ventricular hypertrophy, increased arterial stiffness, and increased carotid intima media thickness are the most prevalent cardiovascular (CV) complications in children and young adults with CKD that contribute to CV morbidity and mortality.[20,21] Pediatric obesity also has a substantial impact on CV risk among children with CKD and

Table 3
Phosphorous management by dietary intake[13]

Phosphorus Point System

My Goal Points: _____ Points Per Day

0 Points	1 Points	2 Points	3 Points	4+ Points
ALL		Corn (1/2 cup or 1 cob)	Green peas (1/2 cup)	
		Mushrooms (1/2 cup)	Baked potato, small	
		Mashed potatoes (1/2 cup)	Avocado (1/2 cup)	
		Sweet potato (1/2 cup or small)		

FRUITS

0 Points				
ALL				

DRINKS

0 Points	1 Points	2 Points	3 Points	4+ Points
Water (8 fl oz)	Coffee (8 fl oz)	Gatorade (8 fl oz)	Soda, dark cola (12 fl oz)	Hot chocolate (8 fl oz)[5]
		Tea, bottled (8 fl oz)	Nepro (1 can)	Milkshakes (8 fl oz) (7 pts)
			Suplena (1 can)	

Dairy & Dairy Alternatives

0 Points	1 Points	2 Points	3 Points	4+ Points
Milk	*Cheese*	*Milk*	*Milk*	*Milk*
Almond milk (8 fl oz)	Parmesan cheese (1 tbsp)	Soy milk (8 fl oz)	Rice milk (8 fl oz)	Milk (8 fl oz)
Cheese	Lite cream cheese (1 oz)	*Cheese*	*Cheese*	Chocolate milk (8 fl oz) (5 pts)
Cream cheese (1 oz)		Unprocessed cheese (1 oz)	Cottage cheese (1/2 cup)	*Cheese*
		String cheese (1 stick)	Shredded cheese (1/2 cup)	Processed cheese (1 oz)
			Shredded cheese (1/4 cup)	

should be a motivating factor to prevent and treat pediatric obesity.[21] However, uncontrolled hypertension remains the most significant risk factor for cardiovascular diseases (CVD). Attained clinic blood pressure less than 90th percentile has been associated with slower CKD progression in children with glomerular as well as nonglomerular CKD.[22] ACEi and ARBs are the preferred antihypertensive agents.[22,23] Although patients with CKD may experience some decrease in GFR at the initiation of therapy with ACEi/ARBs, the change is not substantial (-2.1 ± 6.9 mL/min/1.73 m^2).[7] These medications increase the risk of hyperkalemia when used in patients with advanced CKD and are associated with toxicity to the fetus during pregnancy.

Anemia

Anemia remains a common and challenging complication of CKD in children. Its cause is multifactorial, the primary contributing factors being endogenous erythropoietin deficiency and iron deficiency. Untreated anemia increases the risk for hospitalization, left ventricular hypertrophy, and overall pediatric CKD morbidity.[24] Treatment with erythropoiesis-stimulating agents and iron supplementation has improved outcomes and importantly, has significantly decreased the need for blood transfusion in the CKD and ESKD populations.

Psychosocial need

Advances in the diagnosis, treatment, and disease outcomes have often been associated with the need for psychosocial adjustment of children with CKD and their families. The frequency of medical appointments, increased medication needs, and the requirement for attention to special developmental issues imposes a unique challenge for these individuals.[25] It is for this reason that a multidisciplinary medical team should include psychologists, social workers, and other mental health professionals.[26]

Incidence, Prevalence, and Cause of End-Stage Kidney Disease

Unlike CKD, the incidence and prevalence of ESKD in children is better defined, particularly in developed countries; this is mainly due to the patients' need for dialysis and/or kidney transplantation and the existence of many ESKD registries. In North America, children and adolescents younger than 20 years account for less than 2% of the total ESKD population.[27] Data from the United State Renal Data System (USRDS) reveal that the incidence and prevalence of ESKD in pediatric patients (<20 years) in 2018 were 11.8 and 75 pmarp, respectively.[28] Similar to CKD, the leading causes of ESKD are renal aplasia/hypoplasia/dysplasia, obstructive uropathy, and FSGS; all other causes account for less than or equal to 5% of patients.[29,30]

Management of End-Stage Kidney Disease

Patients with ESKD need continued optimization of nutritional care and growth management, blood pressure control, management of CKD-MBD, and psychosocial support. The underlying principles of ESKD management are the same as in CKD.

Kidney Replacement Therapy

In the United States approximately 75% of all pediatric patients with ESKD receive maintenance dialysis prior to receiving a kidney transplant.[30,31] More than half of the pediatric dialysis patients in the United States receive hemodialysis (HD); peritoneal dialysis (PD) is preferred in younger children. It is of interest to note that the pediatric centers more frequently use PD (65%) as compared with the adult centers that provide dialysis to children (45%).[32] The advantages of HD include the minimal technical assistance required from the patient and family when the procedure is conducted in a dialysis center as well as a shorter treatment time relative to PD. In contrast, the use of PD is associated with less dependence on the dialysis center and increased flexibility for the timing of treatments, which allows greater school attendance. Other advantages/disadvantages of HD versus PD are shown in **Table 4**. Recently, home HD has been used as a treatment option by some families.[33,34]

Hemodialysis
The ability to provide chronic HD to pediatric population mandates the availability of equipment and personnel that can meet the needs of infants, children, and adolescents with ESKD. Although the frequency of HD use increases with age in pediatric patients, even young infants can receive effective HD when it is provided by a multidisciplinary team that includes a pediatric nephrologist, dialysis-trained nurse, social worker, dietitian, child life therapist, and a psychologist.[31]

Permanent vascular access in the form of an arteriovenous fistula or graft (AVF/AVG) is preferred for children with ESKD on maintenance HD, as it is in adults, because of superior performance, longevity and decreased risk of complications when compared with catheters.[33] Preservation of vessels before AVF/AVG placement is important and mandates education of the patient with advanced CKD, as well as the family and health care team about the importance of avoiding or limiting venipuncture/intravenous (IV) placement in vessels that may be the potential candidates for creation of the access.[35] The vascular access for smaller children and infants is an indwelling HD catheter.[36] The most frequent complications associated with HD catheters are infection (eg, bacteremia) and thrombosis, which often requires removal and replacement. Recommendations have been published regarding catheter care practices associated with a decreased infection risk.[37]

In-center HD usually requires the child to spend an average of 12 hours/week on dialysis. Technical decisions start with choosing the appropriate size of the HD circuit and dialyzer. Ideally, the extracorporeal blood volume should not exceed 10% of the child's total blood volume to help maintain hemodynamic stability; a slightly greater extracorporeal volume may be possible in the stable child with a near-normal hemoglobin value. Occasionally, albumin or packed red cell (PRBC) diluted with 5% albumin (to achieve a hematocrit of 35%) may be used for circuit priming if the child is hemodynamically unstable or increased extracorporeal blood volume is needed, especially in infants less than 8 kg in weight. The use of PRBC should be avoided, if possible, because of the risk of sensitization and production of anti-human leukocyte antigen (HLA) antibodies that may preclude early transplantation.[31] A wide variety of lines and dialyzers are available to meet the requirements of most patients. Commonly used catheters for chronic HD are shown in **Table 5**.

Rapid osmolar changes at the time of dialysis initiation can be associated with cerebral edema, disequilibrium syndrome, and the development of seizures.[38] Children are also known to have a relatively low seizure threshold; therefore, limiting the amount of urea clearance to 30 to 40 mg/dL at each of the first few dialysis treatments or the IV administration of 0.50 g/kg mannitol is recommended to minimize osmolar shifts.[38] Small infants in particular need more careful monitoring because the current HD machines have ultrafiltration rate of around 50 to 100 mL, a value that may contribute to hemodynamic instability.[31]

Peritoneal dialysis
Although PD is the most frequent dialysis modality used for children worldwide, the number of children who were started on PD in the United States decreased between 2010 and 2019, and the number who transitioned from PD to HD increased slightly.[28,39] In PD, the solute and fluid removal are achieved by infusion of dialysis

Table 4
Comparison of hemodialysis and peritoneal dialysis as treatment modalities

Hemodialysis		Peritoneal Dialysis	
Advantage	Disadvantage	Advantage	Disadvantage
Minimal technical assistance by family	Need for vascular access and anticoagulation therapy	Potential home-based therapy	Longer and daily treatment time
Shorter treatment time	Advanced and expensive health infrastructure	Better preservation of residual kidney function	Significant technical assistance by family
Precise fluid removal and uremic substance clearance	Increased time away from school and friends	Minimal health infrastructure	Less precise fluid and uremic substance clearance

solution into the peritoneal cavity and its drainage after a dwell time. The dialysis solution comprises electrolytes, calcium, and an osmotic agent (typically dextrose). The contraindications to chronic PD in large part hinge on the availability of a functional peritoneal membrane and are elaborated in **Box 1**. Presence of a colostomy, gastrostomy, ureterostomy, and/or nephrostomy tube does not preclude chronic PD.

The quality of life for both the patient and family assumes great importance in the selection of home PD because of the "burden of care" associated with this therapy. As such, careful evaluation of the family's social, psychological, and economic background by the multidisciplinary dialysis team is mandatory if a fully informed decision is to be made.[31]

A reliable peritoneal catheter is the cornerstone of successful PD. The key elements of the catheter are the intraperitoneal configuration (curled or straight), number of Dacron cuffs (1 or 2), and subcutaneous tunnel configuration (straight or "swan" neck). The number of cuffs may be particularly influential in terms of patient outcome. NAPRTCS study reported a significantly lower incidence of peritonitis with double-cuff catheters (1/21.0 patient months) as compared with single-cuff catheters (1/15.7 patient months).[29,40] Particularly important is the preference to place the catheter exit site as far from a stoma as possible in children with a vesicostomy, gastrostomy, or colostomy to help prevent contamination and infection.[41] Infection (31.4%) and malfunction (39.9%) are the most common reasons for PD catheter revision.[42]

PD modality options include continuous ambulatory peritoneal dialysis (CAPD) and cycler or automated peritoneal dialysis (APD). Although personal preference and lifestyle are the factors that most frequently influence the chronic PD modality selection, individual variation in peritoneal membrane transport characteristics may also influence a patient's suitability for a particular therapy (eg, high transporter: APD; low transporter: CAPD).[42] The PD prescription should be tailored to the needs of the individual patient, with consideration of the medical needs as well as the patient/family quality of life.[43,44] Most children on APD are prescribed a regimen consisting of 6 to 12 exchanges over 8 to 10 h per night, sometimes with a single long daytime exchange. Peritonitis is more common in children than in adults and is the most common reason for technique failure.[28]

Patient survival on dialysis. Data derived from both the USRDS and the NAPRTCS provide age-related patient survival data and confirm the significantly compromised life expectancy of younger children on dialysis.[28–30] In the 2020 report, the USRDS

Table 5 Cuffed hemodialysis catheters[31]	
Patient Size (kg)	Catheter Options
<20	8 French dual lumen
20–25	7 French twin Tesio 10 French dual lumen
25–40	10 French Ash Split 10 French twin Tesio
>40	11.5 or 12.5 French dual lumen

revealed 1-year survival probabilities of 82.3%, 93.8%, 93%, and 97.1% for patients in the age groups of 0 to 4 years, 5 to 9 years, 10 to 14 years, and 15 to 19 years, respectively.[28] The best survival rate for children, seen in those older than 12 years (98.2% at 12 months after dialysis initiation), still shows a modest decrease after 3 years of dialysis (95.4%). Overall, the survival rate for all children receiving chronic dialysis has increased only slightly over the past 15 years. The main causes of death are cardiovascular disease (25.1%), infection (14.2), cancer/malignancy (4.5%), withdrawal of care (4.8%), other (21.5%), and unknown (29.9%).[28] In the NAPRTCS database, younger age and growth failure were predictive of increased mortality in children on hemodialysis.[30]

Kidney Transplantation

As shown in **Table 6**, kidney transplantation improves the estimated life expectancy of children by 2- to 3-fold compared with dialysis. A total of 897 children (<21 years) received kidney transplants (KT) in the United States in 2018, the majority (59.8%) were from deceased donors (DD). In the United States, the percentage of pediatric KT that are derived from a deceased versus a living donor has progressively increased from 55% to 66% over the past 10 years (**Fig. 1**).[28,45,46] In the past decade, the percentage of younger children (<10 years) on the transplant waiting list has also increased (43.3%), and it is predominantly males (61.3%) with CAKUT.[45,46] Almost half of the children on the waiting list in the United States are White (47%), 20.7% African American, and 29.1% are Hispanic.[28,45,46] Finally, after introduction of a new Kidney Allocation System in 2014, the waiting time for children has been favorable, with 52.7% of the children having spent less than 1 year on the waiting list before kidney transplantation in 2018.[47]

Box 1 Contraindications to peritoneal dialysis[31]
Absolute contraindications
○ Omphalocele
○ Gastroschisis
○ Bladder extrophy
○ Diaphragmatic hernia
○ Obliterated peritoneal cavity and peritoneal membrane failure
Relative contraindications
○ Impending abdominal surgery
○ Impending living-related kidney transplantation
○ ack of an appropriate caregiver for home therapy

Table 6
Expected remaining lifetime in pediatric patients with end-stage kidney disease. USRDS, 2020[28]

	Dialysis		Transplant		General Population	
Age	M	F	M	F	M	F
0–14	23.3	20.9	60.3	59.3	70.6	75.4
15–19	21.4	18.7	47.6	49.1	59.6	64.3
20–24	18.5	15.8	43.7	45.2	54.9	59.4

Donor–recipient matching

The current donor allocation system for pediatric KT involves donor and recipient HLA typing, recipient anti-HLA antibody screening, and cross-matching.[48] Among all pediatric deceased donor transplants, only 5.5% of those in the NAPRTCS database matched all HLA loci (6/6), 53.8% had at least one match on either the A, B, or DR locus (3/6), and 10.3% had no DR matches.[48] DR matching is of particular importance because of the recent finding that 2 HLA-DR mismatches in the first KT is associated with higher degrees of sensitization, longer wait times for retransplantation, and worse graft outcomes in children.[49]

Recent knowledge regarding HLA molecules and their associated epitopes, a protein segment composed of amino acids that can trigger an immune response, allow us to better understand the consequences of certain HLA class II (HLA-DR, DQ, and DP) mismatches. In an attempt to decrease donor-specific antibody production and prolong graft survival, pediatric transplant programs have also started to incorporate HLA class II epitope mismatching as part of the organ allocation process.[50]

The therapeutic cornerstone of long-term graft survival is effective immunosuppression, ideally characterized by medication regimens, which provides the desired outcome with acceptable risk of complications such as infection or malignancy. Typically, maintenance immunosuppression consists of a calcineurin inhibitor and an antiproliferative medication with/without systemic corticosteroids.[45,46]

Outcome of pediatric kidney transplantation

Graft survival has progressively improved in United States pediatric kidney transplant recipients. The most recent USRDS data have revealed 1-, 3-, 5-, and 10-year graft survival rates of 97.8%, 91.7%, 82.6%, and 60.6%, respectively, in deceased donor recipients[28,45,46] (**Fig. 2**). Corresponding graft survival data following living donor

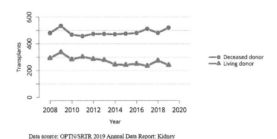

Data source: OPTN/SRTR 2019 Annual Data Report: Kidney

Fig. 1. Pediatric kidney transplants by donor type. All pediatric kidney transplant recipients, including retransplant, and multiorgan recipients.[45]

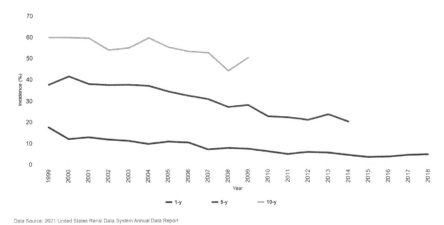

Data Source: 2021 United States Renal Data System Annual Data Report

Fig. 2. Adjusted 1-, 5-, and 10-year cumulative incidence of graft failure in children who received a deceased donor kidney transplant, 1999–2018.[28]

transplant are 99.2% at 1 year, 94.7% at 3 years, 91.2% at 5 years, and 70.3% at 10 years[28,45,46] **(Fig. 3)**. In addition, the USRDS previously demonstrated the poorest outcome to be in adolescent recipients.[28] Nonadherence to immunosuppressive therapy is an important risk factor for graft failure and a critical target for intervention.[51] Pediatric data suggest that routine performance of surveillance transplant biopsies may provide histologic evidence of subclinical, modifiable factors, which if addressed successfully, could favorably affect graft outcome.[52] Overall, 50.7% of graft failures are caused by rejection, with chronic rejection accounting for 35.8% and acute rejection accounting for 13.0% of cases.[28,45,46]

Graft function, as measured by eGFR, has also improved substantially over the past decade. Recent OPTN/SRTR database reported that the proportion of pediatric living donor and deceased donor recipients with an eGFR 90 mL/min/1.73 m² or higher at 12 months posttransplant were 31.3% (increased from 19.7% in 2008) and 28.5%

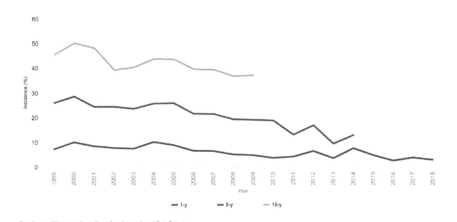

Data Source: 2021 United States Renal Data System Annual Data Report

Fig. 3. Adjusted 1-, 5-, and 10-year cumulative incidence of graft failure in children who received a living donor kidney transplant, 1999–2018.[28]

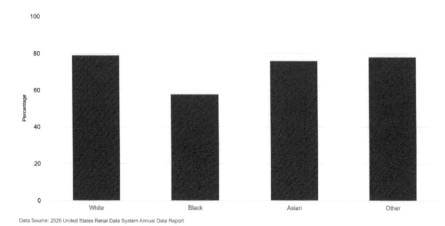

Fig. 4. Percentage of time spent with a functioning kidney transplant among prevalent adult survivors of childhood ESKD by race, 2018.[28]

(increased from 22.3%), respectively.[45] Preemptive kidney transplantation, defined as transplantation before the initiation of dialysis, is conducted in approximately 26% of children with ESKD in the United States, in part because of the frequent availability of a parental kidney donor.[53] These children seem to have some benefit regarding graft survival and overall morbidity compared with children who have received dialysis before kidney transplantation.[54]

Patient survival after kidney transplant. For young adults aged 18 to 24 years with childhood onset ESKD, the "ESKD lifetime" with a functioning kidney transplant was 79% in Caucasians and about 58% in Blacks (**Fig. 4**).[28] In fact, the proportion of young adults with a functioning (first or subsequent) transplant has gradually increased over the past decade.[28] However, with CVD and uncontrolled hypertension continuing to be the leading causes of death in young adult patients with ESKD,[46] accompanied by impairment of quality of life related to growth failure and poor control of CKD-MBD as additional comorbidities,[30] it is evident that the development and successful implementation of better treatment strategies is required to improve long-term outcome.

  Racial and ethnic disparities There is a substantial racial and ethnic disparity in ESKD treatment, as it pertains to access to home-based dialysis modalities and transplantation, as reflected by data from the USRDS.[28] White children with ESKD and receiving HD in the United States have been found to be twice as likely as Black children to receive a kidney transplant (20.8% vs 10.0%). In addition, a substantially higher percentage of Black (57.3%) as compared with White (40.5%) children who required dialysis were initiated on HD. Likewise, Hispanic-Latino children received a kidney transplant at ESKD onset less often than did non-Hispanic children (12.0% vs 20.2%) and initiated HD more often and PD less often than non-Hispanic children between 2015 and 2019.[28] The cause of these disparities is multifactorial, with several influential factors being socioeconomic status, access to health insurance, as well as language barriers.[55] The fact that preemptive kidney transplantation is more common in children from households characterized by higher income (>$75,000) or maternal college education (all more likely among White children) is an example of the influence that socioeconomic factors can have on treatment options.[53]

SUMMARY

Optimal treatment of pediatric patients with advanced CKD requires a multidisciplinary approach, which addresses both the medical and psychosocial aspects of management. Although the complexity of care increases with progressive worsening of kidney function and the need to initiate kidney replacement therapy, prevention or prompt treatment of clinical complications and a philosophy of shared decision-making between the health care team and the patient/family are key components of a successful approach to care.[26]

CLINICS CARE POINTS

- As CKD in children commonly occurs due to congenital anomalies of the CAKUT, initial radiologic imaging should usually be conducted with ultrasound, which avoids the need for IV contrast and the associated risk of nephrotoxicity.

- The use of ACE and ARB therapy for treatment of hypertension in children with CKD should be accompanied by close monitoring of the serum potassium level.

- Consideration for growth hormone therapy to treat growth impairment in children with CKD should be preceded by correction of metabolic acidosis, salt depletion, and poor nutritional status if they exist.

- The family's psychosocial status and level of support requires close evaluation when home dialysis is being considered because of the "burden of care" associated with the therapy.

- Monitoring for medication nonadherence is essential in adolescent kidney transplant patients because of their increased risk of graft loss associated with failure to receive the prescribed treatment.

DISCLOSURE

Judith Sebestyen VanSickle: none; Bradley Warady: Consultant: Reata, Bayer, Roche, Amgen. Grant Support: NIH, National Institute of Health, United States.

REFERENCES

1. Chadha V, Warady BA. Epidemiology of pediatric chronic kidney disease. Adv Chronic Kidney Dis 2005 Oct;12(4):343–52.
2. Levey AS, Coresh J, Lau J, et al, National Kidney Foundation. National Kidney Foundation practice guidelines for chronic kidney disease: evaluation, classification, and stratification. Ann Intern Med 2003;139(2):137–47 [Erratum in: Ann Intern Med. 2003 Oct 7;139(7):605. PMID: 12859163].
3. Ardissino G, Dacco V, Testa S, et al. Epidemiology of chronic renal failure in children: data from the ItalKid project. Pediatrics 2003;111:e382–7.
4. Ahn SY, Moxey-Mims M. CKD in Children: The Importance of a National Epidemiologic Study. Am J Kidney Dis 2018;72(5):628–30.
5. Pierce CB, Muñoz A, Ng DK, et al. Age- and sex-dependent clinical equations to estimate glomerular filtration rates in children and young adults with chronic kidney disease. Kidney Int 2021;99(4):948–56.
6. Warady BA, Abraham AG, Schwartz GJ, et al. Predictors of rapid progression of glomerular and nonglomerular kidney disease in children and adolescents: the chronic kidney disease in children (ckid) cohort. Am J Kidney Dis 2015;65(6): 878–88 [Epub 2015 Mar 19. PMID: 25799137; PMCID: PMC4578873].

7. ESCAPE Trial Group, Wühl E, Trivelli A, Picca S, et al. Strict blood-pressure control and progression of renal failure in children. N Engl J Med 2009;361(17): 1639–50.

8. Ardissino G, Testa S, Daccò V, et al. Proteinuria as a predictor of disease progression in children with hypodysplastic nephropathy. Data from the Ital Kid Project. Pediatr Nephrol 2004;19(2):172–7.

9. Saland JM, Kupferman JC, Pierce CB, et al. Change in dyslipidemia with declining glomerular filtration rate and increasing proteinuria in children with CKD. Clin J Am Soc Nephrol 2019;14(12):1711–8.

10. KDOQI Work Group. KDOQI Clinical practice guideline for nutrition in children with CKD: 2008 update. executive summary. Am J Kidney Dis 2009;53(3 Suppl 2):S11–104.

11. Shaw V, Polderman N, Renken-Terhaerdt J, et al. Energy and protein requirements for children with CKD stages 2-5 and on dialysis-clinical practice recommendations from the Pediatric Renal Nutrition Taskforce. Pediatr Nephrol 2020; 35(3):519–31.

12. Silverstein DM. Growth and nutrition in pediatric chronic kidney disease. Front Pediatr 2018;6:205.

13. Oladitan L, VanSickle JS. Use of a phosphorus points education program to maintain normal serum phosphorus in pediatric chronic kidney disease: a case report. J Ren Nutr 2021;31(2):206–9.

14. Denburg MR, Kumar J, Jemielita T, et al. Fracture burden and risk factors in childhood CKD: results from the CKiD cohort study. J Am Soc Nephrol 2016;27(2): 543–50.

15. Shroff R, Wan M, Nagler EV, et al. European society for paediatric nephrology chronic kidney disease mineral and bone disorders and dialysis working groups. Clinical practice recommendations for native vitamin D therapy in children with chronic kidney disease Stages 2-5 and on dialysis. Nephrol Dial Transplant 2017;32(7):1098–113.

16. Shroff R, Wan M, Nagler EV, et al. European Society for Paediatric Nephrology Chronic Kidney Disease Mineral and Bone Disorders and Dialysis Working Groups. Clinical practice recommendations for treatment with active vitamin D analogues in children with chronic kidney disease Stages 2-5 and on dialysis. Nephrol Dial Transplant 2017;32(7):1114–27.

17. Harshman LA, Hooper SR. The brain in pediatric chronic kidney disease-the intersection of cognition, neuroimaging, and clinical biomarkers. Pediatr Nephrol 2020;35(12):2221–9.

18. Hooper SR, Gerson AC, Butler RW, et al. Neurocognitive functioning of children and adolescents with mild-to-moderate chronic kidney disease. Clin J Am Soc Nephrol 2011;6(8):1824–30.

19. Verbitsky M, Westland R, Perez A, et al. The copy number variation landscape of congenital anomalies of the kidney and urinary tract. Nat Genet 2019 Jan;51(1): 117–27.

20. Mitsnefes MM. Cardiovascular disease in children with chronic kidney disease. J Am Soc Nephrol 2012;23(4):578–85.

21. Brady TM, Roem J, Cox C, et al. Adiposity, sex, and cardiovascular disease risk in children With CKD: a longitudinal study of youth enrolled in the chronic kidney disease in children (CKiD) Study. Am J Kidney Dis 2020;76(2):166–73.

22. Flynn JT, Carroll MK, Ng DK, et al. Achieved clinic blood pressure level and chronic kidney disease progression in children: a report from the Chronic Kidney Disease in Children cohort. Pediatr Nephrol 2021;36(6):1551–9.

23. Flynn JT, Kaelber DC, Baker-Smith CM, et al. Subcommittee on screening and management of high blood pressure in children. Clinical Practice Guideline for Screening and Management of High Blood Pressure in Children and Adolescents. Pediatrics 2017;140(3):e20171904 [Erratum in: Pediatrics. 2017 Nov 30;: Erratum in: Pediatrics. 2018 Sep;142(3): PMID: 28827377].

24. Atkinson MA, Warady BA. Anemia in chronic kidney disease. Pediatr Nephrol 2018;33(2):227–38.

25. Hooper SR, Johnson RJ, Gerson AC, et al. Overview of the findings and advances in the neurocognitive and psychosocial functioning of mild to moderate pediatric CKD: perspectives from the Chronic Kidney Disease in Children (CKiD) cohort study. Pediatr Nephrol 2022;37(4):765–75.

26. Menon S, Valentini RP, Kapur G, et al. Effectiveness of a multidisciplinary clinic in managing children with chronic kidney disease. Clin J Am Soc Nephrol 2009; 4(7):1170–5.

27. Groothoff JW, Gruppen MP, Offringa M, et al. Mortality and causes of death of end-stage renal disease in children: a Dutch cohort study. Kidney Int 2002; 61(2):621–9.

28. United States Renal Data System. USRDS annual data report: epidemiology of kidney disease in the United States. Bethesda, MD: National Institutes of Health, National Institute of Diabetes and Digestive and Kidney Diseases; 2020.

29. North American Pediatric Renal Trials and Collaborative Studies (NAPRTCS) 2011 Annual Report: NAPRTCS.org.

30. Weaver DJ Jr, Somers MJG, Martz K, et al. Clinical outcomes and survival in pediatric patients initiating chronic dialysis: a report of the NAPRTCS registry. Pediatr Nephrol 2017;32(12):2319–30.

31. Sebestyen JF, Warady BA. Advances in pediatric renal replacement therapy. Adv Chronic Kidney Dis 2011;18(5):376–83.

32. Furth SL, Hwang W, Yang C, et al. Relation between pediatric experience and treatment recommendations for children and adolescents with kidney failure. JAMA 2001;285(8):1027–33.

33. Hothi DK, Stronach L, Sinnott K. Home hemodialysis in children. Hemodial Int 2016;20(3):349–57.

34. Fischbach M, Terzic J, Menouer S, et al. Intensified and daily hemodialysis in children might improve statural growth. Pediatr Nephrol 2006;21(11):1746–52.

35. Singh NS, Grimes J, Gregg GK, et al. Save the Vein" initiative in children With CKD: a quality improvement study. Am J Kidney Dis 2021;78(1):96–102.e1.

36. Sheth R, Brandt M, Brewer E, et al. Permanent hemodialysis vascular access survival in children and adolescent with end-stage renal disease. Kidney Int 2002; 62:1864–9.

37. Marsenic O, Rodean J, Richardson T, et al. Standardizing Care to Improve Outcomes in Pediatric End Stage Renal Disease (SCOPE) Investigators. Tunneled hemodialysis catheter care practices and blood stream infection rate in children: results from the SCOPE collaborative. Pediatr Nephrol 2020;35(1):135–43.

38. Raina R, Davenport A, Warady B, et al. Dialysis disequilibrium syndrome (DDS) in pediatric patients on dialysis: systematic review and clinical practice recommendations. Pediatr Nephrol 2021. https://doi.org/10.1007/s00467-021-05242-1.

39. Harambat J, Bonthuis M, Groothoff JW, et al. Lessons learned from the ESPN/ERA-EDTA Registry. Pediatr Nephrol 2016;31(11):2055–64.

40. Chadha V, Schaefer FS, Warady BA. Dialysis-associated peritonitis in children. Pediatr Nephrol 2010;25:425–40.

41. Warady BA, Bakkaloglu S, Newland J, et al. Consensus guidelines for the prevention and treatment of catheter-related infections and peritonitis in pediatric patients receiving peritoneal dialysis: 2012 update. Perit Dial Int 2012;32(Suppl 2):S32–86.

42. Borzych-Duzalka D, Aki TF, Azocar M, et al. International pediatric peritoneal dialysis network (IPPN) registry. peritoneal dialysis access revision in children: causes, interventions, and outcomes. Clin J Am Soc Nephrol 2017;12(1):105–12.

43. Fischbach M, Warady BA. Peritoneal dialysis prescription in children: bedside principles for optimal practice. Pediatr Nephrol 2009;24(9):1633–42 [quiz: 1640].

44. Warady BA, Alexander SR, Hossli S, et al. Peritoneal membrane transport function in children receiving long-term dialysis. J Am Soc Nephrol 1996;7(11):2385–91.

45. Hart A, Lentine KL, Smith JM, et al. OPTN/SRTR 2019 annual data report: kidney. Am J Transplant 2021;21(Suppl 2):21–137.

46. Saran R, Robinson B, Abbott KC, et al. US renal data system 2018 annual data report: epidemiology of kidney disease in the united states. Am J Kidney Dis 2019;73(3 Suppl 1):A7–8.

47. Rao PS, Schaubel DE, Guidinger MK, et al. A comprehensive risk quantification score for deceased donor kidneys: the kidney donor risk index. Transplantation 2009;88(2):231–6.

48. Althaf MM, El Kossi M, Jin JK, et al. Human leukocyte antigen typing and crossmatch: a comprehensive review. World J Transpl 2017;7(6):339–48.

49. Gralla J, Tong S, Wiseman AC. The impact of human leukocyte antigen mismatching on sensitization rates and subsequent retransplantation after first graft failure in pediatric renal transplant recipients. Transplantation 2013;95(10):1218–24.

50. Bryan CF, Chadha V, Warady BA. Donor selection in pediatric kidney transplantation using DR and DQ eplet mismatching: A new histocompatibility paradigm. Pediatr Transplant 2016;20(7):926–30.

51. Foster BJ, Pai ALH, Zelikovsky N, et al. A randomized trial of a multicomponent intervention to promote medication adherence: the teen adherence in kidney transplant effectiveness of intervention trial (TAKE-IT). Am J Kidney Dis 2018 Jul;72(1):30–41.

52. Odum JD, Kats A, VanSickle JS, et al. Characterizing the frequency of modifiable histological changes observed on surveillance biopsies in pediatric kidney allograft recipients. Pediatr Nephrol 2020;35(11):2173–82.

53. Amaral S, Sayed BA, Kutner N, et al. Preemptive kidney transplantation is associated with survival benefits among pediatric patients with end-stage renal disease. Kidney Int 2016;90(5):1100–8.

54. Atkinson MA, Roem JL, Gajjar A, et al. Mode of initial renal replacement therapy and transplant outcomes in the chronic kidney disease in children (CKiD) study. Pediatr Nephrol 2020;35(6):1015–21.

55. Amaral S, Patzer R. Disparities, race/ethnicity and access to pediatric kidney transplantation. Curr Opin Nephrol Hypertens 2013;22(3):336–43 [Erratum in: Curr Opin Nephrol Hypertens. 2013 Jul;22(4):502. PMID: 23508056; PMCID: PMC3950976].

Printed and bound by CPI Group (UK) Ltd, Croydon, CR0 4YY

03/10/2024

01040467-0007